T4-AVF-432

Language Competence

CONTRIBUTORS

Tanis H. Bryan, Ph.D.
Associate Dean
College of Education,
Room 3015
University of Illinois at Chicago
Chicago, IL 60680

Christine Dollaghan, Ph.D.
Department of Communicative
Disorders
Glenrose Rehabilitation Hospital
Edmonton, Alberta, Canada
T5G0B7

John Dore, Ph.D.
Baruch College and
The Graduate School
City University of New York
New York, NY 10010

Judith Felson Duchan, Ph.D.
Speech and Hearing Clinic,
SUNY
Department of Communicative
Disorders
State University of New York
at Buffalo
Amherst, NY 14226

Susan Ervin-Tripp, Ph.D.
Institute of Human Learning,
Bldg. T-4
University of California,
Berkeley
Berkeley, CA 94720

David Gordon, Ph.D.
1814 Sonoma
Berkeley, CA 94707

Betty Hart, Ph.D.
Juniper Gardens Learning
Center
Kansas City, KS 66101

Jon F. Miller, Ph.D.
Department of Communicative
Disorders
University of Wisconsin
Madison, WI 53706

Mabel L. Rice
Child Language Program
University of Kansas
Lawrence, KS 66045

Todd Risley, Ph.D.
University of Alaska
Department of Psychology
Anchorage, AK 99508

Howard M. Rosenfeld, Ph.D.
Psychology Department
University of Kansas
Lawrence, KS 66045

Richard L. Schiefelbusch, Ph.D.
Bureau of Child Research
University of Kansas
Lawrence, KS 66045

Language Competence
Assessment and Intervention

Edited by
RICHARD L. SCHIEFELBUSCH, Ph.D.
University of Kansas

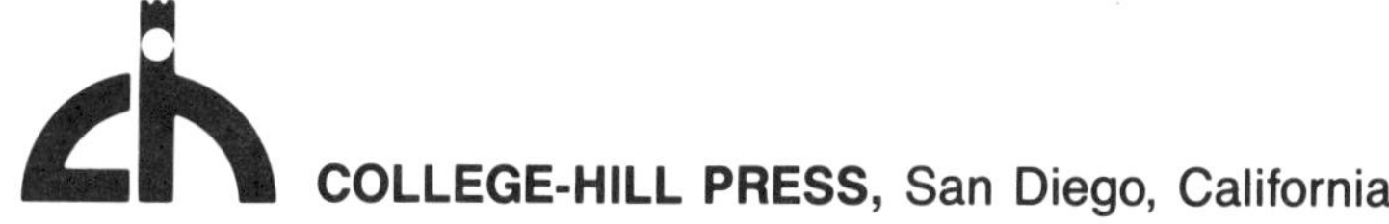
COLLEGE-HILL PRESS, San Diego, California

College-Hill Press, Inc.
4284 41st Street
San Diego, California 92105

©1986 College-Hill Press, Inc.

All rights, including that of translation, reserved. No part of this publication may be reproduced, stored in a retrieval system, or transmitted in any form or by any means, electronic, mechanical, recording, or otherwise, without the prior written permission of the publisher.

Library of Congress Cataloging in Publication Data
Main entry under title:

Language competence.
Includes index.
1. Language disorders in children—Diagnosis.
2. Language disorders in children—Treatment.
3. Competence and performance (Linguistics)
4. Communicative competence. I. Schiefelbusch, Richard L.
RJ496.L35L357 1986 618.92′855 85-24277
ISBN 0-88744-226-9

Printed in the United States of America

CONTENTS

PREFACE

Communicative competence is viewed here from a developmental perspective. The primary focus is on strategies and designs for teaching competencies to children who have developmental delays or special deficits. Such efforts require the specialist to determine the clusters of skills or functions to be taught. Likewise, assessment or evaluation requires the specialist to determine which competencies to describe. Consequently, the reader will find an explanation and a description of communicative competence and an analysis of assessment and evaluation procedures, followed by explanations of intervention procedures. This systematic approach to communicative competence will benefit specialists who seek to do further research and specialists who seek to instruct or guide the development of further competencies.

This is a companion book to *The Acquisition of Communicative Competence* (University Park Press, 1984),* which provides information about developmental factors and functions as well as the knowledge-based dimensions of communicative competence.

Although not designed primarily to provide instruction for parents, teachers, clinicians, and others who guide the development of children, the 1984 volume provides substance about the evolving social competen-

*Now distributed by ProEd of Texas.

cies of children. Their communicative development is traced through the infant-toddler, preschool, and school periods.

The books are not a two-volume series but are instead companion books. Communicative competence is a complex, instrumental area that combines much of the field of child language. The content cannot be easily treated in a single book.

This volume, *Communicative Competence: Assessment and Intervention,* includes practical strategies for assessing and teaching communicative competence. This book is primarily concerned with instruction and intervention tactics. However, the previous book has information for planning programs for children. If the reader wants to gain a better understanding of acquisition issues, the earlier volume has complete content. Either book can stand alone as a source of information about communicative competence. However, they are mutually supportive. The reader of either should consult the other table of contents for relevant topics of interest. Also, the introduction to each book provides content statements. In addition, the introduction to this volume describes how the two contents interrelate.

The editor wishes to thank the authors for their good will and positive approaches to this project. This complex effort was made possible by the cooperation of these and other colleagues: Janet Hankin, formerly of University Park Press; Marilyn Fischer, Robert Hoyt, Thelma Dillon, Mary Beth Johnston, Lori Llewellyn, and Jean Roberts of the Bureau of Child Research; Bambi Schieffelin, University of Pennsylvania; and Marion Blank, Rutgers Medical School, who advised the editor on the selection of authors and topics.

INTRODUCTION

"Communicative competence" was first introduced by Hymes in 1967 in recognition of the continuity of linguistic form with the patterning of social behavior and in view of language as a mode of action. Communicative competence includes all modes of competence in communication. Thus, competence applies to both social behavior and grammar. "Within the developmental matrix in which knowledge of the sentences of a language is acquired, children also acquire knowledge of a set of ways in which sentences are used" (Hymes, 1972, p. 286).

The application of competence to communicative contexts is an expansion of the original meaning of competence proposed by Chomsky (1957). Chomsky said that the speaker possesses knowledge of the rules requisite to appropriate language. Hymes extended this view to include knowledge of how to use language appropriately and effectively in social contexts. Chomsky and Hymes both intended that the emphasis should be on the knowledge of the rules of language whether they pertain to structure or usage.

The shift toward communicative competence marked a radical change in the way most child language researchers thought about language. The language-acquiring child came to be seen as learning not only linguistic knowledge but also the social values and rules underlying language in social interaction. Hymes and others intended to shift the emphasis more to the cultural considerations that shape and modify the child's language. Hymes points out that the dimensional nature of communication contexts can be understood and responded to appropriately through cultural experience. Appropriate comprehension of and response to cultural expectations thus should be part of our definition of competence.

Hymes's assumptions led Slobin (1967) to characterize communicative competence as the totality of knowledge that enables the speaker (1) to produce utterances that are structurally well formed, referentially accurate, and contextually appropriate and (2) to understand the speech of others as a joint function of its structural characteristics and social competence. This is a broad definition of the ways in which children's knowledge of language are applied in communicating with others. However, in considering this definition, we are inclined to add an important conditional element to the term "knowledge." We would add a "knowledge and skill" term, intending thereby to emphasize that speakers not only must know how (from the standpoint of a knowledge base) to use language appropriately in environmental contexts but also should have the skills to perform these functions appropriately and effectively. This use of the term "skill" refers to the mechanics of speaking and the cognitive skills in using language dialectally, and includes the comprehensive knowledge in exchanges within a general range of contexts. This generalized performance skill is in addition to the metacognitive knowledge about how to use language.

Broadening the philosophical issue of competence to include both knowledge and skill is crucial in considering how competence can be taught. Competence includes generalized performance, and the test of this competence is in the child's effectiveness in extending his general understanding of the rules of language into broader contexts. This chosen meaning of competence is at variance with the more popular uses of the term competence within the field of psycholinguistics. Nevertheless, it enables teachers and practitioners in language therapy to be as comfortable with the term competence as ethnographers and developmental psycholinguists are. It is necessary to broaden the field of language acquisition to include the efforts of people who are attempting to teach competence, often to children with less than normal aptitudes for acquisition. We refer to children with impaired sensory intake capabilities and children with impaired motor or cognitive capabilities for developing spoken and written language. The field would also include children who, for whatever reason, do not acquire language in the normal fashion that serves most children.

As indicated in the preface, this book is a companion volume to the 1984 publication *The Acquisition of Communicative Competence,* which is divided into four sections: (1) developmental factors and functions, (2) dimensions of communicative competence, (3) children across cultures, and (4) developmentally different children. Each of these sections includes some special information that is highly relevant to the current volume. In the first section, four chapters focus strongly on early development of communicative competence: Sugarman develops the theme of preverbal communication and its contributions to social development. Snow examines the role of parent-child interaction in the development of communicative abilities. Sachs examines children's play and its role in communicative development. Rice discusses the cognitive aspects of communicative development. These four chapters in combination provide a strong background of understanding about the early stages of the acquisition of communicative competence and how these stages evolve into further competencies that the normal child exhibits during the preschool and school years.

The second section examines the dimensions of communicative competence, particularly the form and force interactions (deVilliers, 1984), the presuppositional usages (DeHart and Maratsos, 1984), the structure of children's requests (Gordon and Ervin-Tripp, 1984), and the grammatical devices that are used in sharing points (MacWhinney, 1984). These chapters introduce a number of important issues that can be studied further on the way to developing a more complete field of communicative competence.

Section three, on "children across cultures," examines the cultural variations in children's conversations and how these variations influence the performance of children in representative social and learning contexts. It is particularly important to consider this work in analyzing the role of bilingual and bicultural influences on children in schools. The adaptation that a child from another culture must make in adapting to school environments is an important theme developed by Schieffelin and Eisenberg (1984).

Section four of *The Acquisition of Communicative Competence* provides some especially valuable information in relation to developmentally different children who may fail to achieve adequate competencies or who may have an incomplete or irregular history in acquiring language. Snyder (1984) is especially interested in children with language disorders, mental retardation, and autism. She discusses their difficulties in acquiring appropriate speech acts dealing with presuppositional assumptions and acquiring conversational skills. Likewise, Urwin (1984) is interested in the acquisitional problems of blind children. She finds that they generally lag behind normal children through early stages of development, and they have some difficulty with imitation and with pronouns and other specific dimensions of syntax.

Overall, the content of *The Acquisition of Communicative Competence* provides a strong background for the further applications of assessment and intervention considered in this volume.

THE PLAN OF THE BOOK

There are two major issues in this book. The first issue bears on how communicative competence is acquired, and the second issue relates to how professional workers and their supporting colleagues can facilitate this development. Acquisition of communicative competence is a developmental consideration; the facilitation of its development relates to assessment and intervention.

Development

How communicative competence is acquired is covered in chapters by Dore and by Ervin-Tripp and Gordon. Each chapter presents an organizing theme and follows it across several developmental stages. The content of these chapters provides many suggestions and implications for intervention planning. The methods used by adults in stimulating and teaching their children from infancy to later childhood are largely congruent with the procedures now advocated generally in intervention programs.

In Chapter 1, Dore focuses on conversational competence and identifies the roles of speakers as agents, ''co-constructing events with others by negotiating their word meanings for their situations at hand.'' His analysis of communicative competence has four interlocking subsystems (or domains of competence) that interact. The basic elements are the *feelings* between participants that motivate the utterance *forms* used to affect various intentional and sequential *functions* relative to the contextual *frames* in which they occur. This approach to competence can be compared with the approach developed by Ervin-Tripp and Gordon in the following chapter. The authors attempt to define conversational competence (Dore) and instrumental language (Ervin-Tripp and Gordon) as a broad set of competencies that involve influences within the context itself as well as the knowledge of the language user. In his feeling-form-function-frame analysis, Dore draws on social theory, linguistics, the philosophy of language, the ethnography of speaking, and other interactive communicative functions. Using a careful observational procedure across several developmental stages, Dore provides a perspective of the issues that can be attended to by parents, teachers, applied researchers or others with an interest in the developing competencies of children. His discussion suggests contextually related tactics for contributing to the language skills of children.

Likewise, Ervin-Tripp and Gordon provide information across several stages of development that enable us to understand how children learn to construct instrumental strategies for environmental effectiveness. They are interested especially in the way children employ strategies in making both direct and indirect requests. They show that the child uses an increasing range of indirect forms that correspond eventually to adult use. In presenting both the social and the linguistic bases of requests, the authors provide specific indicators that can be used categorically in educational contexts. However, the authors fall short of developing a taxonomy of requesting strategies. Their view is that children are not categorically similar across these developmental stages but each child develops strategies within unique cultural and environmental contexts. It is better, therefore, to understand how instrumental requesting evolves than to construct a taxonomy for use with all children.

The reader is urged to supplement the content provided by Dore and by Ervin-Tripp and Gordon with a previous volume by Schiefelbusch and Pickar (1984). In addition there are several publications (Friel-Patti and Louglay-Moltinger, 1985; Snow, Midkiff-Borunda, Small, and Proctor, 1984; and Snyder, 1983) that demonstrate procedures for applying social functions in various instructional contexts. These contexts represent special arrangements for teaching social skills. They suggest important strategies that will guide teachers and clinicians in arranging instruction within various social environments.

Assessment

Dollaghan and Miller (Chapter 3) consider the issue of taxonomies in deciding which features to observe in setting up approaches to measurement. They point out that a general taxonomy could be constructed from existing pragmatics or speech act theory but that it might not be valid for a given observer and a particular child. Instead of proceeding then from a fixed taxonomy, they recommend the observation of variances of the child under study. A special observational period can be used in identifying the observational issues for each child. To facilitate the measurement, however, Dollaghan and Miller suggest three broad clusters of pragmatic issues in the observation of the child. The first cluster includes the child's intentions and the communicative functions used by the particular child in expressing these intentions. The second cluster includes rules for sequencing communicative acts and reflects the child's competency in using the structures and specific functions of language. The third cluster includes ways in which the speaker or listener is able to integrate linguistic and nonlinguistic information in presupposing or foregrounding necessary information for selecting appropriate devices in speaking.

Although the authors recognize overlap among these clusters, they nevertheless provide general guidelines for selecting categories of particular interest for a young child. The focus of observational methods provided by Dollaghan and Miller relates to their plan for observation. Each language intervention specialist or each assessor of communicative competence in the acquisitional study should learn to be a good observer. These examiners provide the steps through which an observational plan must move in arriving at valid data. This approach could be adopted by observers to serve special purposes in language assessments.

In Chapter 4, Rosenfeld extends the observational techniques to a higher level of technical sophistication to help the reader understand the specific methodologies involved in perceiving, recording, analyzing, and interpreting the child's social language behavior. The coding of social information to aid in the storage and accessibility of information receives special treatment. Applying the contents of this chapter might require intensive effort on the part of the reader; however, it is information that can scarcely be avoided if the reader intends to record reliable and valid language information and to use the data appropriately. This chapter suggests that language information is complicated and difficult. Practitioners and scientists must be extremely skillful in handling the data if they are to arrive at a basis of reliable knowledge.

Intervention

Duchan (Chapter 5) develops her framework for intervention from informal assessments and from pragmatics. Her orientation to pragmatics places her within a social and interactional design. However, she draws on several clinical approaches and theories. Her notion of "sense making" emphasizes the social awareness shared by two or more persons if they are to make sense in talking with each other. The speaker and the listener must have some sense of what the other knows and must be able to direct responses toward a common awareness about meaning. The meaning must also include an awareness about the situation, the roles each play, and the events they are attempting to discuss and to negotiate. Duchan also discusses a procedure she refers to as "fine tuning," which is the main strategy of the clinician in helping a client. However, this "fine tuning" is done not by one person acting alone as a communication agent but rather by two or more who may be communicating simultaneously. This later issue places the strategies for language intervention clearly within a transaction framework and suggests that the skills required for communication are in perceiving the meaning of others as well as in providing meaning for others. Sense making and fine tuning provide a framework for clinical activities relating to communicative competence.

Hart and Risley's core incidental strategy in Chapter 6 is less structured and less organizing than is Duchan's approach. They are concerned primarily with the way an adult teacher, parent, or clinician approaches a child to evoke continuing conversation. For instance, they suggest that the adult should prompt the child with questions that encourage the child to name, to describe, or to relate information. They point out that the strategies used incidentally are individually adapted prompts for the elaboration of behavior. Hart and Risley are interested in creating preconditions for incidental strategies in unstructured situations. They teach the adult to recognize occasions in which an incidental teaching strategy can be applied. These applications take place during free play. The primary strategy is to get the teacher to attend to incidental opportunities to get the child to continue talking. Hart and Risley find that getting the child to take another turn is beneficial for language use regardless of the topic or the content of the adult's responses. The skill is in the way the adult attends to the child's feedback. In other words, the teacher learns to focus on the behavior of the child.

In Chapter 7 Bryan establishes the link between learning disability and language deficits. She focuses on social deficits in contrast to deficient literacy functions such as reading and writing. Social skills are examined in relation to the difficulty that learning disabled children have in understanding the in-group language of their peers and in becoming accepted as a member of the "in" group.

These difficulties create problems of social status and social effectiveness for learning disabled children. Consequently, the child may not be able to manage the social contingencies that go with the formal activities of responding to and participating in the learning experience.

Bryan's prescription for intervention is direct, individualized instruction combined with group training programs in more open and naturalistic arrangements. In all instances, instruction should be keyed to the child and maintained within a larger educational experience. The objectives are to help the learning disabled child establish comfortable, effective language use for social and curricular activities.

The last chapter in the intervention section, Chapter 8, focuses strongly on the cultural designs that support the educational experience. Rice explains that her premises relate to cultural knowledge and social cognition. Rice describes the premises usually employed in language intervention work and contrasts these with premises for intervention from a communicative competence model. In doing so she emphasizes the role of inculturation in language instruction. Rice's approach can be compared to Duchan's and to some degree also to the approaches of Bryan and of Hart and Risley.

The four approaches in this section emphasize the importance of social variables in language acquisition. Rice emphasizes cultural issues in addition, but otherwise the authors are similar in philosophy. Where they differ is in how they choose to implement their intervention systems. Duchan's approach to intervention is to concentrate on what the interacting members think is happening and on their sense of shared reality in trying to communicate about something. The interventionist fine tunes that experience to make the child member of the interaction communicate more effectively.

Hart and Risely focus on transaction per se. They cue on the child's initated behavior. They want the child to request or to indicate a need for information, which the adult uses as a basis for encouraging further communication. This approach is instrumental in encouraging the child to engage in further dialogue. They give less emphasis to the language structuring described by Duchan.

Bryan focuses on the social dimensions of language and learning deficiency. She recommends that the learning disabled child receive training to become more effective in the environments where learning takes place. These should include the formal contexts of instruction as well as the social environments of the child's expanding social experience. Rice too holds that communicative competence is primarily social but that the social role-playing of the child is embedded within a cultural system that is larger and more inclusive than is a social experience per se. The emphasis on culture also provides a means for approaching the difficulties of bilingual children who are not fully acclimated in the culture in which the communication is taking place. It provides a means for the teacher, parent, or clinician to help the child become better adjusted. These culturally related contexts contribute strongly to the roles children play and to their experiences in a large range of learning and social activities.

REFERENCES

Chomsky, N. (1957). *Syntactic structures.* The Hague: Mouton.

DeHart, G., and Maratsos, M. (1984). Children's acquisition of presuppositional usages. In R. L. Schiefelbusch and J. Pickar (Eds.), *The acquisition of communicative competence* (pp. 237–294). Baltimore: University Park Press.

deVilliers, J. G. (1984). Form and force interactions: The development of negatives and questions. In R. L. Schiefelbusch and J. Pickar (Eds.), *The acquisition of communicative competence* (pp. 193–236). Baltimore: University Park Press.

Friel-Patti, S., and Louglay-Moltinger, J. (1985, March). Preschool language intervention: Some key concerns. *Topics in Language Disorders, 5*(2), 46–57.

Gordon, D., and Ervin-Tripp, S. (1984). The structure of children's requests. In R. L. Schiefelbusch and J. Pickar (Eds.), *The acquisition of communicative competence* (pp. 295–321). Baltimore: University Park Press.

Hymes, D. (1967). Models of the interaction of language and social setting. *Journal of Social Issues, 23,* 8–28.

Hymes, D. (1972). Models of the intention of language and social life. In J. J. Gumperz and D. Hymes (Eds.), *Directions in sociolinguistics: The ethnography of communications.* New York: Holt, Rinehardt & Winston.

MacWhinney, B. (1984). Grammatical devices for sharing points. In R. L. Schiefelbusch and J. Pickar (Eds.), *The acquisition of communicative competence* (pp. 323-374). Baltimore: University Park Press.
Rice, M. (1984). Cognitive aspects of communicative development. In R. L. Schiefelbusch and J. Pickar (Eds.), *The acquisition of communicative competence* (pp. 141-189). Baltimore: University Park Press.
Sachs, J. (1984). Children's play and communicative development. In R. L. Schiefelbusch and J. Pickar (Eds.), *The acquisition of communicative competence* (pp. 109-140). Baltimore: University Park Press.
Schiefelbusch, R. L. (1984). Assisting children to become communicatively competent. In R. L. Schiefelbusch and J. Pickar (Eds.), *The acquisition of communicative competence* (pp. 525-533). Baltimore: University Park Press.
Schieffelin, B. B., and Eisenberg, A. R. (1984). Cultural variation in children's conversations. In R. L. Schiefelbusch and J. Pickar (Eds.), *The acquisition of communicative competence* (pp. 377-420). Baltimore: University Park Press.
Slobin, D. (1967). *A field manual for the cross-cultural study of the acquisition of communicative competence.* Berkeley, CA: ASUC Bookstore.
Snow, C. E. (1984). Parent-child interaction and the development of communicative ability. In R. L. Schiefelbusch and J. Pickar (Eds.), *The acquisition of communicative competence.* Baltimore: University Park Press.
Snow, C., Medkiff-Borunda, S., Small, A., and Proctor, A. (1984, September). Therapy as social interaction: Analyzing the contexts for language remediation. *Topics in Language Disorders, 4*(4), 72-85.
Snyder, L. S. (1984). Communicative competence in children with delayed language development. In R. L. Schiefelbusch and J. Pickar (Eds.), *The acquisition of communicative competence.* Baltimore: University Park Press.
Snyder, L., and Downey, D. (1983). Pragmatics and information processing. *Topics in Language Disorders, 4,* 75-86.
Sugarman, S. (1984). The development of preverbal communication: Its contribution and limits in promoting the development of language. In R. L. Schiefelbusch and J. Pickar (Eds.), *The acquisition of communicative competence* (pp. 23-67). Baltimore: University Park Press.
Urwin, C. (1984). Communication in infancy and the emergence of language in blind children. In R. L. Schiefelbusch and J. Pickar (Eds.), *The acquisition of communicative competence* (pp. 479-524). Baltimore: University Park Press.

SECTION I
DEVELOPMENT OF COMPETENCE AND PERFORMANCE

Chapter 1

The Development of Conversational Competence

John Dore

The purpose of this chapter is to characterize a conversational version of communicative competence and to demonstrate how such competence changes throughout early development in the child's relationships with other people and in the social contexts in which he or she is involved. In the first section of the chapter, the complexity of the child's competence will be described in terms of conversational subsystems of forms and functions and the contextual frames in terms of which they are interpreted. Changes in competence will be described through analyses of examples from the earliest development during infancy through grade school.

The next section provides background material and concepts and definitions of the elements of conversational competence in terms of the subsystems involved. Emphasis is placed on the units of analysis, the criteria for describing them, the theoretical value of the methods used, and the limitations of each subsystem. The subsystems approach is presented as a descriptive scheme of methods for explicating conversational competence. This approach is useful in showing how utterance forms and functions operate, partly dependent on the social contexts in which they occur and partly determinative of those contexts.

Following sections of the chapter apply the descriptive scheme to four periods of development: the transition from prelinguistic communication to the child's first words; the development during the long one-word period; the nursery school conversation of 3 year old children; the grade school talk of 6 year old children. Analyzing examples from each period in terms of each system will show the shifting preponderance of influence of subsystems on periods of development, that is, the primacy of relationship for the transition to language, of cohesive forms for the one-word period, of coherent functions for nursery school, and of the social contexts for conversation in the grade school phase.

The format for each section is similar. First, certain issues concerning the period are raised. Any additional relevant concepts will then be introduced, the methods and analyses offered, and the results and implications presented. However, the issues discussed and some methods mentioned vary with the period. For example, the affective relationship between mother and infant during the transitional period is analyzed largely in nonlinguistic terms; a case study of one child's lexical development for the one-word period is presented; an analysis of fantasy talk in a play episode among several nursery schoolers is offered; and excerpts from a reading lesson for grade school children is presented. The data for each period come from different projects collected under different conditions for different purposes. Thus, the format is neither a longitudinal study of the same children nor an analysis from a single theoretical viewpoint. Rather, the approach is as an exposition of several levels of interrelated functions of utterance forms relative to their contexts, in which the *critical context* differs with each period of development and the relations among forms and functions become increasingly more sensitive to social constraints on interpersonal activities.

A PRAGMATIC ORIENTATION TO COMMUNICATIVE PERFORMANCES

The analytical criteria for evaluating linguistic competence have been: (1) "*well-formedness*" of a sentence's grammatical structures; (2) the *meaningfulness* of its semantic content in terms of notions like ambiguity, and synonymy presupposition; and (3) the *truth* of the propositions (presuppositions and so on) underlying otherwise well-formed and meaningful sentences relative to the circumstances to which they correspond. On the other hand, the pragmatic criterion for communicative competence has been the *appropriateness* of speech use in context. Whereas many utterances might be appropriate at a given point in a conversation, not all of them will be equally effective. Answering a question with a word for the solicited information may be appropriate, but responding with another question effects quite different purposes. Thus, the differential *effectiveness* of one utterance over another—especially in the different personal consequences for speaker and hearer beyond the sentential information conveyed—is a second criterion of communicative competence. Furthermore, speech is viewed as a means by which speakers influence each other, the ways in which they hold each other accountable to making sense, speaking clearly, maintaining consensus, abiding by rules, and so on can be examined. Communicative effectiveness requires cooperation, and cooperation sometimes requires accountability. Therefore, instead of assimilating communication toward a formal competence model (and searching for distributions, correlations and extralinguistic meanings), a pragmatic performance approach would emphasize the usefulness and effectiveness of forms and the accountability procedures practiced by speakers in negotiating their different scenes.

A thoroughgoing pragmatic approach to speech development thus requires a radical reorientation of theoretical perspective. Ad hoc extensions of the theory of linguistic competençe are inadequate to the data of speech performance. The analytic tools of the structuralist paradigm are incompatible with the nature of pragmatic data, which involve motivation and action in contexts of conversation and concerted activity; that is, the phenomena of intentional and symbolic acts of speech, their functions in conversation, their consequences for participants, and their context-creating power and context-dependent properties are inherently social, dynamic, and dialectical. They are not addressable in terms of the cognitive and monadic constructs of most structurally oriented theories. Indeed, the structuralist and pragmatic approaches address phenomena of a different order: structural approaches to development concern primarily the individual's competence to abstract from, adapt to, and control his or her environment, whereas pragmatic approaches in the wide sense used here concern the organism's development as a person defined in relation to others who deliberately intend the organism's development in conjunction with practical, everyday social concerns.

Structural and cognitive accounts of language typically assume that development is controlled from within the individual (whether by cognitive processes or substantive constraints) and focus on the construction and elaboration of mental products. But pragmatic approaches should begin by postulating that development proceeds from intersubjectively sustained activity to the child's cognitive-linguistic control and should focus on the emergence of self-awareness and the child's personal powers in social interaction. For example, a pragmatic theory of early lexical development cannot begin by asking how meanings are used by the child but must ask, What difference does the use of language make to the child? How do the child's and adult's uses of word forms become meanings for the child? What motivates the child's reorganization of his lexicon? What are the fundamental functions of speech for the child and how do these functions affect the acquisition of structures? How do functions change over time? Some answers to these questions are suggested throughout this chapter.

The study of communicative performance must be oriented to the organized displays of intents and beliefs, as conveyed by actions and speech acts, rather than to the individual's knowledge of grammatically organized propositions and speech acts. It must deal with the actual interpretation of speech across persons in concerted activity in which meanings are *indexical* to the situation and the projected consequences of speech are what motivate its production. Although grammatical knowledge is a guide to the participant's comprehension of the semantic import of sentence type, the *systemic* meanings given by the grammar do not fully determine the many situated meanings of a speech encounter.

Most psycholinguistic accounts view the speaker as somehow pairing concepts and words (propositions and sentences), guided by the processes of attention, perception, and memory, in an effort to describe perceived or potential versions of reality. Pragmatic accounts should view the speaker as an agent interacting with other agents, exercising personal powers in a dynamic attempt to project or eliminate realities or fictions. Instead of beginning with the child-as-monad's construction of symbols, pragmatic approaches should begin by identifying the signals of the dyad's intersubjective experience in confrontation with each other, a confrontation that plays a decisive role in defining the child as well as his conception of the environment. Undoubtedly, the acquisition of linguistic structures does require an underlying category or symbol-making capacity whose purpose is to construct stable conceptual-linguistic representations. But be that as it may, the actual development of speech still depends on the uses of word-symbols in contexts with others whose purposes are to codetermine the status of ongoing activities, to define themselves relative to others and the world, and to deal with the consequences of speech activity.

Morris's (1946) definition of pragmatics as concerning the relationships between symbols and symbol users has often been cited as fundamental to the enterprise. But work has proceeded as if the pragmatic domain were the same in kind as that of syntax and semantics, as though syntactic *structures*, semantic *meanings*, and pragmatic *functions* were homologues of a generic type. On the contrary, the uses to which speech is put are not functional analogues of structural types. The function of interrogative structures, for example, is to ask questions. But this tells us little about the experienced regularities of what, where, when, why, how, and with whom questions are used. Neither does it explain why some interrogative forms fail to elicit answers or why some declaratives are responded to as questions. Nor is there merely a nonisomorphism here between form and function. Rather, uses of speech differ in kind from structures of language. To catalog the functions of language is to try to assimilate the situated uses of speech to a structural perspective and to lose much of the effect of speech from the speaker's perspective. Speech is rich, varied, multivalent, fluid, open, socially sensitive and guided by procedures not listable in advance. The uses of speech, unlike structures, are those parts of messages that remain glued to their contextual backgrounds.

If we are serious about investigating communicative performances, we must identify speech functions in terms of conversational procedures that operate across persons' turns at talk in contexts of different types. Models of linguistic competence are not sufficient nor are taxonomies of speech act types. Short of equating the whole of psychology with pragmatics, we must identify the roles of speakers-as-agents co-constructing events with others by negotiating their word meanings for their situations at hand.

BACKGROUND: SYSTEMS OF CONVERSATIONAL COMPETENCE

Conversational competence comprises four interlocking subsystems (or domains of competence) that interact with one another. The basic elements are the *feelings* between participants that motivate the utterance *forms* used to effect various intentional and sequential *functions* relative to the contextual *frames* in which they occur. The feeling-form-function-frame analyses derive from theories of community, cohesion, coherence, and context as these have been articulated within the disciplines of social theory, linguistics, the philosophy of language, and the ethnography of speaking. Although each element has focused on a different aspect of competence, they can be integrated in a comprehensive description of conversational skills. Their initial separation is for analytical convenience. In actual performance they co-occur and the boundaries among them are not always clear. Moreover, the specific ways they relate to each other change with development.

The relations among participants are important determinants of how a conversation will go. But exactly how relationships affect conversation has received little attention. Here, as background to the analyses, a few notions about relationships will be mentioned, while issues regarding personhood, motivation, and affect will be discussed with regard to infant development. The notion of "community" has been described as varying from a mere random collectivity of individuals, through various types of social groups organized in terms of the reciprocal functions performed by its members, to the personal communion achieved by intimate dyads. With each of these personal and social configurations the notion of "membership" varies drastically. Four kinds of membership are especially relevant to tracking conversational development: the intimate partners in the mother-infant dyad, the younger sibling in the family, the peer relations of play groups, and the pupil status in school.

Whereas the relationships among group members affect many aspects of interaction beyond conversation, the other three subsystems concern the content of a conversational turn at talk proper. Cohesion is the marking by lexicogrammatical forms of semantic and textual relations across turns at talk. Coherence concerns multiple levels of utterance functions across sequences of turns related by propositional and illocutionary phenomena (i.e., belief systems, intentions, and so on), and contextual relations concern the organization of topics, activities, and constraints on conversation, especially how cooperative or competitive talk in a given scene might be. Cohesive ties can range from mere repetition and pronominalization to extensive paraphrases. Coherence covers from minimal backchannel acknowledgements and obligatory pair-parts (such as summons-response) up to the themes of talk as expressed by speaker beliefs, attitudes, implications, and so on. Context may be signaled by deictic references to elements of a scene as well as constrained by culture-wide prescriptions for conducting talk encounters. Most utterances reflect some aspect of all three subsystems. For example, a "me" answer to a teacher's "who" question is a pronominal tie, the satisfaction of an illocutionary expectation of an answer, and a deictic reference to a participant, as well as being indicative of the context of instruction in which it occurs.

Cohesive ties signal a textual relatedness that ultimately accrues to common frames of reference, propositional pools, and shared topics. Coherence reflects interpersonal factors like degree of sincerity, willingness to comply, and the effective sequencing of talk. Context concerns matters such as the ratification of participants, the negotiation of social import, and the shifting of topics and activities. These three strata for constructing a turn's content relate to language in different ways. Cohesion manifests the degree of semantic contingency realized by surface forms; coherence, the extent of common thematic interpretation; and context, that of interactional consensus. The criteria for evaluating each system varies. Of cohesive ties it is asked how well formed and meaningful they are; of coherence, how sensibly connected turns at talk are; and of context, how members hold each other accountable to their shifting consensus. Finally, whereas cohesive ties create a text out of utterance forms, coherently constructed turns give conversation its thematic texture. The context partly determines both but is also partly constituted of both.

Cohesive Ties and Some Functional Analogues

Cohesion has been described most fully by Halliday and Hasan (1976) as the meaning relations among forms that create texts. A "text" is a semantic unit of any length, often realized by sentences but going well beyond grammatical boundaries. In other words, "cohesion occurs where the interpretation of some element in the discourse is dependent on that of another. The one presupposes the other, in the sense that it cannot be effectively decoded except by resource to it" (p. 4). Halliday and Hasan identified five types of cohesive ties in English: reference, substitution, ellipsis, conjunction, and lexical cohesion. Reference occurs when one expression relates to another occurring elsewhere in the conversation; substitution, when another is replaced by a second expression. Ellipsis takes place when an item is omitted that can be recovered from the preceding text, and conjunction occurs when causal, temporal, and other relations are signaled between clauses. Lexical cohesion occurs when items are repeated, synonymous, superordinate, and so on. The amount of interpretation of items that requires reference to other explicit verbal items in a text determines the density of cohesion.

Certain notions from other literatures are compatible with the cohesion model of text and are necessary supplements to it if conversation is to be more fully described. First, nonverbal modalities of expression are often closely analogous to cohesive ties. A gesture may refer to an aspect of the situation, thereby "tying" it to the ongoing talk. Intonational features often signal relations between sentences (in "grammatical cohesion") and between a linguistic and a nonlinguistic element, such as when emphatic stress singles out some contextual element for particular notice. Even the meaningfulness of laughing or crying at certain points can only be interpreted by reference to specific prior events. Body posture can function as a signal of return to some previously established activity. And modalities like gaze and respiration, especially in infants and language-delayed populations, often function as infracommunicational cues to comprehending messages.

A second kind of tie between linguistic and nonlinguistic elements is what Gumperz (1976) called a "contextualization cue." Because sentences are often ambiguous as to which proposition is meant and because speech acts are often equivocal as to what intention is being expressed, additional cues must continually be supplied to express how an utterance is to be taken. These specify the frames for talk. They select which of a potential array of messages suggested by linguistic forms will in fact be heard.

As still another kind of tying, Garfinkel and Sacks (1970) have indicated how conversation is pervasively *indexical* of shared realities. It is not merely that deictic pronouns, adverbs, and other parts of speech express particular persons, times, places, and so on. Rather, virtually all conversation ubiquitously indexes multiple aspects of contexts and can almost always be seen to signal messages such as, "This is what we are doing and meaning now." One type of index is what Garfinkel and Sacks call a "formulation"; that is, the part of a conversation treated as "an occasion to describe that conversation, to explain it, or characterize it, or explicate, or translate, or summarize, or furnish the gist of it . . ." (p. 350). One of their examples concerns a policeman telling a motorist, "You asked me where Sparks Street is, didn't you? Well, I just told you." Here it is not merely the personnel being indexed by the deictics "you" and "me," but the entire activity is indexically formulated by the speech.

Coherence in the Sequencing of Conversational Acts

The coherence subsystem provides ways to sort out and organize the complex and varied elements involved in turns at talk. These elements range from the selection of speakers to the maintainance of thematic relevance. Sacks, Schegloff, and Jefferson (1974) proposed a model of participants' procedures for turn-taking that has two components: *turn-construction*, the selection of linguistic units in formulating one's turn at talk, which has the feature of projectability, such that a listener can anticipate the turn's completion and thus identify a potential transition point for turn-taking; and *turn-allocation*, the technique by which the current speaker selects the next speaker or the next speaker selects himself. But turn-taking is not merely a mechanical matter of waiting for a speaker to finish. Turns have a recipient design. They are constructed in light of an audience, and they are related to surrounding turns. As Schegloff (1971) put it regarding place terms, one must perform a three-part analysis: A *membership* analysis (*who* one is talking to), a *topical* analysis (*what* is being said), and a *geographical* analysis (*where* the location referred to is). Sacks and colleagues (1974) also describe three intra-turn parts: prestarters or links to previous turns, the primary contribution of content, and next-speaker selection. Finally, there are conventional utterance types and sequences. For example, adjacency pairs exist whose first-pair parts can be used to select the next speaker: A summons solicits a response, a question an answer, and so on.

Sacks and colleagues (1974) suggested that the turn-taking system directly affects such crucial factors as sticking to the topic on the floor, accomplishing the purpose of the talk exchange (see also Grice's [1975] maxims) and reflecting a mutual frame of reference. First, the system provides a motivation for listening, for apart from listening out of politeness a speaker must carefully monitor conversation in order to speak next. As Sacks and associates (1974) put it: "The system translates a willingness or potential desire to speak into a corollary obligation to listen" (p. 732). Second, members must attend in order to know what is being done with talk. (Is there a joke, challenge, insult, on the floor?) But the turn-taking system does not provide recognition of such acts (see Dore, 1977, 1978, for such turn content). And third, after securing a turn, the listener displays his understanding of prior turns, which may or may not need redressing. Such immediate feedback displays also give the investigator some access to the participants' own categories of understanding each other because they must continually adjust and make sense of themselves in conversation.

Partners in a conversation must also be able to interpret each other's propositions, the intentions behind the acts performed, and the interactional facts accomplished by these acts. That is, they must be able (1) to use a grammar to parse surface forms into sets of propositions, (2) to determine the kinds of illocutionary acts performed, and (3) to recognize what these acts accomplish socially. Each of these levels influences the others in the process of utterance interpretation.

The unit of the speech act (as formulated by philosophers like Austin, 1962, and Searle, 1969; and as applied to child language by Dore, 1977; Ervin-Tripp, 1977; Garvey, 1975) is a central unit of discourse. It is the unit most capable of conveying propositional, intentional, and interactional meanings simultaneously. This can be illustrated by an example from a reading lesson. When a teacher says to a child, "Read page four!" the proposition consists of an implicit *you* as the subject-noun phrase and *read page four* as the predicate phrase. The teacher's intention is to request the action specified by the proposition. The interactional consequence is to designate the next reader. The child's acceptance of the request commits her to perform the action of reading. Thus, conversational participants determine the kind of illocutionary act performed by analyzing its linguistic form, propositional content, and interactional function.

The performance of an illocutionary act entails certain beliefs, intentions, expectations, and implications on the part of both the speaker and the listener (see Dore, Gearhart, and Newman, 1978, for further details). Some of these entailments are conveyed directly by the linguistic form. For example, the speaker's use of an interrogative mood in English conveys an *intention* to ask a question and an *expectation* to receive an answer. A second group of entailments, however, are not linguistically marked. For example, upon hearing a description, a listener *believes* not only that the speaker's statement is true (i.e., its propositional meaning is true) but also that the speaker believes it is true (i.e., the speaker intends to speak the truth). Such entailments are often called sincerity conditions (Searle, 1969). A third group of entailments are prosodically marked. Thus, an ironically intoned "He's a genius" implies that he is *not* one. Finally, Grice (1975) has suggested a whole array of "conversational implicatures" that can be conveyed beyond the linguistic information given. The production of an illocutionary act—with its entailments and implicatures—shall be called a *conversational act* (or C-act) in analyses proposed below.

However, detailed empirical investigations of the use and interpretation of speech acts have been rare. The most extensive treatment of linguistic acts *and* social frames is Labov and Fanshel's (1977) analysis of therapeutic discourse. They begin with an ostensibly paradoxical view: "Conversation is not a chain of utterances, but rather a matrix of utterances and actions bound together by a web of understandings and reactions" (p. 30). Labov and Fanshel distinguished sharply between the planes of what is said and what is done and claim that the actions performed are more dominant than the forms of utterances: "It is not the linguistic form of the interrogative which demands the linguistic form declarative, but rather requests for action which demand responses to be compiled, put off, or refused" (p. 70). That is, rather than merely questioning and answering one another, participants move on levels of deeper action, and Labov and Fanshel offer many rules of interpretation, showing how different forms may be heard as requests, challenges, and so on as well as rules of sequencing, which show the horizontal relationships across conversational turns that unite utterances and actions in a coherent order.

Participants in a conversation can invoke various kinds of cultural maxims by using contextualization cues. Two sorts of maxims are especially relevant to our scheme. Grice's (1975) conversational maxims for truth, relevance, clarity, and perspicuity in cooperative dialogue constrain the interpretation of illocutionary phenomena. However, there is also a more general kind of social maxim for relating meanings. Sacks (1972) emphasized problems in the "hearing" of utterances, especially on the discourse level across sentences and speakers, that had not been addressed by linguists. For example, in analyzing the beginning of a child's story—"The baby cried. The mommy picked it up."—he argued that the "mommy" is heard as the mother of the "baby" and she is heard as "picking it up" *because* it cried. Such interpretations depend on more than grammatical conventions. They involve what Sacks called "membership categorization devices," (1972, p. 332) such as the "duplicatively organized co-incumbents" of the device "family," and the "category-bound activity" of "crying" for babies via the "stage-of-life" device. Such "hearings" are guided by "viewers' maxims," which specify the relevance of social collectivities to the interpretation of utterances in context. Essentially, then, although lexical systems are preconditions for interpretation, they are not operable without the aid of the social conventions of the sort that Sacks articulated.

Contextual Definition and Interactional Consensus

The term "context" refers to a variety of factors, ranging from physical surroundings to cultural constraints. The sense of context as that which organizes activities of face-to-face interaction is the one that directly influences conversation. Such activities include the scene being enacted, the task performed, the game played, the topic discussed, and the mode of interaction (e.g., serious versus humorous). Several ethnographers of speaking and analysts of face-to-face scenes have contributed notions about a distinct level of immediate social context operating on the turn-by-turn construction of conversation.

The immediate social context can be conveniently analyzed according to the influences that help members to reach consensus and according to the moves they make in communicating. These moves are signaled both by what they say and by the bodily postures and gestures they use. The moves and signals are strongly influenced by the context and, in turn, contribute to maintaining the consensus that constitutes the context.

In 1959 Goffman analyzed how speakers project a definition of the situation on one another and how they achieve agreement as to what they are doing. He called this a *working consensus:* "Together participants contribute to a single overall definition of the situation which involves not so much a real agreement as to what exists but rather a real agreement as to whose claims concerning what issues will be temporarily honored" (p. 9–10).

Garfinkel (1967) also emphasized the procedures that participants use in reaching consensus. These are "members' own methods" (ethnomethods) as opposed to the investigator's categories. Rather than being fully known beforehand and automatically applied, such procedures emerge from the interaction itself. Participants must contingently and reciprocally rely on one another to create and sustain the sense in what they are doing. Prior, shared, and even intimate knowledge is never enough. Interactants must still work to create environments in which they can achieve consensus as to what they are doing together.

Goffman (1974, 1976) suggested that given their understanding of what is going on (the frames), individuals create units of conversation. These utterances are moves that initiate a topic, a problem, or an activity or that reply to or extend ongoing topics, tasks, and so on. Moves characterize (more directly than sentences, speech acts, or speaking turns) what it is that speakers orient to in their interactions.

Information on how moves are signaled come from a number of social analysts. These analysts include Malinowski (1923), Birdwhistell (1970), Scheflen (1973), Kendon (1977), and McDermott, Gospodinoff, and Aron (1978). In their view, social contexts are determinants of what and how meanings are conveyed. Actions, words, sentences, gestures, and similar units do not carry meaning independently of their relation to other such units. The most natural and immediate contexts of communication are signaled by participants' coordinated body motion vis-à-vis one another. For example, Birdwhistell (1970) summed up the kinesic-social connection:

> While body motion behavior is based in the physiological structure, the communicative aspects of this behavior are patterned by social and cultural experience. The meaning of such behavior is not so simple that it can be itemized in a glossary of gestures. Nor is meaning encapsulated atomistically in particular motions. It can be derived only from the examination of the patterned structure of the system of body motion as a whole as this manifests itself in the particular social situation. (p. 173)

So, although concerted body behaviors index fairly clearly what participants signal to each other, not all body movements have the same signal value. As Birdwhistell put it, "Our problem is to describe the structure of body motion communication behavior in a way which allows us to measure the significance of particular motions or complexes of motions to the communicational process" (p. 77).

In particular, Birdwhistell (1970) investigated how linguistic structure is often marked kinesically; he showed how body movements systematically co-occur, and often contrast with, varying levels of linguistic form and meaning. This research makes it clear that reliance on linguistic form alone would be misleading because the meanings conveyed by such forms are regularly qualified, mitigated, neutralized, canceled, and otherwise operated on by the concurrent "body work" of speakers. At the level of closest fit, Scheflen (1973) described how a speaker holds a position while talking:

> A speaker will hold some bodily part such as his head, eyes, eyelids, or hands in one position while he articulates a syntactic sentence, then change the position of this part when he finishes that sentence . . . the terminal body movements and the terminal pitch changes occur in the same direction. (p. 20)

It appears then that we operate with two communicative systems—speech and body motion. But we should be wary of the often-used dichotomy between the verbal and the nonverbal. As Birdwhistell (1970) argued, the linguistic and kinesic modes are only "infracommunicational systems, not directly meaningful in themselves" (p. 173). Their artificial separation for the purposes of analysis distorts the communicative process. Members must interpret utterances on the basis of multimodal framing cues (where mode is not merely isomorphic to each channel but multiple modes exist per channel—lexical and prosodic for speech, gestural and postural for body motion). The problem of interpretation is, as Frake (1977, p. 3) put it, "in locating what cues are being responded to in formulating a particular interpretation."

The complexity of utterance interpretation, apart from social frame determinants, can be glimpsed from Scheflen's (1973) speech-gesture synchrony: "A speaker not only signals the completion of his utterance, but he also provides a signal that informs a listener about the expected response" (p. 20). These signals must obviously interact with the turn-taking system for getting the floor and maintaining the topic in conversation.

McDermott and associates (1978, p. 97) pointed out the individual's contribution to the group's work in signaling mutual contexts: "Each of us had a hand in producing the contexts in which we test our hypotheses about what is going on. Our knowledge turns out to be useful only after we have helped to set up conditions for its use." Exactly how each participant has a hand in defining the working consensus is the substance of the four criteria they offer for the ethnographically adequate description of any concerted activity and its contexts. They show how contexts are in some way (1) *formulated* by the members of the group in words or gestures, (2) *acted out* in form as well as content, (3) *behaviorally oriented to as patterns* by the members at certain significant junctures, and (4) used by the members to *hold each other accountable* for enacting or shifting their formulated orders.

Formulations involve naming in some way what is going on, who is doing what, or any stating of the aspects of the agenda of the moment. But such formulations can be abbreviated as the interaction continues. For example, a teacher may begin a reading lesson by calling on a child to read but later can formulate the same kind of calling in abbreviated fashion by head nods and hand gestures or merely by gazing at a child. "Formulations are used to describe the moment at hand and reflexively to organize the context in which next actions take place" (McDermott et al., p. 248).

As far as *acting out* events, people usually take on postures which are indicative of the task before them, and they usually do this together. McDermott and colleagues (1978) called such bodily configurations *positionings*. These represent "a struggle during which members negotiate their relations with each other. Every person involved carefully monitors everyone else for an interpretation of what it is that is going on" (p. 249). Thus, apart from formulations and the gesturing that mark the speech flow itself, the positionings that members take define their event nonverbally. For example, while reading from a book, children will arrange themselves around a table, but while they are not reading, this positioning about the furniture momentarily disappears.

Members *orient to the patterns* in their formulated order and their postural definitions of it. Two important kinds of patterns are *transitions* from one phase of behavior to the next and *breaches* of the formulated order. When a breach is attended to by someone, it alerts others either to deal with it explicitly or to call everyone back into the positioning appropriate to the business at hand implicitly. At the junctures of reading turns, for example, the children will look up to see who is to read next.

Finally, the most revealing means members have for framing their mutual context is to *hold each other accountable* for accomplishing the formulated order. It would be pointless for people to cue each other into a frame without requiring at the same time that each observe it. Given an operative frame, McDermott and associates (1978) claimed that only certain kinds of behavior are acceptable at certain moments, and the members call upon those who misbehave to change their behavior to fit the dominant version of what that positioning should look like. And this holding accountable often entails the other three criteria: "In order to call each other back to a particular way of behavior, the chastising members must orient to the break in the order of their behavior, formulate what has to be done, and reestablish their bodies into a positioning signaling the formulated order" (p. 251).

THE TRANSITION TO LANGUAGE: THE PRIMACY OF RELATIONSHIP

The infant's first words emerge out of a deeply "dialogical" relationship between infant and mother that precedes the later turn-taking of partners contributing to a conversation. Most of the literature on early language acquisition has emphasized either linguistic inputs or cognitive prerequisites, but most recently interest has grown in the interactional aspects of acquisition. Yet even in this latter enterprise there has been little concern for such notions as interpersonal relationship, motivation, affect, and the states of dialog out of which language emerges. As background to the analysis of earliest language, we shall use a conceptualization of "personhood" and interpersonal motivation for learning language proposed by the philosopher John Macmurray (1961) and then describe some recent work on the intersubjective nature of early development. That background will then allow us to conceptualize the affective dimension of early relationship and to propose how the communicative and pragmatic aspects of language can be seen as emerging out of the mother-infant dialog of affect. The analysis of examples of prelinguistic "conversations" will then be offered in terms of the subsystems in our descriptive scheme.

According to Macmurray (1961), personal development is neither individual nor social in the usual sense of the latter terms. Whereas individual development concerns organic processes of growth and adaptation to an environment and social development is characterized by the organization of activities in terms of roles, functions, and goals, the *personal order* concerns two persons in relation primarily for the sake of being together. So the personal is an order above the material and organic orders, though these two constitute part of the former, and it is prior to and (perhaps) parallel to the social. The personal order is prior in the temporal sense at least, in that infancy is the prototypical personal stage. The infant is defined, develops, and totally depends on his or her relationship with significant others, who are the primary environment. In fact, as Macmurray states ". . . the unit of personal existence is not the individual, but two persons in personal relation . . . we are persons not by individual right, but by virtue of our relation to one another . . . the unit of the personal is not the "I," but the "You and I" (p. 61). For Macmurray, then, the biological analogy of an organism adapting to an environment is an impoverished metaphor for human development.

The random behavior of an infant is gradually interpreted as more and more purposeful in his or her interactions with mother. Macmurray (1961) assumed that the infant's only adaptive behavior is the ability to express needs to those who think for him. But in living this way, the infant immediately partakes of both a loving and rational environment in the form of a caring and thoughtful mother. The infant's existence requires informed cooperation and sharing with her, which in turn requires an ability to communicate: "His essential natural endowment is the impulse to communicate with another human being" (p. 51). His cries of discomfort are treated as calls for help; his comfort sounds, as appreciations of care-giving and caressing. It is the infant's mother who thus endows his behavior with meaning. Therefore, even though the infant may be genetically capable of symbolic behavior, prior to this awareness he receives inputs and after it receives confirmation of his symbol-making attempts.

In this scheme, speech is a complex skill that provides the necessary means of reciprocal communication with others. Macmurray (1961) articulated clearly what has become a familiar assumption of current pragmatics: "Long before the child learns to speak, he is able to communicate, meaningfully and intentionally, with his mother" (p. 60). When and why speech becomes genuinely symbolic is the primary issue. But in order to identify and explain symbol acquisition, we must consider Macmurray's claim that cognition and speech arise in contexts of motivated interactions with others in order to establish, sustain, and reestablish the personal order.

The mother's caring action not only addresses the infant's needs but also modifies progressively as the child's own capacity for action increases. On the child's part, his dependence on his mother occasions the negative motivation of fearing her absence as well as the positive motivation of loving her presence, both kinds of motivation occurring long before the child can reflect on such matters. (For Macmurray, 1961, motives remain largely unconscious, whereas intentions to act in specific ways absorb our attention and become increasingly differentiated with development.) Love and fear remain the fundamental personal motives, and "the behavior they motivate is communication . . . the need which they express is one that can only be satisfied by another person's action. The behavior they motivate is therefore incomplete until it meets with a response from the other . . ." (p. 69). This mutuality of action develops from the child's dependence on others to his interdependence with them, not his independence from them.

Regarding the rudiments of cognition, Macmurray (1961) suggests that they grow out of this primal motivation and that cognition begins with the discrimination of the *general other*, specifically by the *tactual recognition* of the other who responds to his needs. The need to communicate to others "is the absolute presupposition of all knowledge, and as such is necessarily indemonstrable" (p. 77). Knowledge in this sense is the negative dimension of action: knowledge is necessary to inform action which is necessary to commune with others. Caregiving activities (feeding, bathing, changing clothes, and so on) set up a rhythm of withdrawal and return from mother to infant. This induces an initial sense of expectation in the infant and the need to discriminate the *significant other* from all else. Eventually it requires that the child learn to *wait* and to recognize the other as the *same* other. It also induces the need for the emergence of images from a tactual base.

When the child has acquired some locomotive and vocal control, the mother begins to enforce her expectation that he do more for himself, complete more of his initiated activities and, in general, become more responsible. Thus the relationship of pure play, in which the mother provides constant care for his needs, finishes his activities, and caresses him for the sake of being together is changed to a different order. When the child begins to walk and talk he acquires a social role, can perform goal-directed actions, complete his activities, function as a partner, take turns, and contribute to outcomes. The mother's withholding of what she previously provided for the child is both a negative motivational crisis, endangering the child's personal order with her, and an enormous inducement to acquire competence to fend for himself in the newer social order mother is initiating.

When the mother refuses what the child expects in his imagination

> He is forced into a recognition of the distinction between imagining and perceiving. For what he anticipates in imagination is contradicted by what actually takes place, and this institutes the contrast between phantasy and reality. But here we must remember that this happens in action and that the Other is personal . . . The contrast of what is imagined and what is perceived is an aspect of the conflict of wills. It . . . represents, in the consciousness of the individual, the contradiction between his own will and the will of the Other. (pp. 96–97)

This distinction is of course first worked out intersubjectively in terms of feeling and behavior, but it provides the basis for knowledge. When the child begins to resist the action of the personal other, this is necessarily a matter of intention. But the child can never in fact *annul* the relationship with the other. He may act as if his mother's actions were not definitive, but "the most that such negative relation in action can achieve is a *symbolic* annulment; the appearance but not the reality of annulment" (p. 92). Finally,

> There is always an element of illusion associated with the negative phase in the rhythm of personal development . . . In the case of the child whose mother refuses to satisfy his expectation any longer, it only *appears* that she refuses any longer to care for him. (p. 93)

It is this apparent negativity on her part and the child's subsequent symbolic reaction to it that urges the notion that egocentric development is negatively motivated to maintain some continuity in self-image in the face of social constraints. It induces the increasing differentiation of appearance and reality.

At least two postulates for a pragmatic theory of development grow out of Macmurray's account. First, at this critical period of the child's life (around one year), the mother (or other primary care-givers) reorients the child away from the personal order with her and toward a social order with others. In other words, whereas their previous interactions were primarily spontaneous, playful, and relatively unorganized for the sake of being together, the mother now begins to require him to organize his action for practical, social purposes; to act on his own (getting his own ball); to fulfill role functions (feeding himself); to behave well by social standards (not throwing his glass); and so on. This induces in the child the fear of having to perform in terms of social standards, which orient away from the personal order of infancy. It also motivates the learning (a learning *while* doing) of socially accountable behavior; that is, acquiring the communicative competence to become capable of reestablishing a personal order. A second postulate concerns the explanation of symbolization. Learning a shared symbol system is negatively motivated by the fear of maintaining and need to maintain the social order on the one hand and positively motivated by the desire to reestablish a (perhaps more elaborate) personal order with the mothering one on the other hand.

If Macmurray's postulates are correct, manifested in mother-child dyadic behaviors will be the effects of the rhythm of withdrawal and return and, longitudinally, the changes that accompany the dyad's relationship as well as the infant's cognitive growth. Focusing on early infant development, Trevarthen (1977) found Macmurray's "field of the personal" to be a more adequate explanation of mother-infant behavior than the more traditional accounts put forward by behaviorists, psychoanalysts, pragmatists, and Piagetians. Within the first 2 months of development, he found that the infant can fix gaze on its mother, make arm and hand gestures toward her with increasing regularity and strength, and smile and make mouth movements like "prespeech." Mothers reciprocate by waiting for, responding to, and stimulating (in a variety of vocal and nonvocal ways) these infant behaviors. Together mother and infant manifest this "primary intersubjectivity" expressed in the form of mutually fitted, reciprocally functional patterns of vocal and gestural interaction.

Trevarthen and Hubley (1979) describe a "secondary intersubjectivity" that occurs at about 9 or 10 months of age. The following characteristics found in one mother (M) and baby (B) dyad are typical of this profound change in relationship: B smiles at M often during joint activity; B gives M look of recognition in response to M's instruction; B integrates attention to M *and* objects in cooperative activity; M develops B's interest in joint activity in which B now performs complex actions in mutually sustained sequences; while M controls the overall "plan of activity," B imitates M's actions, but also alternates roles in give-and-take games; B is highly responsive to M's directive gestures, such as getting what M points to; B demonstrates triumph in mastery of joint projects and smiles when carrying out an act herself; M's "ordinary speaking . . . attracts B's attention, even when not reinforced by other acts of expression; and B shows she knows the names of some toys" (pp. 210–11).

The Transformation of Affect State to Symbolic Expression

Offered in this section is a two-stage hypothesis about how mother and infant interact during this period and the suggestion that such interaction is a necessary condition for language onset. First, when baby expresses affect in a marked way, mother *matches* it by either *attuning* to the same affect-state, *mismatching* it with a different state, or responding with a *ritualized* form of his behavior. These communicative matches intervene in baby's affect-state in the sense that they "analog" it with a differing intensity and often in a different behavioral channel; they contrast baby's affect with an opposing state; or they reproduce an observable form of behavior that baby comes to recognize as a conventional expression of his or her own affective experience.

A simple example, from early on in this period, will illustrate this hypothesis. When babies in our culture express delight in any way at some unusual sight, mothers typically clap to express joy along with them. How can such a match transform an unmediated expression of delight into an intention to express it? First, baby initiates the interaction by his expression; mother's clapping provides an attunement in an observable form of his own affect. Since baby has been observing mother all along, and may not have identified with it, he can now observe *his* own feeling in *her* behavior. When baby claps in response to mother's clapping, he is not merely imitating some form. At that moment he discovers a gesture for what he is feeling. Since her form matches his feeling, his clapping expresses his own state, not hers, even though his affect had to "loop through" her, as it were to become observable. This may be the original moment of "cognizing" a connection between an internal state and the external sign for it. The behavioral form can then be reproduced when feeling the same affect, thereby allowing both baby and mother to "*re*-cognize" and share the same affect state. Perhaps without her attunement to his state in a conventional form, baby could not become aware of his own state—there would be nothing to observe. This awareness may be the origin of intention—the moment when the motivation for an expression finds an observable form that can be focused on and then reproduced.

But this does not explain why baby would change from expressing to intending. For this postulate that baby is motivated to maintain some state of communion with mother. He needs to adapt to her ways of doing and expressing in order to achieve, maintain, repair, and later renegotiate their relationship. In addition, the emergence of communicative intent is best seen in affectively negative situations.

Conflict arises when mother's communicative mismatch *contravenes* baby's affect-state. For example, when the baby in Table 1-1 tries to mouth a piece of a puzzler, his mother prohibits it; this occasions baby's affect expression of a "protest," with an abrupt, high-pitched, vowellike utterance accompanied arm-flapping in apparent anger. Mother then reprimands baby with an obviously angry, intense, "Don't you yell at your mother!" to which baby responds with a still higher-pitched, indeed violent, protest. Baby here again initiates interaction with the positive affect action of mouthing. Mother blocks that affect, in a sense knowing his pleasure but contravening it. Baby of course can not "cognize" her behavior as a form for his affect. However, his protest is provoked by her prohibition, thereby providing a potential link

Table 1–1. A Prohibition Episode Negotiated Between a Mother and Her 9 Month Old Boy

Mother's Adult Behaviors	Baby's Behaviors	Communicative Functions
Put the leaf in there. That's a part of a puzzle.	(holding piece of a puzzle in hands)	directive comment
	/i:::↗↘/ (raising piece to mouth; hesitates, then looks around to mother)	"pleasure" indexical preventable
No. It's not to eat. (playful tone; shaking head)		preventive
	(puts piece in his mouth)	prohibitable
That's a *leaf.* No /::↗↘/ (pulling piece away with her finger)		prohibitive
	/ŋ:ʔʌ̃/ (flapping arms angrily)	protest-1
Don't you yell at your mother (moving piece away from baby)		reprimand
	/m::m↗↘/ (reaching for piece)	elicitive
I said *NO!* (high, intense, abrupt, angry tone; but she gives the piece back to him)		denial compliance
	(puts piece in his mouth)	prohibitable
(pulls piece out of mouth)		prohibitive
	/æ ↗/ (high pitched; arm flapping)	protest-2
I said no. (low, lax; pulling piece away)		warning
	/æ ↗/ (highest pitch; examining piece)	protest-3
	(puts piece in mouth) /m::m/	"pleasure" indexical
Does that taste good? (rocking head up and down)		accusation
	(takes it out; examines it)	compliance
It's only cardboard.		comment
	(puts it back in mouth)	prohibitable
Huh? Does that taste good?		accusation
Let's put it back! (taking it out of his mouth)		directive prohibitive
	(flaps arm weakly) /ʌ ʔ/	protest-4

between his affect and her mismatch; that is, his protest is an unmediated expression of negative affect that analogs her negative act of prohibition. Moreover, the hypothesis that *mother induces intentions in baby* is seen more clearly in the subsequent round of this interaction. After matching intense prohibitions and protests, mother shifts her tone to a lower pitch with a repeated "I said no" while pulling the puzzle piece away from him again; at this he protests most violently, looking at her. It seems as though at this moment he has become aware, through her contravention, of his own negative affect and can begin to intend to express it for the first time.

But, again, why? If baby's affect is breached by a prohibition, rather than attuned to one, the conflict threatens communion. Anxiety arises. Being able to express his state intentionally allows baby to invite a match of positive affect and to deny negative matches. It allows him to test the state of their relationship. The intent to express becomes the first cognitive tool for communicating about their relative states in their dialog with one another. Because the same affect can be differentiated into two forms and communicated cross-modally, partnership in dialog emerges. But *the analog of affect is the foundation of dialog.*

The second part of this two-stage hypothesis is that mother induces in baby conventional forms for expressing shared affect-states. Given that baby can already intend to express his state, the question arises: how does mother intervene in baby's expressions to change their form? But the mere echoing of forms is not of so much concern as the shared meaningfulness of expressions for the dyad. Now, some degree of meaningfulness must already inhere in baby's intentions to express a shared state, some minimal awareness that a form somehow matches an internal state. Although this requires some cognitive processing, the content of what baby is aware of is not yet a cognitive category; it is an affective match. The problem is then not, as in cognitive approaches, to identify the overlap in semantic features of the baby's first words and his caregiver's. Rather, it is to identify the procedures they use to effect "meaningful" exchanges (i.e., interactions that are effective, consequential, motivating, and so on) and to specify the processes by which word meanings emerge from expressions intended and interpreted as shared affect states.

One possibility here, adumbrated by Vygotsky's (1978) dictum that intrapsychic events first occur on an interpsychic level, would be that *their* conversational procedures become *baby's* psycholinguistic processes: that mother's ways of staging scenes, indicating objects, searching for words to fit them, contrasting meanings, and so forth in their affectively meaningful and shared interactions become his ways of, say, sorting information into distinctive semantic sets. In this way mother would at least highly constrain possible interpretations of their shared affect. The central problem would then become the means whereby affectively meaningful communicative actions *between* mother and baby are transformed into personal meanings-for-words *in* baby. This shifts emphasis away from asking what biological and cognitive categories baby brings to the task of language learning toward asking how categories emerge from interpersonally shared affect states and the behavioral forms by which they are expressed. Word meanings are consequences in baby of what mother and baby feel and express. The dialog they engage in is the interface between his functional intents and her formal requirements for interpretation. Though mother cannot give baby his needs, motives and intents, she does supply him with the forms necessary to express them, which forms in turn contribute to the construction of intents, and so on.

When the mother of the 12-month-old girl in Table 1-2 asks, "Wanna play with the castle?" the baby turns to gaze at her. The mother then points to the pile of "castle" blocks and says "This!" emphatically stressing both her vocalization and her pointing gesture. The baby replies with an unintelligible utterance, low in pitch, volume, intensity and duration, resembling an aspirated stop followed by a back vowel (roughly /hkyɔ/). Mother responds with a high-pitched, rising "No!" in a pleasant tone of surprise. At this baby clearly repeats "No!" with an intense, abrupt tone and emphatic head nod. However, contrary to the expected semantically negative "answer," baby proceeds to knock over some of the blocks anyway.

Describing this complex communicative match, it is clear that the baby intentionally expresses her initial response to her mother, behaviorally manifested by her body orientation to her mother and the blocks, her gazing toward her mother, and her vocalizing to her. Mother interprets baby's unintelligible utterance as negative, but she is either unsure, surprised, or both, so mother produces what might have been baby's "answer." But this is no mere imitation. Mother marks her semantically negative content with positive affect. This simultaneously gives baby's utterance conventional form and solicits clarification. Furthermore, for her part, when baby repeats "No!" it is not with mother's surprised tone but with an emphatic one, perhaps "analoging" mother's emphasis on "This!" earlier. Here is seen a conversion from baby's initial intent to "answer" vocally but unintelligibly to her accommodation to mother's form of answering. Again, like clapping for gleeful affect, here mother *trans*-forms baby's expression to a conventional status.

However, in this case there is no direct affect attunement. Rather, a more complex interplay of affect and form takes place. Baby apparently takes the form of mother's negative content but omits the pleasant tone of surprise on that form and assimilates the emphatic marking of mother's prior "This!" to her own "No!" Moreover, this reply constitutes a move in a conflict of the agendas they are negotiating for baby's behavior: the baby has been playing with a phone while the mother is recommending block play. (In fact, the mother's behavior may be an elaborate distraction from the baby's playing with the real phone, not unlike in principle from our first mother's prohibitions.) Thus we have a degree of tension, if not anxiety, in their agenda clash, motivating baby's apparent rejection. Finally, however, baby's "No" has not quite acquired word status since she does go to the blocks, and during this period there is no evidence that she can contrast "yes" and "no" in a semantically consistent way.

Table 1–2. A Play Episode Between a Mother and Her 12 Month Old Girl

Mother's Adult Behaviors	Baby's Behaviors	Communicative Functions
Boy, there's so much to do.		comment
	/dikədæ . . . / pause /dæ ↗/ (while reaching toward telephone; then turns to A)	elicitive
Yea! (high-pitched, elongated, slow-rising, playful tone)		acknowledgment
	(turns to phone)	
Telephone. /∿⌒/ (slow rising and falling contour)		label
	/dætəkæ ↗/ (samp prosody as mother's "Telephone," with rising terminal contour)	elicitive
Aha.		acknowledgment
	(turns to mother) /dɪkæ ↗/ (emphatic stress)	elicitive
Yea. / ↗ /		acknowledgment
	(walking toward corner) /dəkɪdæ/	accompaniment
Wanna play with the castle?		invitation
	(turns to mother)	
This! (emphatic stress and emphatic pointing)		
	/hkyɔ/ (very low pitch, intensity)	"answer"
NO? (high pitch, "surprise")		clarification
	NO! (high, abrupt tone; emphatic head nod)	answer
Okay.		acknowledgment
	(walks to mother; hesitates; then knocks some blocks over)	accompaniment
	/dəkæ ↗/ ("joyful," emphatic tone)	
Yea. (breathy, laughed)		acknowledgment
Knocked it over, didn't ya? Let's see. Whata ya gonna do with the rest of the castle?		"questionings"
	(turns to phone)	"ignore"
Nothing! ("ironic" tone)		self-answer

The same two questions of this wordlike emergence that were asked of the origin of the intention to express arise: how can a baby do it and why would she or he? The first question has been the concern of most approaches to acquisition; most recently cognitive theories have dominated the market. And, indeed, some degree of cognitive processing must occur if a baby is to contrast positive and negative semantic features in the form of *yes's* and *no's*. Moreover, the infant must be able to adapt and produce linguistically contrastive sounds. Both cognitive and phonological contrastivity are necessary inputs to language. The interpersonal matching of affect is also necessary, and the three together may be sufficient to "cause" word meanings to emerge.

The salience of motivation in this account leads to the conclusion that the dialogical basis of language occurs when dyadic partners match and mismatch each other's affect but express themselves in different forms. Adaptation to each other's affect and form constitutes the dyad's very identity. In Piagetian terms, mother accommodates to baby's affect and assimilates it to her forms; baby accommodates to mother's forms and assimilates them to his affect, cognition, and phonology. Tension always exists from the disequilibrium of their matches, at all levels. Mismatches of both kind and intensity abound in every dyad (see Stern, 1977). After intentionality emerges, the only solution to mutual comprehension in dialog is a shared system of symbols.

Again, to be in communion, to be understood, to be effective in conveying intent and content, the baby must adapt to the mother's forms. Not only uncertainty and ambiguity but also anxiety is reduced by being able to express states, needs, and desires for objects and so forth by unequivocal signals; i.e., words that disambiguate among items desired at the right moment. Words reconstitute the dyad's intersubjectivity. They seem to transform it to a "symbolic intersubjectivity" that allows reproducibility of form and interchangeability of speaker. Thus, words prepare baby for the transition out of the intimacy of infant communion to the public and linguistic communication with others.

The Origin of Conversational Subsystems

Much of the foregoing analysis touched on elements of the conversational subsystems of our scheme. Here the earliest version of the systems will be summarized with reference to Table 1-2. It has been seen how this dyad's relationship is expressed in their matching of affect, despite their agenda conflict. That is, though they seem to be in "communion," there is nevertheless competition between the baby's "telephone" activity and the mother's castle block play. Perhaps because they are so well attuned to each other, they are free to negotiate their joint focus, each member projecting her or his preferred agenda, without a breach in the relationship. Baby's focus on the phone is manifested by her gaze at, handling of, and vocalizing about it. Mother's focus on the blocks is indexed by her invitation, then emphatic pointing, and subsequent comments. However, they also alternate joint focus: They display mutual concern for the telephone in the first four interactive sequences, until consensus shifts to the blocks in the second part of the episode. Each agenda is verbally formulated by mother: the label for "telephone" and the invitation for the blocks. There is also mutual accountability displayed by the talk and by their orientation by joint gaze, posture, and gestures to each agenda.

The coherence subsystem is partly tracked by the communicative functions listed in the right-hand column of Table 1–2. As the literature on prelinguistic communicative development suggests, the infant's greatest contribution is in his "performative acts." Here we see several of baby's prereferential (/dIkədæ:/) "indexical expressions" functioning as "elicitives," in which rising terminal contour, pause, and gaze at mother indicate her expectation of response. Baby can also respond to mother's rising tones with functional "answers," despite that such indexical expressions (see further on) are not yet semantically contrastive. Thus, in Table 1–2, the baby's competence for coherence is demonstrated by her ability to reverse speaker roles like eliciter or responder, and the coherence of this episode is further solidified by the mutual acknowledgements of each partner's efforts.

Finally, the cohesion subsystem, as should be expected before denotation emerges, is the least developed in babies at this stage. Formally, in our example there are two types of repetition of mother by baby: the prosody of "telephone" and the segmental phonemic content of "no." But what is most important developmentally is that both of baby's repetitions were of mother's responses to baby's own similar initiations. In other words, here "telephone" and "no" imitations were preceded by her own idiosyncratic versions of similar forms. This suggests how mother's responses can transform baby's initiations to conventional forms when baby adapts to them. This process also shows how lexical cohesion originates. The term "no" for example usually first emerges as a pragmatic performative such as a refusal or protest, but mothers often treat "no" as the counterpart of "yes," thereby inducing the semantic contrastiveness it eventually comes to have for baby.

THE ONE-WORD STAGE: DEVELOPMENT OF THE LEXICON

A profound reorientation occurs after the child begins to produce words. Whereas there was only minimal cohesion with his mother's forms during the transitional period, lexical development now becomes the focus of his concern, and cohesive ties in his conversations proliferate. The goal of this section is to document, by a case study of detailed changes in one child, the growth of the lexicon during the one-word stage. But first some related issues will be discussed by reference to the works of others who share a similar framework, and then the criteria for describing contexts and conversations will be applied to this period.

Bruner (1978) hypothesized that language emerges out of joint action formats engaged in by mother and child. These are highly ritualized, frequently repeated, and saliently marked (at first only by the mother) routines such as bathing, feeding, and game-playing. Bruner found that, within the context of such activities, and before he or she begins to speak, the infant can secure the attention of another, sustain mutual attention to the joint activity, take turns at vocalizing (as well as turns at performing in games), play role functions such as giver and taker of objects, intend goal-directed actions such as hiding an object from the mother, and in general, integrate his or her attention to objects and people in order to communicate (cf. Sugarman-Bell, 1978). Bruner argued that the child could, on the basis of such experience in action formats, begin to grasp case grammatical notions such as agent and patient.

In a closely related work, Ninio and Bruner (1978) analyzed the dialog formats for the emergence of initial labeling by children in the context of joint reading of picture books. An analysis of mother-child behaviors revealed almost complete alternation pattern of turn-taking and role playing. They found that initial labeling "takes place in a structured interactional sequence that has the texture of dialog" (p. 6). These findings concur with those of Snow (1977), who also noted the early appearance of patterned turn-taking in rule-governed situations involving gestures, eye contact, and vocalizations. Ninio and Bruner also noted that such interactions are thing-oriented, in that the things focused upon serve as topics of the exchanges and in that the child progresses from successful nonverbal participation to the capacity for labeling focal objects. Among many structural constancies in the dialog format, they found that mothers primarily use four utterance types: the attentional vocative ("Look!"), the query ("What's that?"), the label ("It's an *X*"), and feedback ("Yes"). The majority were mother's labels, and the types of labels (e.g., nouns for whole objects, object parts, and so on) used by mothers were almost exactly mirrored by the children's labels. Finally, contrary to the claim that mother's corrections cause words to disappear from children's working vocabularies (Nelson, 1973), Ninio and Bruner found that "correcting a misapplied word . . . increases its chances of being used again" (p. 14).

Still more pertinent, Ratner and Bruner (1978) examined the structure of early games by mother-infant dyads to determine how it facilitates language growth. They found that "the *semantic domain* in which formulated play occurs is most usually highly restricted and well understood or conceptualized by the child"; that such early games "involve a restricted format, a limited number of semantic elements, and a highly constrained set of semantic relations" and a "clear-cut task structure which permits a high degree of prediction of the order of events . . . and a clearly demarcated role structure'' (p. 392). Moreover, the task structure of games ''offers clear-cut junctures at which functionally intelligible utterances can be inserted'' (p. 401). And, most importantly, both task constituents and vocalization types had closely related variant forms, allowing for a reciprocal marking of variation across talk and task. Such findings show the interdependence of social activity and language acquisition. All of the work by Bruner and his colleagues, showing the richness and reciprocality of social and semantic structure, can be construed within a personalist framework.

The Context of Conversation in the One-Word Stage

Because the development in the child's competence for cohesion is illustrated by the growth of his lexicon, the analysis here begins with the contextual factors that function in the child's early conversations. Coherence factors will be mentioned in passing where appropriate.

Consider, for example, one child's development. From about 6 to 9 months the parents played minimal ball-rolling routines with this child. He would push it, they would roll it back to him; he would watch them bounce it, and so on. At 9 months the mother began to routinize a ball game for them. She would *formulate* a game's onset verbally with comments like, ''Okay, let's play ball'' or ''Wanna roll the ball with me?'' and nonverbally by arranging their bodies for the game. She would then *enact the doing* of the game by rolling a ball to him. Moreover, she would sit him on the floor, spread his legs into a V-shape and even get his arm to roll it back to her (thus doing it for him at first) while she too was in the V-position facing him. She would then *orient* to the *transitions* in this routine by waiting for him to roll the ball back and to the breaches in their game's order, such as his breaking of the game's V-posture. Finally, she would *hold him accountable* to playing his role, that is, maintaining posture, performing his function of rolling the ball back, receiving it again, and so on.

Although for certain behaviors it may be problematic to distinguish among formulating, enacting, orienting, and holding accountable, they nevertheless provide initial criteria for describing units of mother-child concerted behaviors in their earliest routines in which the child plays an active part. In fact, what is most useful about his framework is that the child is beginning to do the same things as the mother. He too formulates the onset of the game by pointing to (or getting or, later, labeling) the ball; he performs his role functions; he orients to the routine's structure by displaying waiting behaviors and crying at his mother's breaches (such as when she interrupts the game to answer a telephone); and, verbally, we can see him ''re-envoicing'' his mother's words. Furthermore, such latter behaviors are initial forms of holding her accountable to playing the game. Most importantly, when they synchronize their doings of the game together, both reciprocally and differentially, their own behavioral consensus exists on what they are doing. Thus, a way of interpreting their behaviors relative to their other behaviors within their highly constrained routines is present.

Moreover, these same criteria can be applied to verbal data. Consider the following conversation between mother (M) and baby (B), which took place some months later during the same child's earliest phase of speech:

	Conversation	Activity
M:	Okay, let's go play bally. Wanna play bouncy ball?	(M and B go toward family room)
B:	Ball. /bɔ/	(Falling tone; follows M)
M:	Okay. You get the ball there.	(M points to ball; B gets it and hands it to her)
	Sit down. Here. Like this.	(M positions B in front of her; M spreads out legs in V-shape; B approximates same position)
	Here we go.	(M rolls ball to B; B clutches it)
B:	Ball. /bɔ/	(B pushes ball toward M)
M:	Nice. Good boy, Sean. That a boy.	(M rolls ball back to him)

Notice that the mother formulates the routine by announcing what they should do; that is, she projects what is about to occur. Her instructions to get the ball and sit enact necessary components of the activity. Her verbal accompaniment orients to the first rolling turn in the game's structure, and when he returns the ball, she formulates his accomplishment with her congratulations. A few weeks later, while in the game the child throws the ball at the dog, and the mother exclaims "No! No throwing! Roll it!" This constitutes her verbal orientation to a breach in the order of their game and an attempt to hold him accountable to maintaining their formulated order.

In terms of the child's verbal development, he first plays the game while listening to his mother's use of the term "ball" within their activity and relative to the round object in particular. He then imitates her use of the term. Next, he pointedly indexes either the object or the turn at rolling. But his first uses of the term "ball" relate to the object in their ball-playing routine. He later labels balls conventionally, even when they are in stationary positions. Each of the routine scenes in which the child's terms occur must be analyzed according to these criteria in order to trace developments in the child's ability to perform such activities. The actions can then be correlated with changes in the child's lexicon.

Phases of One-Word Development: Foundations of Lexical Cohesion

Here, because the child's own focus shifts to the choice of word among several options for the circumstance at hand, focus will be on the relations among emerging "lexical domains" as the basis for cohesive tying in conversation. Coherence across turns develops much more slowly and will be treated minimally.

Virtually all of the worklike forms used by the author's son (S) during his one-word stage were recorded, partly by audiotape but mostly handwritten. Four major phases of change were identified. The first phase is one of *proto-communicative signals* characterized by nonconventional, syllabic-like proto-linguistic forms used by infants to perform actions. Halliday (1975) identifies these as having *systematicity* (a stable relation between expression form and functional content) and *functionality* (manifesting a set of semiotic functions). Dore, Franklin, Miller, and Ramer (1976) found similar "phonetically consistent forms" that displayed a quasi-stable form and functioned in several quite specific ways. From his 11th to 15th months S produced six (groups of) forms that were consistently functional for him. However, it should be noted that the "meaning" of proto-communicative signals are not controlled by the child. They are, rather, only interpreted by adults. Table 1–3 lists the forms, functions, behaviors, and tones of signals S produced at this phase.

In the *indexical-sign phase*, terms are more conventional in form and meaning then proto-linguistic forms though not yet denotative. They seem to be tied to sensorimotor schemas (though with no isomorphic relation between term and schema) as suggested by Piaget (1962): "the meaning of a term such as "bow-wow" in the case of J changed in a few days from dogs to cars and even to men." Indexical terms seem always to be related to immediately perceivable elements except when the child calls for something. They are global in that they do not distinguish among parts of overall patterns—that is, objects, actors, actions, locations, and so forth. They are widely overgeneralized, like the *mixed overextensions* discussed by Bloom (1973). At this phase the child has a small repertoire of terms that globally index different sets of action patterns, interpersonal situations, or affective states. The child controls the production of these intentionally, but he does not have semantic control of indexical signs as lexical distinctions.

As examples from S's indexical phase (from 15 to 20 months of age), he produced the terms "mama," "dada," and "nana" relative to his mother, father, and grandmother, though not in strict complementary distribution to them. When one of them was present S would say the

Table 1–3. The Protocommunicative Signals and Functions Produced by S (11 to 15 Months Old)

Forms	Behaviors or Tones	Functions
1. [ijæ], [iji], [ijæjə]	Final syllable elongated Most often loud in volume Occasionally abrupt or rising terminal contour	To call for people, animals, or objects To get attention in general
2. [ʔɛʔ], [ʌʔ]	Pointing, looking at, or grasping for objects or people involved Usually abrupt contour Usually successive occurrences	To indicate some object, action or person To get an object
3. [æ]	Widely varying in length After getting an object	To express joy
4. [məməmə]	While whining or crying Distressed behaviors	To seek comfort
5. [e::], [je::]	Widely varying in length Often with jumping and running to hug the new arrival	To express excitement at someone's arrival
6. [ŋ̩]	A velar nasal of long duration Shaking head in different ways Running away or pushing something away	To reject some action

name, usually whining and wanting to be given something. When one of them entered the house he would say a name excitedly, usually clapping and running to hug them. When hurt, S would call to them for comfort. All of these uses of names involved interpersonal communication, the accomplishment of some action, and a clear display of affect. Similarly, the use of terms in other *proto-semantic domains* were interactive: /ku/ for "cookie," /baba/ for "bottle," and /bɔ/ for "ball," for example, were used when S wanted to eat, drink, or play, respectively, or when these items were involved in some activity ("ball" was used for most games). Table 1–4 lists all of S's indexical signs.

During the third phase of *denotative symbols*, the referents of words were more clearly marked and closer to adult uses, marked not only by more pointed use of forms but also by the accompanying gestures and tones. There is also an expansion of the lexicon and a reorganization of it in terms of more clearly delimited semantic domains, exhibiting clear specifications of some terms and generalizations of others. Communicatively, uses of these genuinely denotative words constitute primitive speech acts, in which meaning and intent (as manifested by configurations of prosodic, kinesic, contextual, and conversational factors) are much clearer than with the proto-speech acts of the idexical phase. The hallmark of this phase is, of course, that the child uses many words displaced in time and space from their referents. Also, symbols are organized in terms of lexical contrasts in meaning.

Table 1–4. The Forms and Contents Produced by S that Constitute His "Protolexicon" During His Indexical-Sign Phase (Age 15 to 20 Months)

Forms	Contents	Forms	Contents
	Animals		*Playthings*
bee	flying insects; birds; airplanes; specks of dirt; breadcrumbs; bleeps across television screen; when table is slapped	/bɔ/	small, round balls; when other objects are rolled; to play
/kiki/	family cat ("KiKi"); or small, furry animals, or toys	key	keys; key chains; small screwdrivers; concerted turning of fingers; car ignition and locks; tinkling noises
	Food		*Vehicles*
/ku/ /kəkə/	cookies, crackers, candies; bags of other sweets or dired fruits; when pantry doors open or close; jars	/bo/	boats; bulky objects floating on water; boatlike plain blocks of wood
			Event-markers
baba	bottles and jars of liquid; glasses, cups, containers	bye-bye	leave-taking; greeting; object rolling away from him
	Relationals		*Personals*
no	refusing objects; rejecting actions	/bubu/	scars, scratches, aches; other people crying; after he is hurt
night-night /nayti-nayt/	related to his going to bed (when in pajamas, while lying down	/dudu/	feces; dirt; anything not in its appropriate place
more	requesting another object (toy) or action (tickle)	/pipi/	anything related to his going to the bathroom (his urine in pottie, while holding his genitals)
	People		*Responses to Questions or Comments*
mama dada nana	for interpersonal purposes (requesting attention, act) accompanied by affect	/ʔɛ/	affirmative in that he wants something at issue
baby	children; small dolls		
/eyə/	to call his sister Angela		
	Onomatopoetics		
brrrr	many engine noises		
grrrr	mimicking monsters		
tsk-tsk	when an inappropriate action occurs (falling, spilling, and so on)		
shhhh	water flowing		
boom	loud noises; noise from falls		

At 20 months S's word uses changed dramatically, precisely after the following incident. A word game that was never successful before was played. We said "mama" pointing to his mother, "dada" pointing to his father, and "baby" pointing to him. He repeated the three-part routine several times accurately, smiling broadly after each. This is the first instance of S using words solely for naming, of using "baby" to refer to himself, and of immediately imitating another's speech upon request. After this he began to label persons and objects without apparent affect or attempting to accomplish an interpersonal act. He practiced the use of labels while playing alone. He also used words to note the absence of persons and objects. Further, S's extensions of a term to new referents came under the control of the physical and functional features of the new referents, and he used the same word to perform different speech acts (see Table 1–5 for referential changes).

Four category changes from the indexical to denotative phase are especially relevant:

1. *Specifications:* "baba" from jars, cups, and so on to *his* bottle only to his bottle only with apple juice.
2. *Generalization:* "ball" generalizes from a small set of small round ones to all shapes, sizes, and colors of balls. Another type is relational, like "more" generalizing from requests for repetition to comments on disappearances and reappearance.
3. *Reorganization:* new terms cover subsets of previously conceived lexical domains: "dog" covers non-cats; "cow," larger animals; "tutu," trains, and so forth. Other types of reorganization include *differentiations* (responses differentiate from positive-negative reactions to specific judgments and identifications) and *contrastives* (pairs like "up" and "down"), which are used to contrast directions of movement, though initially in the context of requests.
4. *Detachment:* words become increasingly more detached from their action contexts: "bubu" detaches from contexts of hurt and is used to remark on past occurrences of someone (including dolls and pets) being hurt. Finally, linguistic relations like synonymy, homonymy, and polysemy among and across lexical domains begin to appear.

Finally, there is the *predicate-syntagm phase* during which the child can say one word and indicate another notion at the same time. For example, the child will say "dada" emphatically while pointing to an object belonging to his father to convey something like "that is daddy's." Also, not only displacement increases but each semantic domain is elaborately partitioned and ramified, and most word uses convey multiple messages. S, for example, would say "bee" and point to his arm where he was stung some time before; he would say "bye-bye," not only as a leave-taking but also as a comment on someone's absence (see Dore, 1984, for more detail).

Table 1–5. The Forms and Referent Classes Produced by S During the Denotative Symbol Phase of His Early Lexicon (Age 20 to 23 Months)

Forms	Contents	Forms	Contents
	Animals		*Playthings*
bee	flying insects; birds; falling leaves	/bɔ/	all kinds of balls, not non-balls
kiki	animals in cat family	key	restricted to keys, key chains
/kæ/	other small animals	/pu/	wading pool; bird bath; puddles
/dɔ/	family dog; some others	/ba/	blocks (of his own sets)
cow	larger animals	/hæ/	his fireman's hat
/ræræ/	monsterlike puppets	brm-brm	his toy fire engine
	Foods	/bʊ/	any book, writing paper, etc.
/ku/	cookies, crackers, chips	/bu/	any crayon
baba	his baby bottle only	/wawa/	water in lakes, ocean, rivers
tea	hot liquids in cup being used by an adult		*Vehicles*
/ænə/	bananas; thin zucchini	/bo/	boatlike objects
/biə/	anything father drinks from glass, mug, or can	/tutu/	trains; trainlike toys
	Relationals: "existence"	brrrr	cars, trucks, motorcycles
no	disappearance; nonrecurrence		*Event-markers*
/tap/	rejecting action; protest	hi	greeting (people and objects)
more	disappearance; reappearance; more than one	bye	leave-taking, going to bed
/tu/	requesting another; more than one		*Personals*
	Relationals: "direction"	/bubu/	his or another's hurt
/mu/	requesting others to move	/pipi/	specified for urine, genitals, pottie, urinating, and the need to urinate
/opi/	request to open door, lid; to describe separation of pieces, top off jar, etc.		*Responses to Questions*
/ʌpi/	request to be picked up; describe vertical movement	yea /ʔʌ/	judgmental yes
/dæw/	request to be put down; to describe vertical movement	no /ʔʌʔʌ/	judgment of negation
bye-bye	when leaving; in car, bed	(object names)	are "Wh-answers to "What's that?" "Where's the ______?" "Who's that?"
	People		*Responses to Comments*
mama, dada, nana	as labels and in relation to their cars, cups, clothing, rooms, etc.	yea /ʔʌ/	agreement
baby	self; sister; other children	no /ʔʌʔʌ/	disagreement; protest
me/mine	for whatever he wanted	Oh	acknowledgment repetition of part of comment signals acknowledgement, agreement or desire for object or action at issue
/ænənə/	to label his sister Angela		
man	all but very feminine adults		
	Onomatopoetics		
moo	imitating or labeling cows		
(slurp)	requesting or labeling liquids		
/iyə/	imitating or labeling cats		

PRESCHOOL CONVERSATION: THE ELABORATION OF COHERENCE

The importance of relationship to the infant's transition to language and of cohesion in the child's initial lexical domains has been stressed. It is during the succeeding preschool years that coherence factors proliferate and seem to dominate development; that is, while beginning to work out new relationships with peers, school authorities, and so on, the child explores the options for getting and constructing his turns at talk and for exploiting the conversational subsystems in negotiating his social power and solidarity.

The primary concern of this section is to demonstrate the extent of the preschooler's competence for coherent conversation. This will be accomplished first by reviewing some issues in terms of the contributions of others, then by introducing the conversational act approach developed in earlier works by Dore, and finally by analyzing a strip of nursery school conversation in terms of the conversational subsystems.

Issues and Models of Nursery School Conversation

Bloom, Rocissano, and Hood (1976) studied the development of relations among utterances between four children and their mothers from Stage 1 (mean length of utterance MLU in morphemes <2) to Stage 5 (MLU 3.5 to 4.0; see Brown, 1973). At first children were more likely to respond to adult utterances than to initiate conversation, as though they followed a simple rule for coherence like ''take a conversational turn immediately following a partner's turn.'' But only about half of the children's responses during Stage 1 were ''linguistically contingent'' (i.e., ''cohesive''). In addition, most of these were cohesive with preceding adult questions. Imitations, noncontingent responses, and no responses more frequently followed nonquestions. Cohesion developed considerably up to Stage 5, and a major development was (apart from decrease in noncontingency) an increase in ''contextual contingency,'' in which children's replies were related to an ongoing joint activity instead of topically related to words in the preceding utterance. However, despite increases in both kinds of contingency, only half of all the children's speech was contingent at Stage 5 when they were more than 3 years old. So even at this point, children find it easier to introduce a topic than to sustain one previously introduced. Similarly, Garvey (1974) found that 3½ year olds in play groups respond contingently to one another only about half the time.

It seems that preschoolers orient to the salient objects and actions in the context, more so than to linguistic form, when responding to adults. However, there are certain kinds of conversational sequences that are well developed before school. For example, Garvey (1977) found that "contingent queries" comprised of three turns—some comment, a request for clarification or specification, and a clarifying response—to be frequent among preschoolers. Another major finding for this group is that by about 4 years of age children can adjust their speech output to their audience. Shatz and Gelman (1973), for example, found that the speech of 4 year olds in the context of giving instructions was much simpler when talking to 2 year olds than to adults or to peers. Similar findings were that, regarding role-play, even 3 year olds adjust for younger listeners (Sachs and Devlin, 1976); although they are good at fantasy play, preschoolers are not adept at negotiating the conditions of play (Gearhart, 1978); and when pretending to be a superior to a peer in play, they use more imperatives than otherwise. So in general, there is a dawning awareness of sociolinguistic rules governing the contextual variation and social constraints on speech.

One model for explaining children's conversational competence concerns the notion of "social scripts." Nelson and Gruendel (1979) described these as cognitive frameworks for representing repeated events, like eating or bathing scenes, in which there are familiar sets of characters, routine sequences of events, and a fairly uniform structure and content. Their claim is that "development of topic relevant dialogue structure may profitably be viewed as a function of building up of scripts" (p. 78). Since these arise first in adult-child communication, it would explain why children are more comfortable and competent in speaking with families (Snow, 1977) and in acting out routine scenes.

A different kind of model, called the "task model of nursery school conversation," was developed by Dore, Gearhart, and Newman (1978). The model was intended to show how grammatical forms convey illocutionary intentions in the service of accomplishing social tasks. It was assumed that illocutionary acts mediate between the grammatical forms that signal them and the interactional tasks for which they are used. One goal of the model was to try to specify rules of the following sort: Utterance U counts as the linguistic act A in context C, where U has a certain content and grammatical form, A is an illocutionary act of a certain kind, and C is the set of shared interactional understandings that determine the conversational status of A. It was hypothesized that the production of an illocutionary act (e.g., a question) is only one individual speaker's contribution, and thus only a *potential* social fact. A listener's orientation to it was what determined the conversational status of the initial act; that is, answering it retrojected the status of question for the prior utterance, making it an operative social fact for both conversationalists. Thus, the initial act provides only the raw material for creating social fact; the performance of the expected effect ratifies the illocutionary material as social fact. Finally, talk accomplishes a task in two ways: sequences of acts constitute what is done; and the sequences display the planfulness of the task as an interactive episode. At the same time, it is the interactively constructed task that provides the participants with a frame for interpreting the text. In this sense, the task determines the text's interpretation, whereas the text pervasively "indexes" the task being accomplished.

Table 1–6 provides a list of the act types used in coding the nursery school data, including the excerpt coded further on. The theoretical basis for the list derives from the three aforementioned sources: the logical and linguistic analyses of utterances as acts by speech act philosophers (Austin, 1962; Searle, 1969); the ethnomethodological analysis of conversational mechanisms (Sacks et al., 1974); and from the application of these two sources to talk by children and their teachers in various educational settings in which slightly different versions of this coding scheme appear (Cole, Dore, Hall, and Dowley, 1978; Dore, 1977; and Dore et al., 1978). Conversational acts (C-acts) are divided into four main classes: requestives, assertives, responsives, and organizational devices. This division reflects that people use utterances to get each other to do things, to state or create facts, to reply, and to control the flow of talk. C-acts are meant to represent the primary illocutionary values conventionally conveyed by utterances as acts, a level intermediate between grammatical form on the one hand and social action on the other. For example, a request for action expresses the speaker's expectation that the listener will do something. But whether it also constitutes an expression of hostility, a supplication, or a challenge depends upon quite different factors.

A Conversational Analysis of Coherence in a Fantasy Episode

An analysis of the conversational competencies of 3 to 3½ year olds should clearly illustrate the limitations in their control of cohesion, coherence, and context relations. Table 1–7 is an excerpt from a play group in a nursery school setting that occurred as a fantasy side-sequence while the children were cleaning up a table after a snack. Notice the cohesion achieved through the use of many pronouns: the many uses of "it" for the "sponge sandwich"; the "yours" and "mine" for sponges; and the "I," "me," and "my" for possessing and "eating" the "sandwich." Notice the tense variations of "Let's have . . ." "We made . . ." "Now we have a sponge sandwich," which formulate what they will do, have done, and are doing. There is ellipsis when Jn answers "I ate it all" to Js's request, "Now give *me* a bite." Here Jn's "it" covers the "sponge sandwich," which Js had not mentioned. There is emphatic stress on *"your, my,* and *me"* and many kinds of lexical

Table 1-6. Codes, Types, Definitions, Sincerity Conditions, and Examples of Conversational Acts

	Code, Type, Definition, (Sincerity Condition), and Examples
	Requestives solicit information or action (S wants H to perform A)
	Questions (S wants H to provide I)
RQCH	*Choice Questions* seek yes-no, either-or judgments of propositions (S wants H to select *a* or *b*): "Is this an apple?" "Is it red or green?"
RQPR	*Product Questions* seek information solicited by "Wh" interrogative pronouns (S wants H to provide "Wh" I): what, which, who, when, and where questions.
RQPC	*Process Questions* seek explanations or extended descriptions (S wants H to provide explanatory I): why, how, what for, what about, and how come questions.
	Requests (S wants H to perform A)
RQAC	*Action Requests* seek the performance of an action by a bearer (S wants H to perform A): "Give me it!" "Read it!" "Can you please do it?"
RQPM	*Permission Requests* seek permission to perform an action (S wants H to allow S to do A): "May I go?" "Can I do it?"
RQSU	*Suggestions* recommend the performance of an action by a hearer or a hearer and speaker (S wants H, or S and H, to do A): "Let's do it!"
	Assertives report facts, evaluate conditions, or establish roles and rights (S believes P is, or will become, true)
	Reports represent existing states of affairs (S states P)
ASID	*Identifications* label objects, events, and so on: "That's a car."
ASDC	*Descriptions* predicate events, properties, locations, and so forth of objects: "The car is red." "It fell." "We did it."
ASIR	*Internal Reports* express emotions, intents, and other mental events: "I like it." "It hurts." "I'll do it."
	Evaluations judge states of affairs (S assumes P)
ASEV	*Evaluatives* express personal judgments or attitudes: "That's good."
ASAT	*Attributions* express beliefs about another's state: "He wants to go."
ASEX	*Explanations* express causal relations, give reasons, or make predictions: "I did it because it's fun." "It won't stay up there."
	Declarations create social facts (S calls P into effect)
ASPR	*Procedurals* invoke norms or rules, set procedures, or define conditions: "It goes here." "That comes later." "We don't do that."
ASCL	*Claims* attempt to preempt rights for the speaker: "I'm first!" "It's mine."
	Responsives supply information in reaction to Requestives or Assertives (S provides I relative to RQ-AS)
	Answers (S provides solicited I)
RSCH	*Choices* judge propositions proposed by questions: "Yes,' no; *a*, not *b*."
RSPR	*Products* provide "Wh" information: "He's here." "It fell."
RSPC	*Processes* provide explanations: "I wanted to." "It wouldn't work."
RSCL	*Clarifications* provide confirmations: "I said no;" repeat utterance.

Table continued on following page

Table 1–6 (Continued)

	Code, Type, Definition, (Sincerity Condition), and Examples
RSCO	*Compliances* express recognition of requests: "OK" "No, I won't."
	Replies (S provides unsolicited I)
RSQL	*Qualifications* add to or alter preceding information: "But I can't do it."
RSAG	*Agreements* agree or disagree with preceding information: "No, it isn't."
RSAK	*Acknowledgements* provide feedback to prior or ongoing utterances: "Oh," "Yes."
	Organizational Devices are nonpropositional, metalinguistic acts that regulate contact and the flow of conversation
ODAG	*Attention-Getters* solicit attention: "Hey!" "John!" "Look!"
ODSS	*Speaker Selections* label speaker of next turn: "John" "You."
ODRQ	*Rhetorical Questions* seek acknowledgement to continue: "Know what?"
ODCQ	*Clarification Questions* seek clarification of prior remark: "What?"
ODBM	*Boundary Markers* indicate openings, closings, and shifts in the conversation: "Hi!" "Bye!" "OK!" "All right," "By the way."
ODPM	*Politeness Markers* indicate ostensible politeness: "Please" "Thank you."
ODEX	*Exclamations* express attitudes nonpropositionally: "Oh!" "Wow!"
ODRP	*Repetitions* repeat parts of prior utterances.

Codes, definitions, and examples of conversational acts, with sincerity conditions given in parentheses. S = speaker, H = hearer, I = information, A = action, and P = proposition. Conversational acts are based on propositional content, illocutionary intent, and conversational function.

cohesion, such as the domains of "sandwich, salad" and "ate, bite." However, there is also hesitation in Jn's ". . . m', y', mine," and K's failure to get cooperation with this ungrammatical "Put top of mine." The episode is more action based than topic elaborated (only Js expands "sandwich" to "salad"): the movement of sponges (the possession of which had been hotly negotiated earlier) motivates the interaction.

Coherence can be seen in that Js's "Let's have . . ." does solicit participation and successfully receive it; commands of the "put your . . ." sort were complied with; but, more cleverly, requests can also be thwarted, as in Jn's response, "I ate it all." Calls for attention ("Look") are heeded, and comments about the "sandwich" that follow one another are coherently related. Contextually, there is both cooperation and competition in the getting and refusing of sponges. Perhaps script knowledge for eating scenes could explain the events of (1) getting materials (sponges), (2) preparing the "sandwich-salad", and (3) "eating." But, unlike adult scenes (or perhaps because it is a fantasy), the "script" disintegrates prematurely. Jn disassembles the "sandwich" abruptly, and he and Js continue fantastically to "bite" separate sponges. What is most striking is the massive repetitions and expansions across turns,

Table 1–7. Fantasy Episode from a Nursery School "Clean-up" Task

Sequence	Turn	Speaker	Utterances and Gestures	C-Act
1	1	Js	Hey,	ODAG
			Let's have a sponge sandwich.	RQSU
			Hey, hey, hey . . .	ODAG
			Put your . . . yours on top of mine!	RQAC
			(Jn puts his sponge on top of Js's but then removes it)	RSCO
2			It needs a salad on it.	ASPR
			(R puts her sponge on his)	RSCO
3			Now put that on!	RQAC
			(Jn puts his back on)	RSCO
4			Look! (holding up the "sandwich" to all)	ODAG
			We made a sponge sandwich.	ASDC
			(Jn takes his sponge back; and Js gives R's sponge back to her)	
5	2	Jn	Now my sponge sandwich.	ASCL
			Put mine on top of m . . . y . . . mine!	RQAC
			(R puts it on)	RSCO
6			Yours on top of mine!	RQAC
			(Js puts his on)	RSCO
7	3	Js	Now we have a sponge sandwich.	ASID
			(Jn pretends to each the "sandwich")	
			Now give me a bite!	RQAC
	4	Jn	I ate it all. (disassembling sponges)	RSQL
8	5	Js	(Takes R's sponge and "eats" it)	
			I ate it all.	ASDC
9	6	K	That's mine. (taking a sponge)	ASCL
			Put top of mine!	RQAC
			(Jn bangs sponge on table, making noises)	

Revised from Dore, J., Gearhart, M., and Newman, D. (1978). The structure of nursery school conversation. In K. Nelson (Ed.), *Children's language, Vol. 1.* New York: Gardner Press.

presumably signaling solidarity: Jn repeats Js's "now" and combines it with a repetition of "sponge sandwich," repeating also "yours on top of mine," and Js repeats his own "now." Finally, Js repeats (but without the same pragmatic effect) Jn's "I ate it all." These echoes reflect that they are doing the same thing together, apart from the physical and topical moves regarding the "sandwich." So they might be described as cohesive ties that function to signal the contextual consensus of "we are fantasizing this together."

THE CONSTRUCTION OF CONTEXT BY GRADE SCHOOL CONVERSATION

Several investigators have reported that there is a radical change in children's language abilities after a few years of schooling; that in becoming literate, they move from a more interpersonal mode to the language of textbooks, in the realm of which the teacher functions as "a mediator of texts" (Olson and Nickerson, 1978). To be sure, quite different rules governing who can say what (how, when, and so on) apply in the formal contexts of classrooms, the goals of which are usually focused on the logical relations among sentences. But recent findings suggest that enormous effort is spent in socializing children for how to converse in educational settings, where the cognitive results are the ultimate products of pervasive social negotiation. Mehan (1978), for example, showed how getting the right to take a turn at talk often involves major manipulations of mutual consent among students and teachers. He also found a typical three-part structure of turns: teacher *initiates* (sometimes informing but often eliciting information), students *respond* (either vying for a turn or avoiding it), and the teacher *evaluates* responses.

Most investigations of classroom talk have concerned teachers' questioning strategies. Mishler (1975) found that question strategies of teachers reflect the social power relations in the school. A typical strategy is "chaining," wherein a teacher uses a child's answer to one question as grounds for her next question. In an earlier exhaustive analysis of "teacher talk" in high school, Bellack, Kliebard, Hyman, and Smith (1966) found almost 50 per cent of the teacher's talk to be "soliciting" moves and 65 per cent of students' turns to be obligatory responses; only 2 per cent of teachers' utterances conveyed personal opinion. Sinclair and Coulthard (1975) analyzed classroom talk in Britain, using a wide array of units ranging from minimal linguistic acts like marking boundaries between turns to large units like lessons. Their primary unit was the "exchange" consisting of a teacher move, a student response, and an extending move of the teacher's. In all these studies the students' contributions are limited to responding in highly specific ways to satisfy the topical and illocutionary demands of the question, with occasional requests on their part.

More closely related to our concern here are studies like that of Olson and Nickerson's (1978), which distinguish Halliday's (1975) interpersonal and ideational functions of classroom talk, the first relating to social relations, the second to logical relations among sentences. They concluded that there is a shift from the child's conversational language to that of "text-related" language, a "realignment of the interpersonal function and the ideational functions of language" (Olson and Nickerson, 1978, p. 121). Similarly, Feldman and Wertsch (1976) found that teacher's interpersonal, or "stance," markers typical of their normal conversation are absent from their classroom talk.

Rather than trying to survey the burgeoning literature on grade school interaction, in this section the C-act approach will be applied to a grade school reading lesson and extended to include a level of social interaction accomplished by the talk. Then, after pointing out some limitations of this approach, a reanalysis of the same strip demonstrates how conversation can be construed in terms of accountability practices. Finally, another strip from the same lesson is analyzed in terms of a more fully contextual model and the implications are discussed. These successive analyses are meant to show how the continual construction of social context by members dominates classroom interaction.

The data are excerpts from a first grade reading lesson in a New York City public school, initially reported by McDermott and colleagues (1978). Six children (with a lower reading ability than other class members) sit around a table and continually negotiate their immediate social context in terms of what to do next. McDermott described their contexts as "positionings" and identified four: roughly, they are (1) reading, (2) getting a turn to read, (3) watching or waiting for the teacher, and (4) "anarchy." He defined these in terms of the shifting configurations of group members' body postures, ranging from the "reading positioning," when the children carpenter themselves around the table and focus on their books, to "anarchy," when no concerted activity across members can be observed. Table 1–8 is a coded transcript of some getting-a-turn-to-read contexts (where read words are in capital letters).

C-Act and Interactional Analyses of a Grade School Lesson

In this scene the teacher calls on Maria to read, as Perry solicits the same turn but is refused. While Maria reads, Perry and Rosa read along with her; but only Rosa is disciplined for it. Then the teacher tries to call on Jimmy, but he challenges the call, and Rosa recommends that Fred read instead. Sequence A is concerned with getting a turn to read, a time during which the children look to the teacher to see who will read next. The talk in the sequence corroborates this in that the teacher designates Maria as next reader while Perry attempts to get the same reading turn. Notice that their talk constitutes (1) an orientation to the transition point between readings in their lesson, (2) the actual doing of the business of getting a turn, and (3) the teacher formulating for the group who (Maria) is to do what (read).

The teacher's "alright" in the first turn (TN1a) is a boundary marker (ODBM) on the C-act level because it occurs at a point between reading turns and it also marks a shift to a new conversational sequence. It is also a new context on the interactional level. Her "let's" (TN1b) is

Table 1–8. One-minute Excerpt from a First Grade Reading Lesson

SQ	TN	SP	Utterances	Prosodic-Kinesic Cues	C-Act	Interactions
		CH	GO OUT AND JUMP		READ	End of prior reading turn
A	1a	T-CH	Alright,		ODBM	Shift in PS and SQ
	b		let's	T nods to M	RQAC	Designates reader
A′	1′	P-T	*Now I read the next page!*	P pounds on table	ASCL	Attempt to get reading turn
A′	2a	T-P	No,		RSCO	Denial of claim attempt
	b		we're gonna read page			accounts for denial, and
			four again.		ASPR	contradicts presupposition
	c		Forget it!	low pitch, falling	RQAC	Disciplines P
A	d	T..	Alright,		ODBM	Subsequence shift
	e	-M	Maria?	high pitch, rising	ODSS	Redesignates reader
	f		Read page four!	T points to page four	RQAC	
				J groans loudly		?dissatisfied somehow?
B	3	P	JUMP		READ	Not designated reader
	4	R	GO		READ	Not designated reader
	5	T-R	/shhh	T looks at R	RQAC	disciplines R (and P?)
	6	R	OUT		READ	
	7	T-R	/shhh	T motions to R	RQAC	Disciplines R again
C	8	M	GO OUT, PATTY . . GO OUT		READ	
	9	P	AND, AND		READ	
	10	M	/AND		READ	
	11	P	/JUMP		READ	
	12	M	/JUMP			
			GO OUT AND JUMP			
D	13a	T-J	Alright,		ODBM	Shift in PS and SQ
	b		let's see you do it!	T nods to J	RQAC	Designates reader
				J turns down and away		
D′	14	R-T	G..go around!	R circles with finger	RQAC	Challenges T's designation
			/			

D	14′a	J-T	*What about Rosa!*	screaming pitch	RQPC	Challenges T's designation
	b		Sh..*she don't get a turn!*	violent body gestures	ASDC	Accuses T of violation
D′	15	R-T	Go *around!*	waves again; whining	RQAC	Challenges T
D′′	16	P-R	You don't get a.. /		?	Sub-subsequence attempt
D	17a	T-J	Jimmy,		ODAG	
	b		you seem very unhappy.	T stares at J	ASAT	Evades challenges, Disciplines J
	c		Perhaps you should go back to your seat.		RQSU	
D′	18	R-T	Go back to Fred, then back to me, back to Fred, back to Anna and Fred and Maria and back to me! /	circling around the table with her finger again	RQAC	Extends challenge
E	19a	T-F	Alright,		ODBM	May be RSCO to R's RQAC also
	b		Fred,		ODSS	
	c		can you read page four?		RQAC	Designates reader
	20a	F-T	Okay.		RSCO	
F	b		GO OUT..PATTY..GO OUT......		READ	
G	21a	T-S	Steven,	loud call across room	ODAG	T disciplining children not in the reading lesson; disrupts F's reading turn
	b		you must do your number paper *before* you look at the library books..		ASPR	
	c		And Paul,		ODAG	
	d		please go to your seat!		RQAC	

From McDermott, R. (1976). Kids make sense: An ethnographic account of success and failure in the first grade classroom. Doctoral dissertation, Stanford University, Stanford, CA.

Key to Coding Symbols: SQ = sequence of speaking turns, labeled A, B, C, . . . consecutively. TN = turn at speaking, numbered 1, 2, 3 . . . consecutively. SP = speaker; CH = all or most of the children; T = teacher, P = Perry, R = Rosa, M = Maria, J = Jimmy, and F = Fred. Slash mark (/) indicates overlap of utterances in speaking turns; each ellipsis dot a second of pause; capital letters for read turns; italics for greater speech intensity; and prime marks (′) for subsequences (e.g., D′) and for overlapped turns (e.g., 1′).

an abbreviated and mitigated action request (RQAC) on the C-act level and the designation of a reader on the interactional level. Although it is abbreviated in linguistic form, its location after a boundary marker and during a turn-getting, along with T's cue of nodding to Maria, are evidence for its RQAC status.

The third utterance, "Now I read the next page!" (TN1), is declarative in mood and thus might be a description. The teacher could be responding to it as a request to read, and it can be taken as a claim (ASCL) to the reading turn. A great deal of evidence indicates it is an attempted claim, an attempt to get the social fact established and accepted that the speaker is to read: (1) It occurs at a turn-transition point, overlapping with the teacher's "alright." But (2) its declarative form suggests it is not a permission request to read, which would almost invariably be in the interrogative mood. (3) Perry pounds the table as he says it, which is less likely to co-occur with a mere description or request. (4) It is intoned with unusually high pitch and intense volume, to underscore the claim, as it were. (5) Its lexical content, especially *I* and *read*, mark the claimed state of affairs. (6) It is not a description on the grounds that he is not in fact reading at the time and that descriptions are not usually denied in the forceful manner the teacher uses this time. (7) The teacher not only refuses to accept Perry's claim but also chastises his attempt (TN2c) to get a turn she has otherwise assigned.

The teacher's "No" in TN2a is a noncompliance on the C-act level, because she refuses to accept Perry's claim and makes a forceful denial of the turn to him on the interactional level. She then supports this by her assertive (ASPR) in TN2b, which states the procedure they will follow. It also has the effect of formally contradicting a presupposition of his claim, namely that they were going to read *the next page*. As with her role of designating readers, she also has the right to determine what is to be read and when. Here she invokes the procedure of reading the page over again. Her "forget it" (TN2c) is clearly an action request (RQAC), that conveys a disciplinary message interactionally. Finally, the teacher marks her shift out of the subsequence with Perry (ODBM), selects Maria (ODSS), and orders her to read (RQAC) in TN2d, e, f. This repeats and reinforces her designation of Maria, at which point exactly the children go down to their books.

The second sequence, B, is taken up by Perry and Rosa reading instead of Maria. Although it is Perry who initiates the sequence (TN3), the teacher chastises Rosa twice for reading, and her "shhh" (TN5,7) is an aggravated form of RQAC, which lends it its interactional force of a reprimand.

It is in sequence D that an abrupt disruption of the lesson's order is seen. The sequence begins, as did sequence A, with a boundary marker by the teacher to signal a shift in both conversational sequence and group positioning, followed by a mitigated (but this time not abbreviated) action request. These RQACs (TN1 and TN13) are mitigated by virtue of the choice of the *let us* forms. The initial reaction to the teacher's designation of Jimmy to read is Jimmy's loud groan and very abrupt body shift out of the immediate context. On the interactional level, Jimmy's groan and gestures can be expanded to an implicit protest. He follows this with a process question (RQPC), aggravated by its screamed intonation pattern, and a description (ASDC) aggravated by the violent hand and body gestures accompanying it. This turn clearly constitutes a challenge to the teacher's designation of him as reader, the implied accusation being that the teacher unfairly skipped over Rosa in allocating turns (and, from the tense of his verb, that she skips Rosa regularly).

After the teacher initiates the sequence with her designation and Jimmy responds with his challenge, the teacher extends the sequence by evading his challenge with a negative evaluation of this emotional state (ASEV) and a mitigated suggestion (RQSU) that he return to his seat in the classroom (i.e., that he leave the reading table.)

By not requiring Jimmy to read nor explaining why she did not call on Rosa, the teacher tacitly accepts their challenges and demonstrates that the children have some considerable say in the interaction. The "alright" in the TN 19a of sequence E can, like the *alrights* of TN 1 and 13, function as a sequence shift. But it also is a canonical form for a compliance (RSCO) to an action request. In this case, it has a double function: it is a RSCO to Rosa's RQAC in sequence D, and an ODBM in sequence E. This latter is a prototypical requestive sequence, with its indirect RQAC and explicit RSCO.

Although this analysis reveals several kinds of relationships holding across conversational units, it has some drawbacks from a more deeply ethnographic point of view. In general, it still relies rather heavily on a computational model of interaction. It assumes that members are fully aware simultaneously of the set of possible options out of which they choose an act for some next moment's purpose. But this kind of approach may very well falsify the member's own experience as well as the analyst's attributions to the member's cognition. It is not likely that speakers remember all options at once. As a purer frame approach would suggest, the sense of context itself automatically eliminates many possibilities for what can be said next. Furthermore, as it stands, this view makes some arbitrary claims about the status of some acts. It underestimates the multiplicity of many utterances' functions and the indeterminate act status of some, and it fails to be sufficiently sensitive to internal contradictions between, for example, simultaneous sayings and doings.

Conversation as Accountability Practice

A more revealing picture of what is going on can be rendered by analyzing this sequence in terms of accountability; that is, members holding each other accountable to something, accountably confirming or blocking such attempts, and giving "accountings" for or against such "accountables." These accountings and accountables include such functions as *projecting* what someone is to do, for example, a feeding forward of what potentially could occur; as *retrojecting* what someone has done, or a feeding backward of what has occurred; as well as preparing for and reacting to such pro- and retrojections. In these terms the teacher's "alright" at the beginning of the excerpt functions to retroject at least that the reading turn has just been satisfactorily completed, that is, to ratify for the group the preceding behaviors as the accomplishment of reading, and her "alright" also accomplishes a transitional shift or a preparation for her projection for a next reading turn. Her "let's . . ." plus a head nod to Maria then projects an attempt to hold Maria accountable to reading next. And, despite its abbreviated form and its being overlapped by Perry's talk, it does feed forward a potential next activity.

Perry's utterance—"now I read the next page"—can be seen as a coprojection or as an apparent attempt to claim the turn for himself, thus competing with the teacher's projection. It also projects a particular agenda for the group's next efforts: that they proceed reading the next page. The teacher's "no" then reacts to Perry's projections, by attempting to block both of them from taking effect. Her "we're gonna read page four again" counterprojects the different agenda that they reread the same page; it may also be said to give an accounting of her "no"-blocking act, and her following "forget it" is accounting that feeds back to him how to treat his projection. Finally, with her "alright, Maria, read page 4" she shifts back to what she was doing when Perry interrupted her, that is, she reprojects the attempt to have Maria read.

The next sequence of talk—a rereading of page four—may be seen as the group's response to the teacher's projection. However, different kinds of accountability work take place, since the projected (designated) reader, Maria, does *not* do most of the reading. Perry, who has not remained accountable to the teacher's projection (i.e., he has not forgotten his own), begins to read with "JUMP." Rosa adds "GO." The teacher then says "shhh" as a means of attempting to hold them accountable to *not* reading. This disciplining is repeated when Rosa shouts "OUT" (her "readings" always being rote repetitions of others). Finally, Maria reads up through the last two words. (Incidentally, as she reads the teacher nonverbally holds Fred accountable to following along by tapping his book.) But Perry again paces her by reading the final two words. Yet the teacher this time suspends accountability. In fact, the teacher's subsequent "alright" appears to retroject that another reading turn has again been satisfactorily completed, thereby implicating that Perry's contribution to the turn did not warrant a singling out as inappropriate. It could be said that, while Perry tacitly remained unaccountable to the teacher's projection and disciplining, she tacitly condoned his unaccountable behavior.

In the next sequence conflicting projections and a confrontation regarding the direction of accountability are seen. With her "alright, let's see you do it" and nod to Jimmy, the teacher projects him as next reader. His first reaction is to avoid this by turning away. But he then violently resists her projection. First, he asks, "What about Rosa," which is a challenge for an accounting of why the teacher skipped over Rosa as a reader in going from Maria to him. Second, his description—"she don't get a turn"—functions as an accusation. His talk therefore is an attempt to hold the teacher accountable to an inappropriate procedure, while at the same time it functions to evade his own accountability to read, as the teacher projected. In other terms, although her designation of him feeds forward to a potential next doing, his description of Rosa feeds back to a violated (hence, accountable) state of affairs. Meanwhile, as Jimmy is trying to hold the teacher accountable to holding Rosa accountable to read, Rosa herself is counterprojecting a different allocation of the turn, one beginning with Fred. So, we have a circle of conflicting directions in accountability—from the teacher to Jimmy, from Jimmy to Rosa, and from Rosa to Fred. This conflict eventually results in the teacher projecting Fred as the reader, thereby suspending accountability toward Jimmy and Rosa.

The teacher's immediate resolution of Jimmy's accusatory accounting is to deal with it obliquely, by describing his internal state ("You seem very unhappy") and by threatening a chastisement ("Perhaps you should go back to your seat"). The first feeds back to a state of affairs that locates the problem in Jimmy; the second feeds forward to a potential disciplining of him. Both utterances have the net effect of avoiding the work of holding him accountable to reading; whether or not he is happy is irrelevant to any group agenda; and, because he is not held to going back to his seat, he is effectively relieved of all accountability.

The Contextual Analysis of a "Pragmatic Counterfactual"

Table 1–8 continues with an 8 second strip from the same lesson. Prior to this excerpt the teacher left the table momentarily, saying: "Alright, let's read it to ourselves, and then raise your hand if you can read it!" Rosa immediately said she could read it, but her remark received no verbal uptake. Then Perry said he was ready, and the teacher acknowledged his remarks. Finally, Perry emphatically repeated twice that he was ready. This background information is crucial because it suggests a possible discourse topic, or what Keenan and Schieffelin (1978) called "the question of immediate concern" that the participant must deal with. Here the potential proposition on the floor is *Perry has the next turn to read.* Not only Perry's repetitions and the teacher's acknowledgements contribute to this potential but also the teacher's initial turn at talk in this excerpt reports Perry's readiness to read. Her "Perry's ready" could constitute elliptically *Perry is ready to read next.*

The linguistic forms of this interaction, however, when taken alone, are multiply ambiguous. The forms "Perry's ready" and "Who else is ready?" are elliptical for *Perry (who else) is ready to ____,* where the blank is to be filled in by some verb according to the grammar of English. Which verb exactly cannot be determined on grammatical grounds. So this is a point at which appeal must be made to the interactional context, namely that these participants are in a reading lesson. The missing verb then could be *read* (as is partly reflected later in Rosa's "I could read it." But this word alone cannot disambiguate these forms.

This group is involved not only in a reading lesson but also in the more immediate context of deciding who is to read next. And there are several ways in which this group allocates turns. Thus, the teacher's remarks could express any of the following propositions: *Perry (who else) is ready* . . . (1) to read next, (2) to call for a turn to read next, (3) to read along silently with the designated reader, or (4) to read together in chorus. The teacher might also intend a combination like Perry is ready to read next, who else is ready to read along? But since she does not say it, the action is negotiable; that is, the agent and the allocating mechanism for the next turn remain open. A positive answer, such as Anna's "me" in Turn 2, commits her to becoming eligible to read. But Jimmy's "not me," although it ratifies his participation in the interaction, disengages him from any responsibility to read.

Rosa's "I could read it" has several formal relations to the teacher's turn. The "I" continues the semantic domain of personal pronouns. Her main verb "read" could manifest the elliptical verb of the teacher's question. But most interestingly, her modal verb "could" is ambiguous. It could state her ability, as in *I am able to read it,* or the hypothetical *I could read it if* . . . (say) . . . *I got the turn.* The underlying proposition, *Rosa read*, introduces a potential propositional topic that could be taken to compete with the *Perry read*, which might be on the table. But Rosa's utterance receives no verbal uptake. Moreover, beyond the structural ambiguity, the utterance is illocutionarily equivocal. It could be an answer to "who else is ready?" "I" could answer the "who"; "read" could fill in the elliptical verb; and "it" could be a pronominalization for *the next page*; the utterance occurs only 3 seconds after the question. But it could also be an indirect permission request to read.

Here is the central problem of illocutionary analysis: how to constrain the multiplicity of speech act functions. But the actual functional efficacy of this remark for the conversationalists is as a *pragmatic counterfactual*; that is, it is taken to mean the opposite of what it literally states. But in order to support this claim, an independent characterization of the context in terms of the speaker's own categories for interpreting it must exist.

In terms of the ethnographic criteria described above, Dore and McDermott (1982) found that members of this lesson often use utterances not for their literal import so much as for their value in organizing their actions for the next social context. Rosa's "I could read it" appears to orient to the issue at hand, namely who is to read next. But its timing renders the remark inappropriate as a substantive commitment to read in that the group consensus has begun to be formulated differently. Perry has begun to read and will in fact have the turn 10 seconds later. Thus, again, Rosa merely appears to be doing the social order of getting a turn.

The nonverbal evidence is compelling.

1. When the teacher reenters the group, as she scans across the students and asks her readiness question, Rosa looks away from her and out of the group.
2. As others begin to respond and the teacher glances at them, only then does Rosa look at the teacher.
3. As the teacher arrives at the reading table, she and Perry do a quite distinct postural dance together, each of their movements co-occurring with and complementing one another (e.g., their torsos turn toward each other, not the table, their arms move complementarily).
4. Anna and Maria watch the teacher and Perry from across the table. This appears to be the first postural indication (if only a hint) toward the consensus that Perry will read.
5. Only near the end of the teacher-Perry dyadic dance does Rosa say, "I could read it," this timing suggesting that the turn has already begun to be otherwise allocated, her remark thus being ineffectual.
6. As Rosa finishes speaking and the teacher begins to gaze toward her, Rosa looks away again, thereby rendering herself unavailable for eye contact, effectively disengaging herself from any commitment to read.

In sum, when Rosa says, "I could read it," others react as if she means that she will not and probably cannot read it and that they should continue as if someone else were going to read. The members of this group use this knowledge about Rosa not just to handle their interaction with Rosa but also to organize their behavior with each other across the whole group. Rosa's utterance accordingly is not just a statement about her affairs, but a tool that group members use to formulate and accomplish their concerted activity. Its truth, on at least a correspondence theory, would be determinable by empirical tests of Rosa's graphic decoding skills. At the moment of its utterance, hearers could have relied on their memories for evidence of the utterance's truth. But this option was not verbalized. No one said anything like "You can't read," and she has never been seen to read, except by rote.

The issue is not whether Rosa's statement is literally true but whether the circumstances of her utterance render it useful in solving the organizational problems facing a teacher and children in a lesson—especially when (1) some of the children do not know how to read, (2) not knowing how to read is an embarrassment and everyone often conspires to hide the stigmatized nonreaders, and (3) ambiguous reader designation procedures allow the teacher the power to assign pages to readers only when they appear able to handle the task. Under such conditions the truth or falsity of Rosa's utterance is less crucial than its function in directing the group to a next step in the reading in a way that allows Rosa's participation in the social order without causing her embarrassments. It provides the appearance of her ability to read, her involvement in the lesson, and her willingness to take a turn, although at the same time its timing and other relations to the social context render it ineffectual as a candidate for a bid to read. This has lead us to describe it as a *pragmatic counterfactual.*

An important implication here is that a primary pragmatic function of talk is both to project alternative realities and to eliminate, for the moment anyway, those realities that do not map onto the flow of concerted activities. In the case at hand, Rosa's utterance projects a potential reality, both personally that she can read and wants the turn and interpersonally that she might become the group's reader. The group's reaction constitutes an elimination of at least the interpersonal reality. Notice here that the context of getting-a-turn induces, or at least encourages, the proposing of competing alternatives for accomplishing reading, as is evidenced by the many propositions momentarily on the floor about who will read. But Rosa's remark goes further. She puts forth a proposition the truth of which is negligible at best and the effect of which is undermined by co-occurring factors.

CONCLUSION: CONVERSATIONAL CHANGE AS CONTEXTUAL COMPLEXITY

This chapter has touched on several ways of looking at conversational interaction, ranging from the "innermost core" (Goffman, 1974) of affect in interpersonal relations to the "outer frames" of institutionally appropriate behavior. Data samples from different developmental stages were selected and subjected to different kinds of analysis. A four-component descriptive scheme was proposed, involving relationships among members, cohesion across their utterance forms, the functional coherence of their sequences of talk, and the contextual constraints on their interactions. Emphasis was placed on one of these components for each developmental stage, implicitly assuming primacy of that component for that stage; that is, although relationship, form, function, and context always operate to some extent, one of these has been taken to dominate (as far as the child's focus of attention is concerned) the others during each stage.

The discussion can now be summarized with reference to our initial question about what exactly changes in the child's language behavior. Given our scheme, the question can be put more specifically: How do relationships and social contexts change such that it leads to changes in conversational coherence and the meaning of language forms? In summing up the answer, the author here proposes an extended hypothesis about the direction of change, selecting for this purpose one critical aspect from each component: those of membership conditions, accountability requirements, utterance functions, and the meaning of words.

The infant's membership in the dyad with his or her mother is one of intimacy. But it would not be quite accurate to call him or her a full-fledged partner, given a necessary dependence on mother. As Macmurray (1961) postulated, and as investigations of affective dialogue suggest, mother and infant participate in a state of communion quite distinct from socially mediated relationships. What Macmurray called a shift from a personal to a social order can be construed as a change in membership of the infant from an almost helpless dependent to a competent family member who has begun to walk, talk, and act responsibly. Certainly the conditions of membership in a symbiotic relationship to an adult caregiver differ drastically from the role of conversational partner who is coresponsible for explicitly constructing a meaning-filled interaction. The switch to such social membership brings with it a set of rights and responsibilities defined by reciprocal functions, such as suggesting the game to play and choosing the materials, performing a part adequately, responding to other's requests, and so on.

Accountability practices partly define such membership status. Whereas mothers tend to interpret most of the infant's efforts as effective (or at least useful for their being together), after the child begins to produce worklike forms mothers shift their accountability requirements. Now the child is expected to use an appropriate word or to try to solicit it; routines for evoking, introducing, or contrasting words are instituted; the child orients to the systematic meanings of words themselves rather than responds directly to the affect motivating word production.

The functions of vocal expressions change. Whereas idiosyncratic forms expressed affect state or, later, globally indexed the situation, words come to denote specific entities. Primitive speech acts convey both content distinctions and expected responses to them. The same form can be used for different functions: for example, "no" for protesting, answering, commenting on disappearance, and even for a kind of "joking-lying" when baby knows the right answer is "yes." This increase in flexibility of utterance function allows for greater complexity of word use, conversational variety, and an unpredictability of response.

Such changes in membership, accountability, and function lead to changes in word meaning. Recall that during the transitional period affect expressions are matched by the adult's conventional behaviors for expressing such affect. The author has hypothesized that this is how a baby realizes that certain behaviors can "re-present" certain states of affairs—that certain vocal and gestural types are *signs* for other internal and external states. Then, after the notion of what a word is is realized, baby's uses of words become increasingly *contrastive*; a system of *symbols* is constructed such that lexical domains are elaborated and differentiated from other domains. Finally, word meaning becomes *predicational*: Entire propositions are produced by commenting, for example, on a feature of an object pointed to. It is tempting to speculate here that the changes in membership to competent and separate partners, accompanied by changes in rights and responsibilities, lead to different uses of utterances and, ultimately, to changes in word meaning. When mother no longer completes baby's efforts, he is held accountable to distinguish for himself among objects, leading to objective reference beyond his subjective state; eventually, he contrasts one symbol with another to indicate his competence as a linguistically flexible and accountable member of the language community.

In nursery school the child's membership again changes drastically to one of a peer among play-group partners. He or she must learn to accomplish tasks and games with members of equal competence—without the aid of an intimate partner and family support system. (Of course, he or she is also finding out that, although social rights are equally distributed, members are not equally talented at exploiting them.) Preschool membership also includes a wider freedom (or at least variation) in constructing interactions. The accountability system for appropriate behavior is correspondingly relaxed. Perhaps this encourages the increase in pretend talk. However, a new relationship, this time to the public institutional authority of the teacher, includes an induction to new responsibilities. Although there is much latitude in play construction, there is no license to become destructive, for example.

Such changes in status and accountability apparently encourage experimentation with utterance functions. Along with the option to lapse into fantasy, the sheer number of response options seems to explode. Relaxed accountability for talk leads to less predictability of response, and contingency across utterance functions easily degenerates. Language is used more flexibly and creatively to project alternate scenes: wood planks are at one moment train tracks and at the next moment skis. A sponge becomes a "sandwich"—a pleasant way to avoid cleaning a table. Again, the teacher allowing this lapse exemplifies both the freedom and unpredictability of talk and action.

The emergence of utterance-function to wield social power is notable. Being able to initiate the "sandwich" fantasy gives Js initial control over the scene. But Jn displayed the equally powerful skill of blocking Js's sponge possession by his stopper, "I ate it all." Such uses of talk to display ownership of playthings, to control a corner of the room, to determine leadership (e.g., who is to "drive" the "bus"), and so on are the great advances in the coherence system during this period.

Regarding word meaning, the increase in fantasy talk shows the ease of alternating between literal and metaphorical meaning. Also, the meaning of a word like "mine" changes in the context of the playroom. Objects are not owned outright as they are at home but are temporarily possessed for play purposes. So, for example, though the meaning of "my sponge" is not metaphorical, yet it has a meaning extended beyond such expressions as "my room" at home; like the adult's use of "my office" at work. Finally, the cohesive relations among forms produced in nursery school settings are much more structurally based. Multiple pronouns, ellipsis, substitution, lexical expansion, and so forth were seen in the "sandwich" fantasy.

In grade school the child's initiation into studenthood involves him with a much wider social milieu, a more structured authority system, an expansion of his relationship to others from peer to educational colaborator and a sense of being one-among-many, perhaps even of being an interchangeable member of a vast institution. Student membership brings with it many new responsibilities for "behaving like a good pupil." Accountability to perform school tasks becomes dominant. The increases in expected competence (to read, write, count, and so on) are enormous. Vast bodies of knowledge lie ahead of the student, like water leaning on a dam. As has been seen, accounting practices become quite explicit and more specific to areas of competence. The business of becoming a competent member of society at large begins.

The influence of such expanded membership and responsibility on language use is profound. It is no longer used merely, or perhaps even primarily, to exchange information or create fantasy. Rather, the child must now negotiate several kinds of contraints simultaneously. He or she must display an intelligence relative to the school task and a relation to the teacher as authority as well as status as member of a larger peer group.

The stigma accrues to the child who adheres too extremely to any one of these constraints, opening herself or himself up to accusations of ''learning disabled,'' ''teacher's pet,'' or ''disciplinary problem,'' and so on.

Utterances must, therefore, serve multiple functions simultaneously, as seen in the illocationary-interactional analyses. Moreover, language becomes a means to ''cover'' oneself, to ''pass'' as a competent member relative to various constraints. In school it is not merely information that is exchanged, but the role of ''normal'' student must be projected; for example, giving the ''right'' answer at the right time, but not being so ''smart'' as to distance him- or herself too much from peers. At worst, the student must project a competence he or she does not have (Rosa's ''I could read it'') and then somehow manage to avoid being held accountable to it. The multiple ambiguity of meaning and equivocality of function built into such ''school talk'' was also seen.

The meanings of terms also seem to take on a new dimension. Just as the ''my'' of preschooler's talk at play signals temporary possession, there is an aspect of ''occasion meaning'' in school talk well beyond what referential and indexical meaning. When a teacher says ''Now we're going to read page four again,'' several contextual qualifications are needed for full interpretation. First, ''now'' means after certain preliminaries are accomplished (such as selecting a reader), and this ''now'' may not come about if the teacher is successfully challenged. Second, ''we'' does *not* include her (because she will not really read), contrary to the lexical definition, and the term ''read'' in this case means something different from decoding novel sequences of graphic symbols; something more like repeating what was already ''read.'' In short, there seems to be a proliferation of different senses of the same term, in which the immediate context disambiguates which sense is meant. Often, some literal feature of a word (like ''we'') is suspended for interpretation on a particular occasion of its use, and meanings can shift constantly across successive uses of a word (like ''read'').

Finally, and perhaps most important for conversational development in general, is the occasional meaning of an entire proposition, ''I could read it.'' This projection of competence to the group ''saves face'' for the speaker (and for the group as constituted of ''competent readers'') but is not intended to express the message that its words literally convey. Rather, its opposite is *heard*, oriented to, and acted upon. The occasion meaning of such an utterance is not of the same sort as facetious, ironic, or similarly ''bracketed'' talk by conspicuous tones or gestures. Rather, it must appear to be serious and literal in order to achieve its nonliteral effect. Such an example of occasional meaning is perhaps the best example of the overall hypothesis of this chapter: shifting membership conditions, along with their accountability requirements for particular social contexts, determine the functions that utterances perform and, ultimately, the meaning words can have for members.

One more note about future directions for this line of research. Converation has been described in terms of accountability practices that constitute struggles to achieve consensus about immediate contexts. This requires not only a considerable amount of cooperation (along the lines of Grice's, 1975, principles) but also a good deal of competition (as we saw in efforts to get and avoid turns to speak and read). McDermott and Tylbor (1983) have described these same data in terms of collusion. They argue that, beyond propositional information and illocutionary intention, institutional constraints require conversationalists to "play along" with one another as if they were enacting contexts such as "We are all reading now." Thus the group's treatment of Rosa's "I could read it" is a moment of collusion: a way to allow a member to appear to be able to read while proceeding in an opposite direction.

However, Dore (in press) suggests that a complement to such a collusive tendency exists in the form of a kind of "confession:" that is, if members conspire (consciously or not) to collusively project agendas, there are also moments when they tend to reveal a "truer" state of affairs. For example, Jimmy's challenging the teacher for not calling on Rosa to read can be seen as such a "countercollusive" move (while at the same time "covering" for his own evasion of the turn to read). This level of description concerns somewhat "deeper functions" of dialog than the cohesive, coherent, and contextualizing practices this chapter began with, and it serves as a way to specify just how cooperation and competition toward consensus can be worked out. But an enormous amount of research will be needed to make this view of conversation convincing. Yet, it seems worth the effort, and at least something of this sort seems necessary to achieve a deeper, pragmatic account of what motivates developmental change in children's language practices.

REFERENCES

Austin, J. (1962). *How to do things with words.* New York: Oxford University Press.

Bellack, A., Kliebard, P., Hyman, R., and Smith, F., (1966). *The language of the classroom.* New York: Teacher's College Press.

Birdwhistell, R. (1970). *Kinesics and context.* Philadelphia: University of Pennsylvania Press.

Bloom, L. (1973). *One word at a time: the use of single word utterances before syntax.* The Hague: Mouton.

Bloom, L., Rocissano, L., and Hood, L. (1976). Adult-child discourse: developmental interaction between information processing and linguistic knowledge. *Cognitive Psychology, 8,* 521–552.

Brown, R. (1973). *A first language.* Cambridge: Harvard University Press.
Bruner, J. (1978). From communication to language: a psychological perspective. In I. Markova (Ed.), *The Social Context of Language* London: Wiley.
Cole, M., Dore, J., Hall, W., and Dowley, G. (1978). Situation and task in young children's talk. *Discourse Processes, 1,* 119–176.
Dore, J. (1977). 'O them sheriff': a pragmatic analysis of children's responses. In S. Ervin-Tripp and C. Mitchell-Kernan (Eds.), *Child Discourse.* New York: Academic Press.
Dore, J. (1978). Conditions for the acquisition of speech acts. In I Markova (Ed.), *The Social Context of Language.* London: Wiley.
Dore, J. (1984). Holophrases revisited, dialogically. In M. Barrett (Ed.), *Children's single-word speech.* London: Wiley.
Dore, J. (in press). *Dialog, conversation and language development in children.* Cambridge: Cambridge University Press.
Dore, J., Franklin, M., Miller, R., and Ramer, A. (1976). Transitional phenomena in early language acquisition. *Journal of Child Language, 3,* 1–11.
Dore, J., Gearhart, M., and Newman, D. (1978). The structure of nursery school conversation. In K. Nelson (Ed.), *Children's language, Vol. 1.* New York: Gardner Press.
Dore, J., and McDermott, R. (1982). Linguistic indeterminacy and social context in utterance interpretation. *Language, 58,* 374–398.
Ervin-Tripp, S. (1977). "Wait for me, rollerskate!" In S. Ervin-Tripp and C. Mitchell-Kernan (Eds.), *Child discourse.* New York: Academic Press.
Feldman, C., and Wertsch, J. (1976). Context dependent properties of teacher's speech. *Youth and Society, 7,* 227–258.
Frake, C. (1977). Plying frames can be dangerous. *Quarterly Newsletter of the Laboratory of Comparative Human Cognition.* New York: The Rockefeller University.
Garfinkel, H. (1967). *Studies in ethnomethodology.* Englewood Cliffs, NJ: Prentice-Hall.
Garfinkel, H., and Sacks, H. (1970). On formal structures of practical actions. In J. McKinney and E. Tiryakian (Eds.), *Theoretical sociology.* New York: Roland Press.
Garvey, C. (1974). Some properties of social play. *Merrill-Palmer Quarterly, 20,* 163–180.
Garvey, C. (1975) Requests and responses in children's speech. *Journal of Child Language, 2,* 41–59.
Garvey, C. (1977). The contengent query: A dependent act in conversation. In M. Lewis and L. Rosenblum (Eds.), *Interaction, Conversation and the Development of Conversation.* New York: Wiley.
Gearhart, M. (1978, March). *Social planning: Role play in a novel situation.* Paper presented at the biennial meetings of the Society for Research in Child Development, San Francisco.
Goffman, E. (1959). *The presentation of self in everyday life.* Garden City, NY: Doubleday.
Goffman, E. (1974). *Frame analysis.* New York: Harper and Row.
Goffman, E. (1976). Replies and responses. *Language in Society, 5,* 257–313.
Grice, H. (1975). Logic and conversation. In D. Davidson and G. Harmon (Eds.), *The logic of grammar.* Encina, CA: Dickenson Press.
Gumperz, J. (1976). Language, communication and public negotiation. In P. Sanday (Ed.), *Anthopology and the public interest.* New York: Academic Press.

Halliday, M. (1975). *Learning how to mean.* London: Edward Arnold.
Halliday, M., and Hasan, R. (1976). *Cohesion in English.* London: Edward Arnold.
Keenan, E., and Schieffelin, B. (1978). Topic as a discourse notion. In L. Li (Ed.), *Subject and topic.* New York: Academic Press.
Kendon, A. (1977). *Studies in the behavior of social interaction.* Lisse: deRidder Press.
Labov, W., and Fanshel, D. (1977). *Therapeutic discourse.* New York: Academic Press.
Malinowski, B. (1923). The problem of meaning in primitive languages. In C. Ogden and I. Richards (Eds.), *The meaning of meaning.* New York: Harcourt, Brace & World.
MacMurray, J. (1961). *Persons in relation.* London: Faber.
McDermott, R., Gospodinoff, K., and Aron, J. (1978). Criteria for the ethnographically adequate description of activities and their contexts. *Semiotica, 24,* 245–275.
McDermott, R., and Tylbor, H. (1983). On the necessity of collusion in conversation. *Text, 3,* 277–297.
Mehan, H. (1978). *Learning lessons.* Cambridge: Harvard University Press.
Mishler, E. (1975). Studies in dialogue and discourse: An expotential law of successive questioning. *Language in Society, 4,* 31–52.
Morris, C. (1946). Foundations of the theory of signs. *International encyclopedia of unified science.* Chicago: University of Chicago Press.
Nelson, K. (1973). Structure and strategy in learning how to talk. *Monographs of the Society for Research in Child Development,* 38.
Nelson, K., and Gruendel, J. (1979). At morning it's lunchtime: A scriptal view of children's dialogues. *Discourse Processes, 2,* 73–94.
Ninio, A., and Bruner, J. (1978). The achievement and antecedents of labelling. *Journal of Child Language, 5,* 1–16.
Olson, D., and Nickerson, N. (1978). Language development through the school years: Learning to confine interpretation to the information in the text. In K. Nelson (Ed.), *Children's Language, Vol. 1.* New York: Gardner Press.
Piaget, J. (1962). *The origins of intelligence in children.* New York: Norton.
Ratner, N., and Bruner, J. (1978). Games, social exchange and the acquisition of language. *Journal of Child Language, 5,* 391–401.
Sachs, J., and Devlin, J. (1976). Young children's use of age-appropriate speech styles in social interaction and role-playing. *Journal of Child Language. 3,* 81–98.
Sacks, H. (1972). On the analyzability of stories by children. In J. Gumperz and D. Hymes (Eds.), *Directions in sociolinguistics: the ethnography of communication.* New York: Holt, Rinehart & Winston.
Sacks, H., Schegloff, E., and Jefferson, G. (1974). A simplest systematics for the organization of turn-taking in conversation. *Language, 50,* 696–735.
Scheflen, A. (1973). *Communicational structure.* Bloomington: University of Indiana Press.
Schegloff, E. (1971). Notes on a conversational practice: formulating place. In D. Sudnow (Ed.), *Studies in social interaction.* New York: Free Press.
Searle, J. (1969). *Speech acts.* Cambridge: Cambridge University Press.
Shatz, M., and Gelman, R. (1973). The development of communication skills: Modification in the speech of young children as a function of listener. *Monographs of the Society for Research in Child Development,* 38.

Snow, C. (1977). Mother's speech research: from input to interaction. In C. Snow and C. Ferguson (Eds.), *Talking to Children: Language input and acquisition*. New York: Cambridge University Press.
Stern, D. (1977). *The first relationship*. Cambridge: Harvard University Press.
Sugarman-Bell, S. (1978). Some organizational aspects of pre-verbal communication. In I. Markova (Ed.), *The social context of language*. London: Wiley.
Trevarthen, C. (1977). Descriptive analyses of infant communicative behaviour. In H. Schaffer (Ed.), *Studies in mother-infant interaction*. London: Academic Press.
Trevarthen, C., and Hubley, P. (1979). Secondary intersubjectivity: confidence, confiding and acts of meaning in the first year. In A. Lock (Ed.), *Action, gesture and symbol*. London: Academic Press.
Vygotsky, L. (1978). *Mind in society*. Cambridge: Harvard University Press.

Chapter 2

The Development of Requests

Susan Ervin-Tripp and David Gordon

In his introduction to this book, the editor describes the contents of *The Acquisition of Communicative Competence*. In that companion volume* to this text, the authors analyzed requests according to the social and situational variables that determine their instrumental effects, and considered the conventional and nonconventional (indirect or "strategic") nature of the instrumental moves that children make, emphasizing the acquisition of requests. How instrumental language provides a major intersection of knowledge of linguistic forms with social beliefs and skills was discussed, and explanations of the instrumental nature of requests within a developmental perspective were provided.

This chapter concerns basic aspects of development during four chronological periods (under two years of age, between 2 and 4 years of age, from 4 to 8 years of age, and over 8 years of age) and issues of social and linguistic development that are relevant to those periods. Those four periods are characterized by important changes in skills. For other summaries, see Becker (1981) and Shatz (1983).

---

*Gordon, D., and Ervin-Tripp, S. (1984). The structure of children's requests. In R. L. Schiefelbusch and J. Pickar (Eds.), *The Acquisition of Communication Competence*. Baltimore: University Park Press.

SOCIAL AND LINGUISTIC BASES OF REQUESTS

The development of instrumental language raises questions concerning the relation of language to action and to social knowledge: (1) In the case of action, how does the child learn to understand instrumental language and make appropriate responses to it? How does the child learn to produce instrumental language to achieve behavioral goals? (2) In respect to social knowledge, how does the child come to understand the social information contained in instrumental language? How does the child learn to vary what to say in order to maintain good relations or to achieve particular social goals with different persons?

Five skills are necessary for effective instrumental acts:

1. *Attention.* The speaker must have or gain the attention of the addressee who is to carry out the desired act.
2. *Clarity.* The speaker must identify by gesture or word what is desired whenever the goal or action wanted is not apparent in the context.
3. *Persuasion.* If the desirability or necessity of the action is not obvious to the addressee, the speaker must explain, persuade, or threaten to move the addressee to action.
4. *Social Relations.* Because instrumental speech acts are at the same time social moves, the speaker must choose appropriate social markers.
5. *Repairs.* When the first move fails, the speaker must identify the reason and make a correction for a second try.

What is the role of social and linguistic knowledge? Getting attention is possible without much in the way of linguistic knowledge. Social knowledge is required because the child must assess where the attention of the addressee is engaged. Deficiencies in clarity are sometimes cognitive, as will be seen, and may sometimes reflect a lack of linguistic resources. With older children, as with adults, the sacrifice of clarity arises from the conflict with social motives. One of the major indicators of strategic skill is the ability to control concrete action and social relationships at the same time. The expression of persuasive arguments may call for complex linguistic resources such as contingent statements and subordination. But the most important foundation for effective persuasion is an understanding of what motivates behavior. Social relations can be marked by very routine forms, thus linguistic bases for social marking of politeness or aggravation are not difficult. What changes with maturity is the ability to adopt the viewpoint of someone else in manipulating information to change behavior, in recognizing when one is being intrusive, in assessing when to use social markings, and in avoiding intrusiveness without loss of effectiveness.

The Language of Instrumental Moves

The distinction between requests and the more general notion of instrumental language needs to be elaborated. Requests are conventional means of getting others to do things. A request such as

Example 1. Could you close the door?

may be expected to get ist hearer to close the door because it is (in part) recognized as a request to do so. On the other hand, an utterance such as

Example 2. It's freezing in here.

may be expected to prompt its hearer to close the door not because of being asked to, but for some other reason suggested by the statement—because the addressee does not want the hearer to be cold or uncomfortable, for example, or because the addressee may feel cold, too, and is encouraged to act for the benefit of both.

It might be expected that an utterance such as Example 2 is not an attempt to get the hearer to take specific action but to do whatever might remedy the situation or make the hearer feel better. In some contexts Example 2 might be reported as a request or command ("James, it's freezing in here"), in others as an exclamation or simple expression of discomfort.

Example 3. It's 12:10.

Example 3 may prompt a hearer to stop speaking and adjourn a discussion that is running into the lunch hour or to start speaking and convene a bag-lunch meeting. In either case, it would not seem appropriate for an observer to say that the speaker asked, told, or *requested* the hearer to start or stop doing something. We would expect that whatever the hearer did after hearing Example 3 would probably be a response to the information it contains rather than a result of being asked to do something.

The point that Examples 2 and 3 make is that speakers may use language to achieve instrumental goals without using requests and without intending to be interpreted as making requests. Among the various reasons for such language are motives to maintain some features of social relationships (Brown and Levinson, 1978; Ervin-Tripp, 1976). Because such instrumental forms are not conventional requests, they will not be referred to as indirect requests but as nonconventional instrumental moves, or NCIs. Children often hear NCIs and undertake an appropriate action without perceiving the utterance as a request intended to lead to action.

In the case of older children and adults, the motivation for compliance with an NCI may not be different from the reason for carrying out a conventional request. Expressions similar to Example 2 may be immediately interpretable as requests, and the conventional request Example 1 may be complied with because the reason behind it (namely, that it is freezing) is immediately recognized. Speakers may combine utterances such as Examples 1 and 2 to produce justified, socially appropriate requests:

Example 4. Could you close the door? It's freezing in here.

One way to distinguish between requests and NCIs is to examine how they are learned. Conventional requests usually require only a simple grammatical specification or a simple formula in which lexical substitutions are made. In the case of American English, these might include imperatives or certain modals plus the desired act ("Can you. . . ?" "Could (Would) you. . . ?" and so on). But unconventional means require specifications having little to do with either grammar or specific lexical items. In order to treat Example 2 as a "conventionalized" or rule-generated way of getting someone to close the door in an appropriate context, specification of the rule will require finding an adequate reason for the hearer to act, such as stating a problem that the act might solve. This is why the development of effective social control acts depends on cognitive and social strategies rather than a linguistic repertoire.

Instrumental Strategies

Once instrumental language is thought of as relying on strategies for getting others to cooperate with a speaker's goals, the planning behind conventional requests and NCIs can be investigated. One such strategy is to simply ask for cooperation, and this is what is found in conventional request forms, in which the form of the utterance makes explicit the call for cooperation (or obedience). This strategy can be combined with other strategies in the formulation of NCIs. The strategies used by children in making requests and in dealing with denials of requests have been examined in previous research (Bates, 1976; Garvey, 1975).

At the most general level, there are probably two basic approaches:

1. Identify a reason or cause for the hearer to carry out the desired action and make the hearer aware of it (e.g., "It's your turn").
2. Anticipate an obstacle to the hearer's cooperation and neutralize it (e.g., "If you give me *X*, I'll give you *Y*").

It is unlikely that young children have general procedural rules of this nature or that adults have such rules for NCIs either. These approaches are descriptive frameworks under which the more specific instrumental strategies may fall. (For an elaboration of instrumental strategies see the section on Instrumental Language in Gordon and Ervin-Tripp, 1984.)

Social Variables

The social information reflected in instrumental moves can be divided into three overlapping classes. The first class represents power, distance, status or role, rules and rights, and permanent possessions. These tend to be enduring features of the relationship between the speaker and the other members of the social group. In most contexts the relationships will be presupposed, although in some contexts the nature of the situation and the activity determine or alter them on a temporary basis. In role play, for instance, power relations and rights and possessions may all be temporarily changed.

The second set of social meanings relates to the situation at hand and involves shorter-term conditions. These include rights and obligations in temporary roles, intrusion on the addressee's attention, disruption of the addressee's activity, and the value or difficulty of what is requested. These are negotiable and not as likely to be presupposed as is the previous set. They often require sensitivity to the perspective of a hearer and are particularly likely to reflect changes of age and cognitive development.

The third dimension is attitudinal and conveys information about friendliness, irritability, insistence, playfulness, cooperativeness, and so on.

Given the social features mentioned above it is possible to evaluate the social "cost" (Brown and Levinson, 1978) of an instrumental goal. This gives us a means of relating the social variables to the choice of strategy, act, and form. For adults, the higher the cost, the more polite or formal, or indirect, the instrumental language. For example, if a person of lower status wants a person of higher status to do something, asking for it involves a high social cost, which may be "paid" for through an expression of deferential politeness. Asking for something that it is one's right to have involves lower cost—and generally less deference.

As Brown and Levinson (1978) have shown, an assessment of cost allows one to account for a speaker's selection of instrumental language in terms of politeness, informality, and indirectness. It also allows, from the hearer's point of view, an evaluation of how the speaker has assessed the price of the task and the quality of social relations with the hearer. The analysis of children's instrumental language needs to take both the hearer's and the speaker's "calculations" into account.

The following section reports research on the development of instrumental language in children (with much of the information coming from the author's research). Specifically it is drawn from three studies: (1) naturalistic studies of children ranging from infancy to 8 years old (white middle-class families); (2) 142 American children's (aged 3 to 8 years) interpretations of instrumental language, and (3) an adaptation of the second study with seventy-five 4 to 12 year old children in Europe, primarily English- and French-speaking children.

THE DEVELOPMENT OF INSTRUMENTAL COMMUNICATION IN THE FIRST 2 YEARS

In each of the age category sections in the following pages, information derived from both production and comprehension tasks is presented. The production information precedes the comprehension information section in each age category.

Production

The child's earliest intentional communications are gestures toward the end of the first year. At this point, the prototypical instrumental move (Bates, 1976) involves (1) reaching toward a desired object and at the same time (2) looking toward the desired agent who is to act as a mediator. Such gestures are often accompanied by vocalizations or cries to gain attention or express affective states. Both Carter (1974) and Halliday (1975) noted the development of generalized vocalizations for different types of requests and an early naming of desired goal objects as the one-word stage was entered.

Attentional Foregrounding. The earliest instrumental speech appears to express primarily what the child is attending to at the moment. The work of investigators such as Haselkorn (1977) and Veneziano (1981) show how the verbalizations in early one-word requests are selected. Haselkorn noted that the earliest words added to gestures often do not add information to what is gesturally or situationally evident to an observer. Verbalizations are often redundant with already evident "need" states, desired objects or goals, and intended means or agents of action. Veneziano found that children initially tend to verbalize what is to them "new information," which consists of (1) absent or not visible objects more often than visible ones, (2) objects or people further away from the child, or (3) new or unexpected agents whom the child wants to carry out some desired action. To get a ball, a child might say "Ball" on an occasion when the ball is out of sight or across the room and say "Papa" when both her parents are present and the ball is visible. Later, as the child begins to attend more closely to processes and means, actions are mentioned along with objects (goals) or agents, and two-word instrumental moves are formed.

Clarity. The earliest requests, like other speech in this period, tend toward brevity. Therefore the variety of forms described earlier is simply not yet available. The formal range in the early speech includes the following:

1. *Vocatives.* Without first getting attention, most control moves would fail. Children of age two do not usually separate attention-

getting from requesting itself. Indeed, they rarely seek attention vocally before launching an instrumental move.

Attention-getting strategies were discussed in McTear (1979). These include "smiling, gazing, laughing, touching, tugging, poking, turning towards or approaching the intended addressee. . . . Verbal means include the use of vocatives, attention-getters such as *look, hey, wait, see,* etc., or attention-getting questions such as *you know what? guess what?*" (p. 10).

The addressee's name alone ("Mom!"), like other attention-getters, can be an effective directive when the hearer is cooperative. But the listener has to figure out the intent.

2. *Refusals and Prohibitions:* for example, "No."
3. *Ellipsis: Goal Objects, Goal Locations, End States:* for example, "Up," "Here," and "More juice." Haselkorn (1977) noted that at first goal objects are redundant with gestures but later other possibilities develop; for instance, holding out a bottle while saying "Milk."
4. *Imperatives Specifying Means.* These tend to develop later than goal words. "Gimme," "Blow," "Wind," "Book read," "Sweater off," and "Apple me."
5. *Hints: Problem Statements:* for example, "He's stuck," "Carol hungry." Although these look like hints, they seem to be generated by a simple verbalizing of the child's attentional focus. They are not intentionally off-record like the hints of children of six and older.
6. *Explicit Claims Stated as Possessives:* for instance, "that mine," "my book."

The forms used by children at this age are not always clear and explicit about the hearer's task. The child depends on a listener to figure out why the addressee is being called, what is to be done about a named object, what is the goal object for the imperative, or how to solve the problem that is identified. When requests fail, repairs are limited to repetition. Clear examples of verbal persuasion or social differentiation are awaiting the growth of more complex language.

Comprehension

Caregivers' earliest requests to infants are accompanied by gestural support. Shatz (1975) reported in her study of five families that there was sensorimotor support for all the mothers' direct imperatives and 87 per cent of the mothers' question directives (e.g., "Are there any more suitcases?"). Gesture attracts the child's attention to the desired interaction with the caregiver, and gesture directs the child's attention to relevant parts of the environment. Gesture remains an important component of caregivers' requests for a couple years or so before declining markedly. Zukow, Reilly, and Greenfield (1978) give details on the decline with age of gestural support.

The presentation to the child of gesture and speech at the same time provides a basis for relating words to objects and actions and for recognizing the patterns of words that constitute requests. As Zukow and coworkers (1978) state, "During the transition from sensorimotor to linguistic communication, one would expect that the simultaneous presence of a message on both the sensorimotor and linguistic levels would be the key to the new linguistic forms."

It is to be expected that the child's initial understanding of instrumental language is supported from an early age by four factors: (1) the caregivers' use of gestures that call the child's attention to relevant components of context, (2) the repetition of behavioral routines that give the child a basis for expecting and carrying out specific activities (Bruner, 1975, 1982, in press), (3) repetition by the caregivers in a more explicit way when their initial requests are not understood, and (4) the timing of new information to fit the child's behavior.

THE DEVELOPMENT OF INSTRUMENTAL LANGUAGE BETWEEN 2 AND 4 YEARS OF AGE

To reiterate, in successful requests, a speaker must solve five problems: getting attention, being clear, being persuasive, maintaining desired social relations, and making repairs. There is a sequential structure between these components that we will not detail here but that Garvey (1975) and McTear (1979) have addressed.

Production

The problems provide convenient subheadings in the production sections of subsequent age categories. Information from several sources is included to address these problems.

Getting Attention. Effective instrumental moves require having the hearer's attention. Two to 4 year olds are still hampered by lack of success in this area. In our video data, 89 per cent of the times when 2 year olds addressed somebody who was already busy with something else they made their requests without first attempting to gain attention. For 3 year olds the percentage declined to 78 per cent; for 4 year olds it was still as high as 57 per cent (Ervin-Tripp, O'Connor, and Rosenberg, in press). The attention-getting forms of this age group tend to be less specific than those of older children (e.g., they call "Hey" instead of

"Hey, Joe"). Furthermore, young children seemed to face an insurmountable barrier of "ignorability." At every level of relevance, their interruptions were more likely to be ignored than those of older children.

Clarity. Between ages 2 and 4, children develop a full array of basic forms for making instrumental moves, although their use of them remains very different from adults' use. Clarity ceases to be their major problem. Newcombe and Zaslow (1981) gathered 800 requests from nine 2 and a half year olds during play sessions with one of the children, the child's mother, and two researchers.

They found that in their production of question and declarative NCIs 2½ year old children (1) referred to the desired action or object (e.g., "Where's a place for me?") 67 per cent of the time, (2) "identified a problem requiring adult expertise or assistance" (Newcombe and Zaslow, 1981) (e.g., "I can't sit anywhere!") in 36 per cent of examples (1 and 2 are not mutually exclusive), and (3) used other types of NCIs in only 5 of 115 cases, four of which were produced by one child. Thus, NCIs that are not identifications of problems and that mention neither the desired action or object are rare at 2½ years, although not nonexistent. Although these requests are interpretable in context, many of them do not make verbally explicit what the action of the hearer should be.

The major changes taking place thus have to do with explicit formulation of hearer acts and with explicit social marking. Read and Cherry (1978), using an elicitation task in which requests were made to a puppet, found that the only age change between 2½ and 4½ years were an increase in conventional requests, which, like imperatives, are clear about agent, action, and goals. The major changes taking place thus have to do with social marking.

Social Distinctions Reflected in the Use of Instrumental Language. By age 2½, children begin using auxiliaries in English that give them the possibility of adding polite questions to mark social contrasts in instrumental acts. The forms used by young children to make social distinctions are almost entirely requests imbedded with "please" and intonation. By age 2, children's speech already makes some distinctions on the basis of who is being spoken to. MacWhinney (1976) studied the speech of a Hungarian child who by the age of 1 year and 8 months used imperatives to other children, a form analogous to "please" for making requests to the mother, and a markedly polite request form to other adults. Lawson (1967) studied a 2 year old child who used different forms to her father and to her mother and altered her speech to children at nursery school depending on whether they were her age, 3 years old or 4 years old. The 2 year olds received imperatives, and older children received either imperatives or imbedded requests with "please" or "OK?"

Example 5. Child (age 2) to parents:

Child: (to father):	What's that?
Father:	Milk.
Child:	My milk, Daddy.
Father:	Yes, it's your milk.
Child:	Daddy, yours. Yours, Daddy?
Father:	OK, yours.
Father:	OK, it's mine.
Child:	It's milk, Daddy.
Father:	Yes, it is.
Child:	You want milk, Daddy?
Father:	I have some, thank you.
Child:	Milk in there, Daddy?
Father:	Yes.
Child:	Daddy, I want some, please? Please Daddy, huh?
Child: (to mother):	Mommy, I want milk.

(*C. Lawson*)

In this example, the politeness markers used are please, OK, the repeated naming of the father, and, of course, the long devious build-up.

In our videotapes, the children used significantly more imperatives to mothers than to fathers. The only imbedded requests used by 2 year olds were addressed to the visiting researchers. At ages 2 and 3, 60 per cent of directives to outsiders were polite, whereas only 1 per cent of instrumental moves to mothers and 14 to 24 per cent of control acts to other children showed politeness.

Example 6. Nursery school child (age 5.5) to adult visitor: Do you think you could put your foot right there?

(*B. A. O'Connell*)

Why should mothers be at such a disadvantage? The mothers in the families in the sample are *assumed* to be always available for services to a child. Older children are not, and certainly visitors are not. As shall be seen later, these assumptions about rights are fundamental. In cooperative play between children, just as in cooperative activity between adults, the unmarked routine form for an instrumental act is used. In the case of children, this is an imperative or a statement of want or need. One indication that children make these assumptions about mothers is seen in a threat by a much older child to his mother:

Example 7. If you don't give it to me now I won't want it later.

Besides presumptions about rights derived from role or status, children by age 2 have a sense of rights of possession. *Requests for the goods of another* were typically polite. The only instances of 2 and 3 year olds' polite speech to the mother involved possessions. When they wanted a younger sibling's toys, they chose polite forms 44 per cent of the time;

otherwise, 9 per cent. They are clearly sensitive to ownership or "territory." A common choice in these cases is a "Can I" permission request:

> Example 8. Nursery school child to peer: Can I have one of the reds (wheedling tone)?
>
> (*B. A. O'Connell*)

The preceding example indicates that children between 2 and 3 years make distinctions between addressees on the basis of age (or size or *power*), familiarity (researcher versus family), role (mother or father), and territory, or "rights." Power or authority, familiarity or social distance, role, territory, and rights are the major social variables addressed in adult speech. One might think here—although it is not the interpretation advocated—of a nascent politeness system in which the implications or meanings of each social variable are filled out during the course of development. This could also account for 2 and 3 year olds' choices of instrumental form in terms of a system of "costs" that is a simplified version of the cost system of adults: commands (imperatives or "I want" statements) for low-cost goals, questions (e.g., "Can I have . . . ?" "Would you . . . ?") for high-cost goals (when explicitness is needed for clarity), and, perhaps for intermediate costs, imperatives combined with softeners such as "Please?" "OK?" or modulated intonation.

The previous description of the 2 and 3 year olds' instrumental language treats it as if it were simply a reduced version of adult language (Ervin-Tripp, 1976). The authors do not think this is the case because the child's conception of politeness and social interaction must undergo major changes before the reasons underlying a choice of form come to match those of mature speakers. Such changes are reflected in the use of NCIs and the elaborations and explanations that older children add to their basic requests. But the simple polite markers seen at first, such as "please," "can you," "can I," and "d'you wanna," may not just be markers of the status or rights of the addressee. Instead, they may just indicate that the child separates those cases of presupposed, presumed cooperation from the cases in which compliance cannot be assumed. These include involvement with fathers who do not usually supply food, outsiders who do not attend to the child's needs, and owners who do not have to give up property.

Bates (1976) raised the question of when children begin to modify their instrumental moves on the basis of politeness rather than efficiency. When do children have a general concept of politeness? "To make a command more *efficient,* one generally increases either its information content or its attentional pull. But to make a command more *polite,* one must consider the possibility that the listener might be offended, or prefer a more modest approach by the speaker" (p. 279). Bates concludes from her research on Italian children that children's speech adjustments (use of "please," intonation patterns, minimizers such as only, just, a little) by age 2.6 show some ability to follow instructions to be more polite. This is some extension beyond what is deliberately taught. It is not until years later that children produce instrumental forms (e.g., imbedded requests and hints) that are intended to be indirect and to give the hearer options not to comply.

Persuasion. Although basic instrumental forms are present early in children's speech, 2 and 3 year olds infrequently provide spontaneous explanations or justifications for their requests. Children at these ages in our naturalistic video data did so for only 6 per cent of their requests and NCIs. This rose to 14 per cent for 4 year old children. Such "adjuncts" are frequent in adult speech and provide a different understanding of how requests and social interaction work.

There is a major cognitive basis for a rise in justifications. Around age 3, children begin to *question* adult refusals and directives with "Why?" An increase in justifying is related to the growth of "because" clauses, which Campos, de Castro and de Lemos (1979) have shown started with justifications offered for the *partner's* requests, prohibitions, or refusals. Later, these justifications were conjoined to the child's own instrumental acts and became persuasive adjuncts. This history shows that justifying starts in the child's search for rationality in the move of others. This in turn may be derived from adult modeling of justifications. If so, a good deal of social variation depending on adult practices would be expected.

Repairs. Bates (1976) indicates that intentional politeness in young children can be ascertained by looking at children's second tries after an initial instrumental move has failed. Haselkorn (1979) found that at the one-word stage children's remedies for failure were mainly to increase clarity, that is, to specify what they wanted more clearly. In the family research the authors found that the younger children made second tries by repeating over and over what they said the first time. The older the child, the larger the reformulations used in making repairs.

Bates's (1976) notion is that the initial elicited demand of a 2½ year old is likely to be direct, and on a second try politeness markers will be added if the child has developed a politeness rather than an efficiency strategy. Bates's data support her finding of politeness strategies in children of 2½ years. The younger children in her study typically changed to question intonation when asked to make their request "nicer."

More recently, Newcombe and Zaslow (1981) have looked at second tries in the spontaneous speech of 2½ year olds and found that fewer than 7 per cent of their second tries moved in the direction of increased politeness. They clearly do not believe politeness increases efficacy, and they are right. The authors' family research found no effect of children's politeness on compliance, when "cost" is controlled (Ervin-Tripp et al., in press).

These studies of second tries suggest that at this age children assume their failures arise from not being explicit and intelligible enough. They do not think the repairs should make requests more polite unless instructed to do so.

Comprehension of Instrumental Language Between 2 and 4 Years of Age

Young children's comprehension has been studied by noting their responses to directives. Comprehension has also been studied contextually by interpreting communication interactions and social (politeness) markers.

Action Responses to Directives. Shatz (1975, 1978) has looked at children's responses to directives. In her 1975 study early 2 year olds were presented imbedded "can" requests (e.g., "Can you talk on the telephone?") in two contexts, one of which called for the action to be carried out and the other of which asked for information only, since the preceding items ("Can Mommy talk on the telephone?") could not be directives. Two year olds and 5 and 6 year old language-disordered children (Shatz, Bernstein, and Shulman, 1980) carried out the actions in action contexts but also tended to carry them out half the time in information only contexts. The more linguistically mature children (those who used more than three words per utterance) made a large contrast but still gave 29 per cent action to informational contexts. In her 1978 study, Shatz looked at the interpretation by children between the ages of 1½ and 3 of different types of control moves in action versus information contexts. The youngest children correctly responded in action contexts but also acted in information contexts. The most advanced children in the sample still carried out actions in information contexts 28 per cent of the time. "Why don't you . . . ?" uniformly elicited actions in highly weighted information contexts, and even noninstrumental forms starting with "May you . . . ?" were effective in triggering action, much as if they had been "Can you?" or "Would you" requests.*

On the basis of such findings Shatz reports that "in a neutral controlled situation the children showed a strong bias toward action re-

*Luria (1961) pointed out long ago in his studies of verbal mediation that the discrimination of action from nonaction by verbal mediators was compromised by the child's tendency to treat all verbalizations as signaling action. For instance, if children were taught to press a bulb when a light went on, any verbalization led to pressing. If they were to say to themselves "now" or "press" for a red light, and "don't" for a blue light, even more pressed with the blue light than when they were silent. Luria believed that after 4½ years of age, words change from triggers to impulsive responses and become differentiated signals.

sponding'' and concluded that children must learn *not* to respond when the context implies an informational interpretation rather than action interpretation.

The more advanced children in Shatz's 1978 study (Mean Length of Utterance [MLU] 3.2 to 4.0) were less likely to carry out actions in information-only contexts. Children at this age may be starting to compare the form and content of an utterance with the context in which they occur before responding rather than relying primarily on their own immediate expectations about behavioral routines or appropriate actions.

The child's "set" to respond to an utterance with an action (discussed by Shatz) has also been observed in research on children's imitations. In the course of an imitation protocol Ervin-Tripp (1970) obtained the following sequence:

Example 9: E: Say, "Under his foot was a snake."
Ch: Under his foot was a snake. (Child waves cup in the air.)
E: Say, "Put the cup down."
Ch: Put the cup down. (Puts cup down.)
E: Say, "What is your favorite color?"
Ch: What is your favorite color? Red.

One way of interpreting the imitation behavior and Shatz's findings is to say that the young or language-delayed child is limited in the ability to maintain two contexts in mind at once. They have trouble in learning to subordinate local cues and to favor the instructions. For the child, an utterance may suggest an immediate action-context that overrides the more distant instructions. The limitation here is probably cognitive.

When reference is made to an action set in 2 to 4 year olds it should be recognized that this set is really a function of the child's nonlinguistic orientation to activities that are in themselves either interesting or meaningful. In an experimental situation in which the child is not engaged in any other activity, the child may be ready to carry out a behavioral response to speech, but when the child is already engaged in an activity the availability of such an interpretation strategy is quite restricted. Thus Urzua (1977), in a study of the directives of four middle-class mothers to their 2 year old daughters, found that question requests were frequently not recognized as parental control moves. This is shown in the following episode in which a mother continues the use of ineffective question directives:

Example 10. (Child messes up records.)
Mother: Where do those go when . . . do they go somewhere?
Child: All gone. (Continues messing up records)
Mother (after 15 seconds): Where do you want them to go?
(Child kicks records.)

Mother: Well. That isn't very nice to the records. Want to put them back here? (Begins putting away. Child watches.)

The evidence from Urzua's (1977) study and the authors' own research (discussed further on) suggests that in such instances the child is not just ignoring what she or he recognizes as an instrumental move; she or he does not realize in the first place that an attempt to guide behavior is being made. In the authors' illustrated narratives (Ervin-Tripp, 1977), subjects often did not recognize NCIs as requests. For example, in the helping situation in which a mother with groceries in her arms asks, "Is the door open?" many subjects had the children in the story open the door for her, but when asked why the mother said this, they typically responded, "She just wanted to know." ("Then why open the door?" "To get the groceries in the house!")

Shatz (1978) found that children often treated a conventional form as a request for action when in the larger context it was not. The authors have found in their picture stories study that children over 4 years old respond with action as well as independently answer NCIs even when they do not recognize them as intentional requests. In this view of the children's interpretive processes the questions can call for answers and also draw attention to states of affairs that lead the children to change their actions. But the relationship between the answers and the action is not direct.

The authors found that the 3 year olds answered the questions and that there was no relation between answering and helping or complying with the request. The older children also answered question NCIs and independently complied even when they did not recognize them as requests in intent. Bates (1971) in her sample of communication from ages 2 to 4 also found incongruence between verbal and action responses. Interrogative request forms did not show an increase in compliance with age, but there was an increase in verbal replies to them. She argued that the discourse and action aspects of the response were difficult to handle at once for 2 year olds, so they did one or the other, not both. This reflects basic processes in the way children understand and use language. Verbal processing is not on a linear path to pragmatic interpretation but parallel to it.

Language Embedded in Experience. Language is interpreted in context on the basis of previous experience and expectations about possible activities, social interactions, and communication. In hearing speech, the child of 2 years already brings many expectations into play. Some of the factors that set up such expectations and facilitate appropriate responses to speech are:

1. Objects have intrinsic action norms that are likely to be carried out by young children even in the absence of directives.
2. Ownership and norms of location can be recognized. Calling attention to out-of-place objects (e.g., "Are those your shoes in the middle of the room?") can lead to remedies.
3. Activities have internal structure. A child who rides a tricycle goes somewhere. Blocks get piled up. People carrying groceries put them in the kitchen and into the refrigerator.
4. People have normal roles in the activity system. It may be the mother who puts the groceries in the refrigerator in one family; in another it may be assumed that the child does it. Under cooperative conditions, participants carry out their normal roles in getting the activity completed.
5. Some activities are prohibited to everyone or to some persons.

In the context of this much knowledge, language can be thought of as drawing the listener's attention to something in the setting, and allowing the child's nonlinguistic norms to work on producing a plan of action. In this way, not only familiar language formats such as imperatives but also embedded and implicit request forms can function as if explicit and direct when they are linked to contexts and expectations with which the child is familiar. In the prohibition situations in stories in one of the author's studies (Ervin-Tripp, 1977), subjects were asked what the story children's response would be after the mother's utterance. All 3 year olds recognized that the portrayed activities were prohibited, and they regularly said the children's response to the mother's utterance would be to stop the activity, regardless of what the mother actually said, whether it was a softly spoken "Are you fighting?" or something silly or irrelevant. If the mother was silent, 3 year olds still said the mother "wanted" the story children to stop their activities. Thus, in such situations the action norms are so obvious that very young children are strongly affected by them and even subtle verbal forms may appear to be effective control acts.

Shatz's finding (1978) that children have an activity set in response to language is understandable. Children are "set" to act in any event, with or without language. The child structures a great part of the work in terms of activities and knowledge about activities, as indicated previously. Objects are used (thrown, worn, manipulated, and so on) or experienced (seen, tasted, heard, and so forth); people do things and allow, facilitate, or prevent activities and can be used (for instrumental purposes) and experienced (heard, seen, played with). This structuring of the child's reality is made up of expectations not about context-free activities but of "situated" activity: of sequences of "scenes" containing settings and the activities that are appropriate to the scene or that lead from one setting to another. Language, for both child and adult, calls up, and is used to call up, scenes, sequences of scenes, and expectations about their organization and the activities and roles that are a part of them (cf. Nelson and Gruendel, 1979; Schank and Abelson, 1977).

Language is not only interpreted in context, it also creates the contexts in which it is interpreted. Tone of voice, for example, may let us know if the context is one of friendly or hostile interaction. An expression such as "Did you hear the one about. . . ?" or "Hi, how are you?" tells us that we are going to be offered a joke (thereby defining a familiar kind of social interaction and level of rapport) or at least a passing conversation as part of validating or defining a social relationship. The less known about the forms and nuances a language provides, the more a person must fall back on nonlinguistic expectations. In the author's picture narrative studies, "realistic directives," which varied in form and involved real responses to requests or hints made by experimenters, were included. The variation was from explicit conventional requests such as "Can you reach my purse?" to less clear forms not specifying agent ("I can't reach my purse,") to NCIs ("Is my purse over there?" "My purse is over there." "Oh, my purse." A few anomalous forms were also included: "My purse is white." The 3 year olds gave help to 90 per cent of the conventional requests and to 50 per cent of the partly explicit forms. Help of the 3 year olds declined steeply for NCIs, which are far less explicit. When NCIs like "Oh, my purse" were used in the "real-life" part of the authors' interpretation experiments in Switzerland, it was found that English-speaking school children were more likely to carry out helping actions than Genevan school children—apparently a function of culturally different assessments of the experimental situation or of interactions with adults. English-speaking children were even more helpful when they were tested in French than in English. It would seem likely that in hearing French these children could not be as confident of their linguistic interpretations, and therefore relied more heavily on searching the context and their own social behavioral expectations for an interpretation of what was said.

The young child learning a first language is less socially mature at the same stage of language development and cannot be relied on for pragmatic interpretation so easily. Thus it was found that in the realistic helping situations it was the youngest, the 3 year olds, who were the most dependent on verbal explicitness and the least responsive to hints.

Examine briefly the child in Urzua's study at play with the records (Example No. 23). The child is clearly "set" on her own action. In such contexts it is to be expected that children will hear most speech in terms of their own interests or immediate activities. If there is no connection, the speech will be ignored. Certain signals will cause the child to attend to what is said: a preemptory tone of voice, for example, or perhaps an imperative syntactic form combined with appropriate request or command intonation. Such signals serve as instructions to interrupt or look away from the immediate focus of activity. Just as the young child must learn to secure a hearer's attention in order to make successful moves, the child must learn to attend to the speech of others, independent of immediate preoccupations.

Understanding Social Markers. Bates (1971) developed the first tests for 2 year olds for relative politeness. Later she extended these methods in Italy with 60 children aged 2 years 10 months to 6 years 2 months (Bates, 1976, pp. 295–315). Children were asked first to generate polite forms to get a cookie. Then they were asked to judge which of two frog puppets should get a cookie. This method allowed paired comparisons between request forms. Although the method is context-unspecified, the presence of the experimenter presumes speech to an older addressee. The discrimination between the use of "please" and its omission and between harsh and soft speech was significant before age 4. Although little work has been done on social interpretation on such young children, there is evidence of budding discrimination.

In many languages it is common to displace the agent, that is, to say "we" when the speaker means "you," as in, "We have to take our naps now." "We" is a typical mitigator when talking down in rank. This distinction was detected by Bates (1971).

INSTRUMENTAL LANGUAGE BETWEEN 4 AND 8 YEARS OF AGE

Children experience a greater range of social participation during this age period. Consequently, their instrumental moves must be more effective. This shift is noted in the research information reported here.

Production

The information on production suggests that children aged 4 to 8 years old make extensive gains in strategies for getting attention, in knowing when to clear, in how to achieve social appropriateness, in how to use persuasion, and how to make repairs.

Getting Attention. During this age period, children both increase the specificity and effectiveness of attention forms ("Hey, Mary") and increase the likelihood of noticing the need to attract attention when listeners are preoccupied. At age 4 years, 57 per cent failed to try for attention, but at ages 5 and 8 years only 31 per cent failed in our sample of four families. This age change is related to children's ability to take the role of the addressee and identify the focus of the partner.

Knowing When to be Clear. Early requests derive their form from the child's focus of attention rather than from the informational needs of listeners. Young children are not good at attending to the cognitive states of listeners.

Stalder (no date) has based several studies on the increases at this age in the children's awareness of the knowledge of others. Children aged 4 to 7 years were in a room with structured toys with missing parts; the missing parts were in another room. Typically the children's first requests were polite requests, but the second requests were abbreviated to hints and elliptical forms, especially to the mother and especially by the older speakers.

In a second experiment an adult stranger was noncompliant half the time. Stalder questioned the children about their beliefs concerning the listeners' expectations. Basically, the children decreased explicitness and increased NCIs if they correctly surmised the listener expected a request and also after the stranger-addressee refused to comply. Why after refusals? Because the justifications accompanying refusal increased the child's awareness of what the listener knew. *Explicitness occurs when the child thinks the listener does not expect a request.*

A number of studies have shown that NCIs increase in the school years, presumably affected by awareness of the listener, as Stalder has proposed (e.g., Liebling, 1981; Montes, 1981).

These changes show that the child's enlarging social awareness permits the intentional modification of clarity. These modifications have two goals. One is brevity, which takes into account the knowledge of the hearer and is strongly valued in our culture among adults, as an evidence of solidarity. The other is deviousness, in the interest of avoiding being intrusive and demanding, a classic social motive for hinting. Specific examples are given below.

Social Appropriateness. Younger children are sensitive to *relative status* and to *rights and possessions,* and these will remain important features after age 4. In the authors' family videotapes, the 5 to 8 year old speakers had a conventional pattern of status differentiation, with adults receiving more deference (polite markers) than children, and older children more than younger. Significantly more imperatives were addressed to mothers and more mitigating explanations were addressed to fathers. Some studies have compared speech to mother and to peers. Yet, as pointed out previously, mothers are expected by children to comply with their wishes, and they do comply much more to "high-cost" requests than either children or other adults do. Because mothers, like cooperating peers, are expected to comply and receive imperatives, mother versus peer contrasts are not appropriate for discovering children's social differentiations in deference.

Wood and Gardner (1980) observed the play of nursery school children paired by dominance. They found that when age was controlled, the dominant partner both gave more directives and used more imperatives, and the subordinate partner gave more imbedded imperatives and mitigators. They also found that the successful directives of subordinates were significantly more polite. Because family studies found no differential compliance by the politeness of children's directives (relative age, and for everyone but mothers, cost, seem more involved than form), it is assumed that it must be in the relatively more egalitarian conditions of peer play that these nuances are reinforced. Perhaps this is how they are learned rather than by modeling alone.

Role-play data are rich in showing the social meaning of directives. As Mitchell-Kernan and Kernan (1977) have suggested, directive forms are used "to establish a relationship of dominance-submission between the characters." Corsaro (1979) found imperatives composed 60 per cent of the speech of nursery school superordinate role speech to subordinates. "Let's" was also a feature of dominant role speech, whereas subordinates responded or asked permission. Andersen (1977) elicited role-playing in which the child played two parts in three-character scenes with puppets, such as doctor-nurse-patient or mother-father-child. She included children of 4 to 6 years. The "father" gave more imperatives than the "mother" and the "mother" more hints. In the oldest group, the husband gave more than twice as many directives to his wife as the reverse. The 4 year olds depicted the children as giving 42 per cent imperatives to the mother and 14 per cent to the father. Doctors gave imperatives, nurses hints. Hollos and Beeman (1978), who studied elicited requests in Norway, commented that though Norwegian children generally favored indirectness, with the mothers they were not only direct but even rude.

The high frequency of formal reflections of status when the speaker's own property is at issue was demonstrated by James (1978) with picture eliciting. James tested 4 and 5 year old children, who tended to hypercorrect and prefer highly explicit polite formulas. They proposed "please" 29 per cent of the time to a younger child, 59 per cent to a peer, and 92 per cent to an adult in retrieving rightful property. The elicited and role-play data make clear that status on its own affects the form of requests.

The youngest children were sensitive to rights. James' eliciting study showed that the contrast in politeness by rank was greatest in the low-cost condition, but not when a favor was asked, which involved the others' property. Favors even to a younger child contained "please" 45 per cent of the time. Under the "rights" condition, even to an adult stranger, only 49 per cent were questions.

In the following example, a request that presumes on the territory of the other gets a conventional polite form. Presumably telling his sister what to do is not his right:

> Example 11. Four year old to 2½ year old sister: Addie, why don't you show Gina what you wore. OK?

Social markers in relation to social features have been examined in eliciting or memory studies with an adult or child addressee or rights versus favors as content. For example, Hildyard (1979) studied recall of requests and found children "corrected" the recall so that conventionally polite forms were preferred for favors and for peer or adult addressees. Direct commands were reconstructed to younger children when demanding a right.

A nice feature of Hildyard's (1979) recall study was that it showed evidence not merely of making forms more polite but of keeping commands direct in appropriate conditions. The adult norm is not that direct commands go to subordinates but rather that they accompany rights, possessions, and the presumption of cooperation. The second graders followed this pattern. Kindergarteners "hypercorrected" and changed commands to polite requests sometimes even when the speaker's rights were involved.* This finding suggests that kindergartners in eliciting by adults are most concerned with being correct about "politeness" to strangers and have not yet worked out the fine tuning of appropriateness.

In the family interaction, even the 4 year olds seemed to be concerned with using polite markers whenever cooperation could not be assumed because the other was more powerful or because their goods were involved. Parsons (1980) found in a puppet eliciting experiment that 5 to 9 year old children were more polite in soliciting a favor from a puppet addressee that they expected not to comply than to one who had been compliant before. The forms used were conventional questions and "please."

By 5 to 8 years, children in the authors' family sample also became sensitive to the interruption of the listener. They were polite 12 per cent of the time when the listener was already cooperating with them but 54 percent of the time when compliance would interrupt an activity or plan

*In Hildyard's recall study, declarations of rights ("That's mine!") were not usually rephrased but were left as adequate, confirming the finding by Montes that in conditions in which the listener has taken the speaker's possessions, children presuppose that the listener expects a directive, so a hint is clear enough. But other NCIs declarations of fact, justifications, or hints for favors were rephrased as imbedded requests. In the author's family studies, children routinely made claims to property instead of explicitly requesting its return.

of the other. Imperatives decreased from 60 per cent to 27 per cent under conditions of interruption.

Age changes in dealing with interruptions have also been explored in an experiment in which children on several occasions had to ask busy adults for a letter or a marker pen (Gordon, Budwig, Strage, and Carrell, 1980). Children in the kindergarten through second grade were compared with children in grades three to five. Both groups avoided imperatives. They did not differ in the frequency of conventional forms like permission requests. The younger children used somewhat more obvious forms that do not supply an excuse or option for the hearer. Their typical forms were "I need a blue marker" "Where's the marker?" or "The marker's broken." Sometimes they might add a justification: "The marker's broken, I need a new one."

By the end of this period, then, children not only use politeness modifications for issues of status and rights as they had used at 2 years, but have added sensitivity to their intrusions into the activity trajectory and conversations of others. This seems to be a clear case of the growth of social perspective taking. They have also developed a sense of cost that identifies overpoliteness as inappropriate.

Are these conventional kinds of politeness aspects of being persuasive? The authors' data suggest that politeness in the family is not rewarded by greater compliance. On the other hand, the role-playing data show that children regard the formal contrasts as a way to identify social features. This seems to be unambiguous evidence that beyond any attempt to be persuasive such forms have acquired a symbolism.

Do these forms have an semantic content other than their social features? Clearly some forms, like "please," are just formal markers. This becomes an urgency indicator, with an aggravated voice.

Example 12. Give it to me *please*!

Many of the formal politeness markers are analyzable and have to do with reasons for refusal. For example:

Example 13. Can you help?
I can't help. I'm busy now.

Probably most of the cases of use of these forms are formulas or idiomatic routines. But their continued survival in unreduced forms suggests that speakers sometimes attend to their literal meanings. Garvey (1975) has shown that nursery school children's excuses have the same semantic range as their requests: dealing with features of willingness, ability or permission, and reasons and rights.

However, the older children have begun to use speech that is not formulaic. These kinds of forms genuinely imply options for the listener and are often creative. The forms used to mark social relationships have extended from fixed formal markers like "please" and embeddings to justifications and hints.

Persuasion. Garvey (1975) found only 67 conventionally polite requests in her study of 4 and 5 year old peer dyads, but 111 adjuncts, or supportive remarks, many of which supplied reasons or checked willingness. The adjuncts she found included causes, norms, goals, needs, and wants. These justifications are reasonably oriented to the child's view of social rights. For example, "I want it" or "I need it" are common intensifiers on second tries. They seem to be viewed by children as self-contained and sufficient explanations, as are the wants of others.

The first examples found of frequent justifications are in instances of an attempt to stop another's activity. In these cases, the context does not supply a clear reason for compliance, so the child seems to be asking for a favor. The kinds of explanations may refer to rights or to reasons. The reasons are intensified on second tries, according to Montes (1981). Children allocate these adjuncts according to the social features of the addressee. Caregiving roles, for example, may be appealed to in addressing adults:

> Example 14. Beth (age 5) to mother: Mommy, I want you to open all of them, the paint, so I won't have to trouble.

> Example 15. Lisa (age 4) to researcher: OK, we don't know all these pages, so you read 'em.

Norms, goals, or facts about the world may be appealed to with younger children.

> Example 16. Eight year old to 4 year old: We only have a little more, OK? So don't use one on every Valentine.

> Example 17. Four year old to 2 year old: Get out of my space. This is *my* space.

Older speakers eventually use the justifications or preconditions alone as requests.

Montes (1981) has experimentally looked at instrumental moves and justification adjuncts in nursery and grade school, using an eliciting technique based on questioning about getting back a child's valued possession from a named friend or teacher. This was a condition of claiming rights, in which explicitness was not necessary because the request could be expected. She found that in first grade the ratio of imbedded requests was at a maximum. By third grade, the preferred forms were the hint, which presupposes the listener expects a request, and provides a justification, or an imperative plus justifying reason. (A hint can be seen as an adjunct alone without the explicit directive.) Altogether persuasive adjuncts in this case of claiming rights increased from 34 per cent in nursery school to 50 per cent in kindergarten and 79 per cent in third grade. These figures of course represent the artificial conditions of the eliciting experiment and should be compared with the authors' frequency of 14 per cent adjuncts in the family videotapes. In addition, forms that soften the force of a request rose from 17 per cent in nursery school to 49 per cent in third grade. Forms of increased urgency or demand went from 17 per cent to 31 per cent between nursery school and the third grade. These findings indicate that during the period from 4 to 8 years there are important developments in the child's ability—or wish—to modulate the precise force of instrumental moves and the impression they make on hearers.

A major development at this time is the use of reframing as in the use of pretense. This is a way of making a desired move of the addressee more acceptable by redefining the activity in which it is to occur. Negotiation has already appeared:

> Example 18. 42 month old to peer: If you give me this for a while, you can have this for a while.
>
> (*Ervin-Tripp*)

The details of the evolution of persuasive tactics cannot be described here.

Repairs. Grimm's (1975) study of German children's remedies in making requests to a puppet showed that kindergarteners with increased urgency became more intense, but second graders turned to more persuasive tactics like obligation, justification, and bribery. In the Montes (1981) experiment, if children failed on the first try, nonverbal strategies increased, intensifiers or aggravation increased, and offering of justifications (except for rights) increased. There is little evidence that mitigation by making requests more polite is a spontaneous routine at this age for remedying failures. Like the younger children, these children aggravate and intensify requests. But more important, they find additional forms of persuasion and justification.

Comprehension of Instrumental Language Between Ages Four and Eight

Recognizing Requests. In young children, comprehension appears to be affected by three factors: the familiarity of the routine, brevity, and grammatical complexity.

It can be expected that as children come to anticipate situations in which directives are likely, they will more readily recognize hints as directives. American middle-class mothers gradually become less explicit. They move from imperatives to imbedded imperatives to NCIs with the age of the child, becoming more explicit in the case of repairs (Bellinger, 1979; Schneiderman, 1983). Shapiro's (1978a, 1978b) work in classrooms suggests that teachers follow the same principles. For example, newcomers were given more imperatives and explicit directives by kindergarten teachers at the beginning of the school year. Later, as the children learned the routines of the classroom, the teachers could be less explicit. Liebling (1981) found that first and third grade children had trouble understanding hints about picture narratives but fifth graders did not.

More evidence of the importance of familiarity with a form of indirection is found in the study (Gordon and Ervin-Tripp, 1984) of conversational dares in Geneva. These were used in problem situations so obvious that even 3 year olds recognized they were transgressions. When children were throwing food in the living room in the picture narrative, for instance, the mother came in and said, "Beautiful, go right ahead!" On the European continent, such sarcasm by parents and teachers is familiar, but English and American children in the Geneva sample judged it to be lying since it is literally untrue. American and English children who were 4 years old or more, when tested in Switzerland or France, readily recognized the intent of the corrections in French, though they did not recognize them when tested in English until after 8 years old.

In the picture narrative research, concern centered not only with age changes in ability to understand NCIs (such as "Is the door open?") but with how the children did it. It was found that children older than 4 years of age proposed helping about 80 per cent of the time. But when asked what the speaker wanted, only about 60 per cent said the speaker wanted help. The others said the speaker just "wanted to know." When pressed about why the child in the picture offered help, the children pointed to a state of affairs that called for a remedy. In our view, even with adults, many hints work by drawing attention to a state of affairs that calls for a remedy if one is cooperative. But inferring intention may not be necessary.

Young children are not good at attending to the state of mind of others. In the picture narratives, it was found that the younger children did not even think about the adult speaker's point of view. They seemed to identify with the children in the stories. For narratives of naughty actions the 3 year olds' responses were identical to the visible silent mother and the invisible audible mother. They reacted simply to "mother in the vicinity" without distinguishing what the mother might know (like a child playing in hide-and-go-seek who hides only his or her head). By the age of 7 years it was found that when the pictures with the stories did not show the mother, the children often lied about naughty actions, saying the mother could not see what was going on. So awareness of the partner's point of view appears after 4 years.

There is some data on brevity comparing normal children with children whose progress is not normal. Browning's (1974) study of 7 and 8 year old schizophrenic children found that long expressions were not understood. Browning used phrases such as "Steve, it is too noisy. Please close the classroom door." In contrast, four-word directives were more easily understood. Normal children by this age can understand both. Studies of the interpretation of particular linguistic structures by normal children have been carried out by Leonard, Wilcox, Fulmer, and Davis (1978) and Carrell (1981).

Understanding Social Relations. The period after 4 years of age appears to be a time in which the social meanings of formal markers begin to be interpreted by children in terms of dimensions like "politeness" and social categories of speakers. Bates' (1971) tests of Italian children's *judgments of politeness* revealed that while Italian children themselves routinely used question intonation in their own speech to mitigate, they did not judge it as nicer or more polite until after age 4½. The Italian formal pronoun and the conditional tense were not judged differently until a year later.

Another way to assess recognition of social features is to ask children to *identify possible speakers*. Becker (1981) asked children to pick a doll who could have spoken a request and found children of 4 years were able to identify conditionals, mitigated tone, and hints as spoken by a younger or lower-status speaker. The older children even discriminated "can" versus "may," title versus first name, "I need" versus "may I have," and even "Will you give" versus "Do you have any left."

THE DEVELOPMENT OF INSTRUMENTAL LANGUAGE AFTER 8 YEARS OF AGE

Age 8 years appears to mark general changes in instrumental language and in awareness of the perspective of others. This is the age when the intention of other speakers is taken into account. Even English monolinguals could recognize conversational dares or sarcastic directives. They also began to identify lying as a possible strategy of the children in our test narratives, when the recognized the different informational state of others.

Social Appropriateness

Prior to age 8 children have acquired the instrumental forms that make up adult speech and can combine these with adjuncts and politeness markers to modulate features such as urgency, force, friendliness, and demand.

However, in an experiment (Gordon et al., 1980) in which children had to get marker pens and letters from busy adults, there was a clear difference between children below the third grade (under 8 years old) and in third grade and above.

The speech of children below the third grade in most cases expressed an assumption that the adult addressee had the marker (or letter) desired:

Example 19. I need a blue marker.

Example 20. Where's the marker?

Example 21. Can I have the letter to my parents?

Forms such as Examples 19 and 20 tend to assume compliance. Example 21 does not, but it places the burden of noncompliance on the hearer.

The forms the older children used revealed a different sense of the simple interaction:

Example 22. Are there any more markers?

Example 23. Do you have a green marker I could use?

Example 24. She told me to get a letter for my parents.

Examples 16 and 17 acknowledge the possibility that the hearer might not comply with the request, and Example 18 recognizes that the child may be intruding and deflects the responsibility to another.

From data such as that given and informal observations of the authors' video data and narrative experiments, it can be suggested that at about age 8, or at the third grade level, children's speech begins to address the viewpoint of the hearer, recognizes problems of intrusiveness as a social issue, and acknowledges options for noncompliance with requests.

Some cultural variation in how much children are encouraged to avoid explicitness may be found. For instance, Hollos and Beeman (1978) found that 4 to 5 year old Norwegian children would use their mothers as intermediaries to strangers, whereas 9 to 10 year olds, like the older children in our sample, could say to a storekeeper, "Have you chocolates?" or to a neighbor, "That cake is very good" when they wanted some.

Mitchell-Kernan and Kernan (1977) adduced evidence that children aged 7 to 12 were sensitive to *cost* as a factor in formulating directives. Since imbedded imperatives were infrequent in the dramatic role-play data, they looked to natural conversations for evidence and found that polite marking increased

1. When the speaker was estranged from the peer group.
2. When the speaker interrupts the addressee's activities.
3. When the task was difficult.

Polite requests then appear to be alternatives to imperatives that compensate, much as Brown and Levinson (1978) have described in their reports of facing-saving devices.

Hints in Mitchell-Kernan and Kernan's data (1977) seemed to occur specifically to avoid some negative implications in polite conventional requests. They are strongly related to group norms about the child role.

The changes that take place around age 8 bring children's use of language close to that of adults in many respects, but there are still important developments that have not taken place. Children at this age are usually still limited in their ability to recognize the intentions behind many NCIs even when they respond to them appropriately. Thus, Ervin-Tripp (1977) points out that even a routinized form such as "Is your mother there?" spoken on the telephone to a child as old as 10 years may still be interpreted literally as a request for information. It also appears that young adolescents often do not recognize the intention behind NCIs such as

Example 25. Aren't your parents going to be worried about your being out so late?

which was spoken by the parent of one teenager to a visiting teenager in the hope of getting him to leave, without having to ask directly. At the same time, we have examples such as

Example 26. We haven't gotten our allowances yet. Hint, hint.

Here a young teenager has produced an NCI, realized that the intention behind it was transparent to the hearer, and self-consciously responded to show his awareness of this and the request implications of his utterance.

In another case, a visiting 12 year old overdoes all the politeness markers available in an effort judged as "uncomfortable" by a peer:

Example 27. Do you have any water I could drink?

Here an explicitly polite permission request, "Can I drink water?" is embedded in a routine obstacle question that seems odd because it has no realistic foundation: "Do you have any water?" By avoiding commitment about the person who will get the water and by displacing to the conditional, the visitor achieved a very delicate but extreme politeness.

Unsystematic indications such as the preceding example suggest to us that it is during the period of early adolescence that self-consciousness and a complex orientation to the intentions and attitudes of others is being worked out and dealt with in speech. During this period the "presentation of self" and concern for social face (that is, a positive social appearance) and the face of others is developed to the point of correspondence with adult social perceptions and understandings. Conveniently, and not coincidentally, it can be assumed, the changes taking place around age 8 and at adolescence correspond chronologically with the cognitive changes Piaget (1926) has described in terms of concrete and abstract reasoning.

Persuasion

The major changes in persuasive tactics derive from the capacity of children over the age of 8 years to take the perspective of their partners. Two examples will illustrate this change.

> Example 28. Sister to brother, age 4: D'ya wanna be Santa Claus? Here, take these toys to the basement. (Ties her laundry in her nightgown and he carries it to laundry.)

In the second example, the boy was becoming whiny because he wanted to cram his tricycle in a station wagon already full of bicycles. He was wearing a Batman cape.

> Example 29. Sister to brother: Batman, you don't need a bike. You can *fly* over everyone faster than the bikes! (He accepted her proposal.)

On both occasions, the request was part of a proposal for play in which the boy had a desirable role. This method accommodates his perspective and borrows the familiar pretense strategy. Reframing makes cooperation flow out of the natural trajectory of the new activity. It is successful if the recipient's motives are taken into account and if the recipient feels cooperative. It calls for perspective-taking the younger children cannot manage.

ISSUES FOR FURTHER INVESTIGATION

In a consideration of issues for further investigation, this chapter will emphasize cultural differences and will also raise several questions relating to development.

Cultural Differences

Cultural and social differences may have a major effect on the use of language. Research on the relations among culture, family style, and language is important and desirable. Most of the research has been carried out with American and European middle-class children, leaving little reason for confidence in the generalizability of our findings. Here some of the cultural issues that should be explored are indicated.

As Schieffelin and Eisenberg (1984) point out, aside from important differences in social structures, there are major cultural differences in how children's competence is seen and in how much verbal exchange adults undertake with young children. If children are not engaged in focused interaction, their learning of style variations in requests and their interpreting of the meaning of indirection will have to come from observation alone. As a result, there will be considerable cross-cultural difference in the extent to which children learn social uses of language through direct participation and through observation.

Within a single culture area there may be wide variations in types of interaction. Children differ in their interaction networks and in their exposure to varying types of language, such as talk between adults of different status. There are also major structural differences among familial organizations. The following list of factors may differentiate both family milieux within a culture area, in heterogeneous and complex cultures, and apply generally to differences between independent cultures such as the Kaluli and the Hopi.

1. *Reliance on Situational Routines.* If a series of routines is repeated often the child rapidly comes to recognize and anticipate them. Predictability reduces the need for explicit verbalizing of directions. As a result, although initial occurrences may require explicit instructions about what the child is to do, later repetitions may call for only limited cuing. A set of such routines may result in a subtle system that is less apparent to outsiders than systems based on explicit verbalizations.
2. *Adult Usage to Children.* In some families, highly direct forms are regularly used with children. In others, there is a high frequency of imbedded forms such as "can you" and "will you." In some families, as a result of situational training, hints are frequent and effective. We know very little about family relations and how they influence the forms used and understood by children.
3. *Teaching to Expect Hints.* In some cultures children are taught very early to recognize the intentions in implicit hints and indirect forms. In Japanese families (Clancy, 1980) a small child might be explicitly asked, "What did he want when he said . . . ?" In such cases there may be accelerated understanding of hints, although within cultures there is a variation in the extent to which families use indirect forms.
4. *Explicit Teaching.* In some cultures children are explicitly taught the forms they should use for asking. Italians are unwilling (Bates, 1976) to accept "I want" unqualified by conditionals or other softeners and consistently correct the child's misuses. Kaluli mothers (Schieffelin and Eisenberg, 1984) instruct children to imitate and then model appropriate moves. Apparently whereas the Italians wait for

an error to occur and then correct it, the Kaluli constantly anticipate and model.

5. *Status-, Person-, or Group-Orientation of the Value System.* These values (e.g., Bernstein, 1972) will affect how important it is to give identifying reasons and justifications for control acts that do more than simply assert the authority or power of the speaker. Reasons for compliance differ among status- and person-oriented systems and a third type of system, which is group oriented. Children in a group-oriented family learn that the smooth functioning of the family is the primary justification for behavior, and family goals are shared. Here, individualized justifications and excuses or refusals would have less legitimacy than in person-oriented, atomized, or highly individuated families.

Developmental Questions

Much of this discussion of the development of instrumental language, indirect speech acts, instrumental strategies, and so forth, has been speculative, based on suggestive rather than assured data. The views presented by the authors are given not because of confidence that they are correct but because it is hoped that such an approach to these matters may indicate lines along which future research into social development and instrumental language can be carried out. Some questions that need to be taken up in the future are:

1. What contexts do children recognize? How do they change with development? Do children construct the same basic contexts and instrumental categories for themselves, or is there individual variation? What do the child's instrumental moves tell about the child's social understandings?
2. Within a context or type of instrumental goal, what forms are in alternation? Are these forms conventional requests or NCIs? What "meanings" do these forms have for the child? How do the meanings change: Do old forms for making requests come to express new social meanings, and new forms express already established social concepts, as found in syntactic and semantic development? Do children tend to acquire and use the same forms in the same order, or does this vary widely between families?
3. How does the child's concept of politeness develop and change? How does an understanding of social face develop and find expression in language? How does a child learn to monitor what he or she says in advance in order to convey social information about himself or herself?

The changes in the use of language around age 8 years and again around adolescence may reflect cognitive changes associated with these ages. What social and sociolinguistic changes would a more differentiated approach find during the Piagetian periods of preoperational thought and concrete and formal operations? Approaches are needed that go beyond blanket assessments of developmental periods that span a number of years. In general it can be asked, What strategies do children develop for gaining compliance, and how are these related to such concepts as "face," "egocentrism," social reasoning, and mental operations? The answers, however, clinicians would like to know in detail.

Modern research in psycholinguistics began with questions about the child's acquisition of grammar, and the central issue was how the child learned to form and recognize "appropriate" utterances in respect to linguistic organization: grammaticality. The basic research issue was defined in linguistic terms. the development of the child in terms of the grammatical structure of language. As the scope of psycholinguistics enlarged to include semantics and the way linguistic structures related to the world of the child and the child's concepts about the world, issues of cognition became increasingly important. But cognitive issues could still be treated in terms of a wide range of linguistic issues because the structure and vocabulary of a language are so closely tied to the needs of articulating concepts and cognitive processes.

However, the expansion of psycholinguistic research to include pragmatics (the relation of language to social interaction and the functions served by speech) raises very few new linguistic issues. Although there are conventional forms in all languages for some communicative functions at the speech act level of requests, offers, promises, and so on, these conventional linguistic forms (e.g., imperative form, "polite" forms using can and could, will and would) are generally simple paradigms that are limited in the functions they serve (often, primarily as "politeness" markers). The structure and lexicon of a language must, of course, be capable of serving social communicative functions, but it does not appear that these functions are codified "in" these structures as much as expressed "through" them. Thus the basic issues in the child's acquisition of socially appropriate speech are social, not linguistic, and pragmatic research in the future must look less to questions raised by linguistic research than to issues of social development.

REFERENCES

Andersen, E. (1977). *Learning to speak with style.* Unpublished doctoral dissertation. Stanford University, Stanford, CA.

Bates, E. (1971). *The development of conversational skill in 2, 3, and 4-year-olds.* Unpublished master's thesis, University of Chicago, Chicago.

Bates, E. (1976). *Language and context: The acquisition of pragmatics.* Academic Press, New York.

Becker, J. A. (1981, April). *Preschoolers' judgments of speaker status based on requests.* Boston, Massachusetts. Paper presented at the Biennial Meeting of the Society for Research in Child Development.

Bellinger, D. (1979). Changes in the explicitness of mothers' directives as children age. *Journal of Child Language, 6,* 443–458.

Bernstein, B. (1972). *A sociolinguistic approach to socialization; with some reference to educability.* New York: Holt, Rinehart.

Brown, P., and Levinson, S. (1978). Universals in language usage: Politeness phenomena. In E. Goody (Ed.), *Questions and politeness* (pp. 356–389), Cambridge: Cambridge University Press.

Browning, E. R. (1974). The effectiveness of long and short verbal commands in inducing correct responses in three schizophrenic children. *Journal of Autism and Childhood Schizophrenia, 4:* 293–300.

Campos, M. F., de Castro, P., and de Lemos, C. (1979). Pragmatic routes and the development of 'causal' expressions. Wassenaar, Netherlands: *Sciences Child Language Seminar.*

Carrell, P. L. (1981). Children's understanding of indirect requests: Comparing child and adult comprehension. *Journal of Child Language, 8:* 329–346.

Carter, A. L. (1974). *Communication in the sensorimotor period.* Unpublished doctoral dissertation, University of California, Berkeley.

Clancy, P. M. (1980). *The acquisition of narrative discourse: A study in Japanese.* Unpublished doctoral dissertation, University of California, Berkeley.

Corsaro, W. A. (1979). Young children's conception of status and role. *Sociology of Education, 52:* 46–50.

Ervin-Tripp, S. (1970). Discourse agreement: How children answer questions. In J. R. Hayes (Ed.) *Cognition and the Development of Language.* New York: Wiley.

Ervin-Tripp, S. (1976). Is Sybil there? The structure of some American English directives. *Language in Society, 5:* 25–66.

Ervin-Tripp, S. (1977). Wait for me, roller-skate! In C. Mitchell-Kernan and S. Ervin-Tripp (Eds.) *Child Discourse.* New York: Academic Press.

Ervin-Tripp, S., O'Connor, M. C., and Rosenberg, J. (in press). Language and power in the family. In C. Kramerae and M. Schulz (Eds.) *Language and power.* Urbana, IL: University of Illinois Press.

Garvey, C. (1975). Requests and responses in children's speech. *Journal of Child Language, 2:* 41–63.

Gordon, D. P., and Ervin-Tripp, S. M. (1984). The structure of children's requests. In R. L. Schiefelbusch and J. Pickar (Eds.), *The acquisition of communicative competence.* Baltimore: University Park Press.

Gordon, D. P., Budwig, N., Strage, A., and Carrell, P. (1980, October). *Children's requests to unfamiliar adults: form, social function, age variation.* Fifth Annual Boston University Conference on Language Development, Boston. (ERIC Document Reproduction Service No. ED 205–053)

Gordon, D., and Lakoff, G. (1971). Conversational postulates. In D. Adams, M. A. Cambell, V. Cohen, J. Lovins, E. Maxwell, C. Nygren, and J. Reighard (Eds.), *Paper from the Seventh Regional Meeting of the Chicago Linguistic Society.* University of Chicago, Department of Linguistics, Chicago.

Grimm, H. (1975). *Analysis of short-term dialogues in five- to seven-year-olds: Encoding of intentions and modifications of speech acts as a function of negative feedback loops.* Third International Child Language Symposium, London.

Halliday, M. A. (1975). *Learning how to mean: Explorations in the development of language*. London: Edward Arnold.

Haselkorn, S. L. (1977). *The relationship of verbal to preverbal strategies for making requests*. Second Annual Boston University Conference on Language Development, Boston.

Haselkorn, S. L. (1979). Success or failure: Does it affect young children's request strategies? *Papers and Reports on Child Language Development, 17:* 73–80. Department of Linguistics, Stanford University, Stanford, CA.

Hildyard, A. (1979). *Remembering requests: The interaction of conversational rules and politeness*. Mimeo draft from the office of R and D, Ontario Institute of Studies in Education, Ontario.

Hollos, M., and Beeman, W. (1978). The development of directives among Norwegian and Hungarian children. An example of communication style in culture. *Language and Society, 7,* 345–356.

James, S. (1978). The effect of listener age and situation on the politeness of children's directives. *Journal of Psycholinguistic Research, 7:* 307–317.

Lawson, C. (1967). Request patterns in a two-year-old child. Unpublished manuscript, University of California, Berkeley.

Leonard, L. B., Wilcox, M. J., Fulmer, K. C., and Davis, G. A. (1978). Understanding indirect requests: An investigation of children's comprehension of pragmatic meanings. *Journal of Speech and Hearing Research, 21:* 528–537.

Liebling, C. R. (1981). *Comprehension of the directive pragmatic structure in oral and written discourse by children ages six to eleven*. University of California, Berkeley. Unpublished doctoral dissertation

MacWhinney, B. (1976). *Some observations on requests by Hungarian children.* Hungarian research on the acquisition of morphology and syntax. *Journal of Child Language, 3,* 397–410.

McTear, M. F. (1979). Hey! I've got something to tell you: How preschool children initiate conversation exchanges. *Journal of Pragmatics, 3*(4), 331–336.

McTear, M. F. (undated). *Getting it done: The development of children's abilities to negotiate request sequences in peer interaction*. Working papers in language and linguistics, Belfast.

Mitchell-Kernan, C., and Kernan, K. (1977). Pragmatics of directive choice among children. In C. Mitchell-Kernan and S. Ervin-Tripp (Eds.), *Child Discourse* (pp. 189–208). New York: Academic Press.

Montes, R. (1981). Extending a concept: Functioning directively. In *Children's functional language and education in the early years*. Final report to the Carnegie Foundation.

Nelson, K., and Gruendel, J. M. (1979). At morning it's lunchtime: A scriptal view of children's dialogues. *Discourse Processes, 2:* 73–94.

Newcombe, N., and Zaslow, M. (1981). Do 2½-year-olds hint? A study of directive forms in the speech of 2½-year-old children to adults. *Discourse Processes, 4:* 239–252.

Parsons, C. L. (1980). *The effect of speaker age and listener compliance and noncompliance on the politeness of children's request directives*. Unpublished doctoral dissertation, Southern Illinois University, Carbondale, IL.

Piaget, J. (1926). *The language and thought of the child*. New York: Harcourt, Brace and Company.

Read, B. K., and Cherry, L. J. (1978). Preschool children's production of directive forms. *Discourse Processes, 1:* 233–246.

Schank, R. C., and Abelson, R. P. (1977). *Scripts, plans, goals and understanding*. Hillsdale, NJ: Lawrence Erlbaum.

Schieffelin B., and Eisenberg, A. (1984). Cultural variation in children's conversation. In R. L. Schiefelbusch and J. Pickar (Eds.), *The acquisition of communicative competence* (pp. 377–420). Baltimore: University Park Press.

Shapiro, E. R. (1978a, September). *Structural relations among teacher directive child comprehension behaviors, and teacher relations.* Third Annual Boston University Language Development Conferences.

Shapiro, E. R. (1978b). *Teacher directives, child responses, and teacher reactions: A factor analytic study of classroom interactions.* Ellenville, NY: Northeastern Educational Research Association.

Shatz, M. (1975). How young children respond to language: Procedures for answering. *PRCLD, 10,* 97–110.

Shatz, M. (1978). Children's comprehension of their mothers' question directives. *Journal of Child Language, 5,* 39–46.

Shatz, M. (1983). Communication. In J. Flavell and E. Markman (Eds.), *Handbook of child psychology, Vol. 3.* New York: Wiley.

Shatz, M., Bernstein, D., and Shulman, M. (1980). The responses of language disordered children to indirect directives in varying contexts. *Applied Linguistics, 1,* 295–306.

Stalder, J. (no date). *Effects of knowledge about the addressee on children's process request behavior.* Mimeographed.

Urzua, C. G. (1977). *A sociolinguistic analysis of the request of mothers to their 2 year old daughters.* Unpublished doctoral dissertation, University of Texas, Austin.

Veneziano, E. (1981). Early language and non-verbal representation: A reassessment. *Journal of Child Language, 8,* 541–564.

Wood, B., and Gardner, R. (1980). How children get their way: Directives in communication. *Communication Education, 29,* 264–272.

Zukow, P. G., Reilly, J., and Greenfield, P. M. (1978). Making the absent present: Facilitating the transition from sensorimotor to linguistic communication. In K. Nelson (Ed.), *Children's language, Vol. 1.* Halstead, NY: Gardner Press.

SECTION II
ASSESSMENT OF COMMUNICATIVE COMPETENCE

Chapter 3

Observational Methods in the Study of Communicative Competence

Christine Dollaghan and Jon Miller

Observational methods are fundamental and pervasive in the study of communicative development and disorders. Every person who has ever studied some aspect of communicative behavior has, knowingly or unknowingly, employed observational methodology. While observational data for theoretical, diagnostic, and management purposes has burgeoned over the last few years, there has been surprisingly little attention to an examination of the observational process itself or the ways in which the quality of information obtained through observational techniques can be improved. This lack is particularly evident in the area of communicative competence, which presents a host of potential pitfalls to the unwitting or unwary investigator. This chapter is intended to address the need for additional scrutiny of our observational methodology by providing an overview of the nature, advantages, and disadvantages of observational methods and a discussion of the use of such methods in the study of communicative competence. It seems an inescapable conclusion that improving our understanding and implementation of observational methodology will improve the quality of both theoretical and clinical efforts in the area of communicative competence. This chapter will engage the reader in some "consciousness-raising," with the aim of making the already widespread use of observational methods a more conscious, planful, and goal-directed activity for clinician and researcher alike.

The plan of the chapter is as follows. First, an overview of the issues of reliability and validity in observational methods is presented. Next, the sequence of stages in planning a successful observation is discussed. Finally, each of these stages is considered as it relates to observational investigations of three general categories of pragmatic phenomena.

OBSERVATIONAL METHODS

Webster's New Collegiate Dictionary (7th Ed.) defines observation as "the act or practice of noting and recording facts and events." By this definition, any technique for gathering information is observational. However, the phrase "observational methods" is most often used when human beings, rather than automated instruments, quantify phenomena of interest to them. Thus, according to Sackett (1978), a primary feature of observational methodology is the necessity for human perception and judgment in the measurement process.

Although Sackett (1978) further specified that observational methods are used to quantify behaviors when few or no constraints are imposed by the investigator (i.e., when the setting and task are allowed to remain as "naturalistic" as possible), this view of observational methodology is too restrictive. Observational methods can be used regardless of the "naturalness" of the setting or the degree to which the client's responses are controlled by the investigator. Decisions about setting and subject response characteristics can be made quite independently of the decision to use observational methods for data collection. For this reason a broader definition of observational methodology as any information-gathering endeavor in which the data of interest are quantified through the perceptions and judgments of a human observer will be used in this chapter.

It is self-evident that the available data on communicative competence have arisen from observational methodology; the authors of this chapter are aware of no "communicative intent transducers" that would circumvent the need for a human observer to note, categorize, and interpret communicative phenomena. However, the use of human observers to quantify communicative (or any other) phenomena requires particular attention to the two crucial constructs of reliability and validity. Information derived from observational methods must be both valid and reliable to be of use, particularly when clinical judgments of an individual's communicative skill may have extraordinary consequences for him or her.

Reliability in Observational Methods

Reliability refers to the dependability, stability, or consistency of data collected, whether through observational or instrumental means. Kerlinger (1973) distinguished two types of reliability, one of which concerns the accuracy of information obtained; that is, the extent to which events or phenomena are correctly identified and recorded. The other type, in the more usual sense of the term "reliability," concerns the degree to which repeated uses of a data collection method yield identical results; in other words, the replicability of findings from a data collection procedure.

The reliability of information obtained through the use of human observers is directly related to the level of abstraction of the phenomena being measured. At the heart of this issue is the relationship between observations and inferences (Boehm and Weinberg, 1977). Duncan and Fiske (1977, P. 6) noted that the observation-inference distinction is captured by the terms "etic" and "emic": "An 'etic' descriptive system is one that remains as close as possible to raw physical description of the behaviors involved. . . . Contrasting with an 'etic' system would be an 'emic' one representing a hypothesis as to the essential elements of particular . . . codes under investigation." An emic description is at a higher level of abstraction, because it seeks to account for the inferred system underlying the observable physical events described at the etic level. Thus, "phonetic" descriptions aim to specify the acoustic characteristics of speech signals, while "phonemic" descriptions attempt to account for the phonetic facts in terms of an underlying system. A simple record of the utterances produced by a speaker is more 'etic' than an interpretation of those utterances as requests for information, contingent queries, or topic initiations would be.

Ways to Increase Reliability

Because all attempts to characterize human communication are to some degree abstractions from the most basic phsyical events, so the etic-emic distinction is best viewed as a continuum. However, it is usually the case that descriptions closer to the physical end of this continuum (i.e., etic descriptions) will be most reliable, for they typically require fewer subjective judgments from the observer. As the observer makes judgments based on information that is increasingly distant from the observable physical events, the difficulty of obtaining acceptable levels of reliability increases.

Recognition Rules. Duncan and Fiske (1977) suggested that one way to increase the reliability of observations is to separate, as much as possible, the actual physical events from the inferences that are based on them. In order to obtain accurate, reliable observational data on which theorizing about more abstract relationships can be based, they discussed the human observer's need for "recognition rules." Recognition rules isolate and define the observable events of interest. Duncan and

Fiske distinguished between explicit recognition rules based on formal definitions of the phenomena of interest, and implicit recognition rules based on ostensive definitions. An explicit recognition rule for identifying a communicative event (e.g., "question") might consist of a list of its formal syntactic characteristics (e.g., "A sentence with inversion of the subject and first verb in the verb phrase, commencing with a question word, or ending with a question tag" Crystal, 1980, p. 294). An implicit recognition rule, on the other hand, could be developed through repeated demonstrations ("ostensions") of phenomena that the investigator wishes included as questions, such that observers eventually agree in their identifications of them. An explicit recognition rule for identifying an "utterance" in transcribing a language sample might be, "A stretch of speaker talk bounded by silent intervals of more than two seconds." An implicit recognition rule would be established by having observers listen to a number of examples of the kinds of units that the investigator wants counted as distinct utterances, until acceptable levels of agreement are reached.

The level of abstraction of the events being quantified often determines how explicit their recognition rules must be. As Duncan and Fiske (1977) pointed out,

> Although fully explicit recognition rules are a goal for social science, use of implicit rules is not necessarily a major obstacle for the achievement of interjudge reliability and the generation of useful data. For example, raters may have little trouble in agreeing on what is a smile or a head nod or a hand gesticulation, even when these events are defined implicitly. (p. 16)

Thus, observers may not need explicit recognition rules to reliably identify events that are common features of everyday experience (such as the smiles and head nods referred to). However, many pragmatic phenomena are far removed from the shared, conscious knowledge of observers, and recognition rules must be written in specific terms to enable observers to identify them reliably. Thus, although observers may not need detailed recognition rules to consistently identify certain events as "words" in transcribing a language sample, reliable identification of more abstract constructs such as particular speaker intentions or discourse functions is likely to require recognition rules that are quite explicit.

Other Tactics for Increasing Reliability. In addition to their suggestion that reliability among human observers can be improved by making recognition rules as explicit as possible, Duncan and Fiske (1977) recommended several other tactics for increasing the reliability of observational data in light of human information processing constraints. First, observers should make judgments on only one kind of event at a time, in order to ensure a narrow focus of attention. For example, observers are not likely to succeed in simultaneously identifying both the formal syntactic characteristics and pragmatic functions of utterances; their attentional resources would probably be exceeded in attempting to monitor two such different types of phenomena, leading to reduced levels of reliability. Second, Duncan and Fiske recommended that observers not be assigned tasks that require them to sum their judgments over time, particularly if these judgments are being made "on-line." For example, phenomena such as nested contingent query sequences (Garvey, 1977), or successive speaker moves that first appear to be independent but later are revealed to have been related efforts toward a particular communicative goal, may be very difficult to identify reliably on-line. When the data are preserved on videotapes or audiotapes, human information-processing limitations pose fewer threats to reliability.

Accuracy

As noted previously, reliability implies not only that observations are replicable but that they are accurate. Although accuracy, like replicability, is likely to be related to the level of abstraction of events being identified, it is important to distinguish between these two notions, for it is quite possible to obtain judgments that are reliable but accurate. This could occur, for example, if two observers consistently misclassified an event; they might have high levels of agreement in judging the event, but their judgments would be in error. Thus, in addition to demonstrating that observers agree in their judgments and that their judgments are consistent and replicable, the accuracy of their judgments must also be evaluated. Accuracy of observations can be established through thorough training procedures that produce expert observers and through periodic accuracy checks by other expert observers to reduce the likelihood of "observer drift" (the slight, gradual modification of judgments that can occur as an observer makes repeated observations over time).

Documenting Accuracy

How can replicability and accuracy of judgments be documented? Interobserver reliability is evaluated by computing the percentage of agreement between two or more observers. Intraobserver reliability is determined by computing the percentage of agreement for a single observer making judgments at different times (e.g., in successive weeks) or under different conditions (e.g., on-line or from a tape recording). To compute the percentage of agreement in either case, the total number of judgments is divided into the number of identical judgments. For example, to computer interobserver reliability for two observers who have counted the requests for information in a transcript, one observer would be taken as the reference point, the number of judgments this observer made would be determined, and the number of identical judgments made by the other observer would be counted. If Observer 1 identified 15 requests for information, and Observer 2 identified 13 of these, the percentage of agreement between them for judging this particular event would be 13/15 = 87 per cent. A similar procedure would be used to determine whether an observer's on-line judgments were as reliable as his or her judgments from an audiotape. In this case, the observer would count requests for information on-line but would also tape the session and later identify requests for information from the tape. The intraobserver reliability would again be equal to the number of agreements divided by the total number of judgments; a sufficiently high percentage in this case would allow the observer to confidently dispense with audiotaping and later relistening, and to make these judgments on-line instead.

Determining the accuracy of judgments requires the computation not just of overall percentages of agreement but of percentage of "point-by-point" agreement. In percentage of point-by-point agreement, each of an observer's judgments is examined for its correctness, as compared with an expert's coding of the same set of events. Rather than simply demonstrating that two observers identified 13 and 15 requests for information, for example, each event identified by the two as a request for information would be examined to ensure that it meets the criteria specified in the recognition rules. Thus, if only 10 of the requests for information identified by the first observer were accurate instances of this category, and the correctly scored transcript contained 14 of these events, the percentage of point-by-point agreement would be 10/14 = 71 per cent. Notice that this percentage is lower than the percentages of agreement based on judgment of numbers of events (87 per cent). Point-by-point agreement is a more stringent reliability measure, for it reflects both consistency and accuracy of observer judgments.

How high should percentages of agreement be? How much reliability is enough? These questions do not have an absolute answer; as Shriberg and Kent (1982) pointed out, the required degree of reliability varies depending on the uses to which the data will be put. If small differences are being used to make important clinical decisions, high reliability levels are critical; however, lower levels of agreement may be perfectly satisfactory in making rough, preliminary estimates. It should be emphasized, however, that the strength of confidence in observational data is directly related to its reliability. Data that are inaccurate or inconsistent cannot support either clinical or research conclusions.

Thus, to ensure that observations of pragmatic phenomena are accurate and reliable, a number of steps must be taken. After deciding which events the observers are to identify, recognition rules must be written in terms that are sufficiently explicit to allow observers to reach acceptable levels of accuracy and agreement in their judgments of these events. For abstract events, recognition rules will generally require a quite detailed, explicit form; even if the events of interest can be identified implicitly, explicit recognition rules can lead to increased reliability. When recognition rules have been adequately specified and observers have been given practice in implementing them, levels of accuracy and agreement among observers, and for the same observer over time, will be acceptably high. However, ensuring adequate reliability is only one of the tasks in using observational methodology, as shall be seen.

Validity in Observational Methods

The question of whether something can be quantified consistently or accurately is quite different from the question of whether it is worth quantifying at all; the latter is a question about validity. A valid observational procedure is one in which the events being quantified do in fact serve as meaningful indicators of the phenomenon being studied. For observational data to be valid, the variables that are isolated for measurement must provide a "true" reflection of the phenomenon under investigation.

Problems of Validity in an Observation

Two elements of an observation are most vulnerable to problems of validity. The first is the selection or construction of a system of categories (a taxonomy) for quantifying the phenomena of interest. In deciding which events will be identified and classified, the investigator makes judgments about their relevance to the goal of the observation, or their "content" validity. These decisions are subjective, and the investigator must constantly be alert to the possibility that his or her categorization of the events may not be the most valid one. In the "participant observer" method common in ethnographical research, the investigator becomes extensively involved with the situation and subjects to be observed prior to selecting an observational taxonomy in an effort to ensure that the categories are truly relevant from the the subjectively valid perspectives of the participants rather than being externally imposed by the investigator (Rist, 1977).

Judging the validity of a taxonomy used in observation is a subjective process (Kerlinger, 1973). The perceived validity of a taxonomy or measurement procedure depends in large part on its comprehensiveness, or on the degree to which it addresses all of the events relevant to a particular theory. The test of the content validity of an observational instrument lies not in an objective criterion but in the degree to which its users perceive it to be an accurate, logically and theoretically motivated reflection of the phenomenon of interest. Content validity, then, is not an absolute phenomenon; it is assessed with reference to the purposes of the measurement tool and the most current theory and evidence available.

The second aspect of an observation in which questions of validity must be addressed concerns the generalizability, or "external validity," of findings. Numerous factors may affect external validity, including variables in context, participant, and task. Thus, results obtained from one observation cannot be assumed to hold for other settings, subjects, or tasks. This is particularly true for observations of communicative competence, because language serves so many purpose (e.g., expressive, directive, phatic, metalinguistic, and stylistic Hymes, 1974); capabilities in one domain cannot be generalized to the others. Elucidating the ways in which pragmatic phenomena are context dependent is one goal of the study of communicative competence in normal and disordered individuals, and it is necessary to systematically vary subject, setting, and task variables to obtain the most representative picture of a subject's communicative skill.

Relationship between Validity and Reliability

Validity and reliability do not exist in isolation from one another; from some perspectives they actually appear to conflict. Maximizing the reliability of an observation generally requires minimizing the subjective input of the observer to the measurement process. On the other hand, establishing maximally valid categories for an observational taxonomy clearly requires subjective judgment.

Several terms have been associated with the apparent conflict between those observational approaches that demand that the observer divorce his or her subjective impressions from the task and those that emphasize the observer's subjective judgments. Some of these terms are listed with their definitions in Table 3-1. However, as Rist (1977) pointed out, it is naive to suppose that reliability is more important than validity, or vice versa. Neither validity nor reliability is an end in and of itself; both are essential to the adequate investigation of a phenomenon. Demonstrating that observations are reliable in the absence of validity is vacuous, whereas observations that appear to be valid are unconvincing if they cannot be demonstrated to be reliable. The two emphases are probably better viewed as complementary, each being differentially important at different phases in the observational process. For example, Tukey (1977) pointed out that scientific investigations typically consist of initial exploratory and subsequent confirmatory stages. During the exploratory stages, establishing the validity of observational measures is the primary concern; during the confirmatory stages, the focus is on establishing the reliability of the valid information obtained.

Table 3-1. Some Polar Terms Associated With the Apparent Conflict Between Reliability and Validity

Approaches Emphasizing Reliability	Approaches Emphasizing Validity
Objective: Divorced from personal feelings or prejudices	*Subjective:* Relies on individual's own attitudes, beliefs, or opinions
Quantitative: Emphasizes surface, observable events	*Qualitative:* Emphasizes subjective understanding, insights derived through introspection
Etic: Describes raw physical events	*Emic:* Describes system inferred to underlie physical events

Adapted from Duncan, S., and Fiske, D. (1977). Face-to-face interaction: research, methods, and theory. Hillsdale, NJ: Lawrence Erlbaum Associates, and Rist, R. C. (1977). On the relations among educational research paradigms: from disdain to detente. *Anthropology and Education Quarterly, 8,* 42–49.

Planning an Observational Investigation

Table 3–2 presents some key steps in planning an observational investigation, and this section examines these stages and the factors that predispose an observational investigation to success.

Step 1: Specify the Observational Objectives

The first step in an observational endeavor is that of explicitly defining its goals: specifying the amount and kinds of information to be obtained and the uses to which the information will be put. This step is absolutely crucial, yet its importance is frequently underestimated. An investigator who is unable to clearly and concisely define the objectives of an observation in advance is likely to gain very little useable information from it. This does not imply that all observations must be aimed at collecting highly specific bits of information. As noted earlier, both etic and emic data can be collected validly and reliably, and if the investigation of a phenomenon is at an initial exploratory level, it may well be crucial for researchers to immerse themselves in the situation being observed in order to derive maximally valid categories for the subsequent confirmatory phases of the investigation. Whether the observational objectives involve fairly general or fairly detailed information, however, the successful observer will spend a considerable amount of time formulating a well-specified description of the phenomena of interest and will also possess a clear understanding of the ways in which the observational data will be used. Familiarity with theory and evidence regarding the phenomena under investigation will facilitate this initial phase of the observational endeavor. An investigator who undertakes an observational study of "conversation," for example, without first reviewing

Table 3-2. Steps in Planning an Observational Investigation

1. Specify Observational Objectives

What kinds of information are to be obtained? How much information is needed? How will the information be used?

2. Select or Construct an Event Toxonomy

What categories of events reflect true distinctions for the subjects being studied? Is a period of exploratory observation needed to determine whether the taxonomy is a valid one?

3. Write Adequate Recognition Rules

Will observers use implicitly or explicitly defined criteria to identify instances of events? Do observers meet acceptable levels of accuracy and agreement in implementing recognition rules?

4. Select a Data Recording System

What are the information processing demands of recognition rules (e.g., abstractness, subtlety, frequency, the rapidity of events to be observed)? Can observers make reliable and accurate judgments on-line? What recording format requires the least attention from the observer?

5. Structure the Observational Context

What type of context will provide data most relevant to the observational objective? Which contextual features must be specified in advance? Is the observational process overly intrusive? What instructions will be given to subjects and observers? Will subject behaviors be restricted? Will steps be taken to facilitate particular events?

---

available theories and hypotheses about the components that define a conversation, the ways in which these components relate to one another both within and between speakers, and so on, is likely to spend a great deal of unnecessary time and effort in this initial phase. To rephrase a useful thought from Kerlinger (1973) substituting "observe" for "test": "To observe without knowing at least fairly well what and why one is observing is usually to blunder" (p. 13).

Step 2: Select or Construct an Event Taxonomy

Having defined the objectives of the observation, the investigator's next step is to construct or select a category system for quantifying the events of interest. Content validity is a key issue at this stage, for, as noted previously the judgments of the investigator determine the taxonomy by which observed events will be classified. Again, the current literature can assist the investigator in deriving or selecting a theoretically defensible taxonomy for categorizing the events of interest.

The trend in studies of the communication characteristics of disordered populations has been to implement taxonomies derived from studies of normal subjects. Although the literature on normal development is a reasonable starting point for developing a taxonomy, its validity must be carefully evaluated in light of the characteristics of the subject population as well as the objectives of the observation. Most studies have focused on discovering differences between normal and disordered populations; though such questions justify the use of taxonomies describing normal performance, one suspects that such taxonomies fail to capture numerous aspects of the performance of the disordered subjects. Our understanding of the communicative skills of disordered populations would be better served by investigations that not only document the existence of differences between normal and disordered subjects but also present valid taxonomies reflecting the performance of the disordered subjects.

If the investigator is aware of a taxonomy that appears to be valid for subjects similar to those being observed and if the categories appear to truly capture the distinctions among the communicative events of interest, then this step in the observational process is fairly easily accomplished. However, the fact that a taxonomy exists in the literature is no guarantee of its content validity; investigators must view all taxonomies with a certain amount of skepticism until experience proves that their categories accurately and adequately capture the phenomena of interest.

If the observation is aimed at exploring phenomena for which a valid taxonomy does not already exist (which may often be the case for communicatively impaired individuals), the investigator will be required to construct his or her own taxonomy. In this case, the investigator will undoubtedly need to spend a significant amount of time in an exploratory phase of "informal observation" (Rosenblum, 1978) to obtain primary data from which a valid taxonomy can be derived. Of course, even in this exploratory phase it is important to state the observational objectives as specifically as possible. Many trials and revisions will likely be needed to construct taxonomy that will specifically provide the information of interest to the investigator.

Step 3: Write Adequate Recognition Rules

After deciding on the set of categories for classifying the observed phenomena, the next step in the observational process is to develop recognition rules for each category. At this stage the investigator specifies the criteria that the observer will use to identify instances of the phenomena included in the taxonomy. As mentioned previously, adequate recognition rules define the observable events that will serve as indicators of the phenomena under investigation, such that observers can reach acceptable levels of accuracy and reliability in their judgments about them.

The investigator must make a number of decisions in order to write adequate recognition rules for the categories of the taxonomy. If the taxonomy includes a category called "repetition," for example, the investigator must answer a variety of questions prior to writing a recognition rule that will successfully distinguish repetitions from other events (e.g., Do repetitions follow other utterances immediately or can there be a time delay? Must they be exact reproductions of a preceding utterance? How will reproductions having pronoun changes and word omissions be handled?).

Like the stage of formulating observational objectives, the importance and time required of this step are often underestimated. Investigators frequently fail to realize the extent to which their definitions of phenomena are intuitive or subjective until they attempt to obtain agreement with other observers. In addition, investigators must spend a considerable amount of time anticipating the marginal cases, which are bound to occur, in order to make the recognition rules sufficiently detailed that decisions about these questionable cases can be made rapidly and accurately.

One reason that the process of writing recognition rules is rarely addressed in the study of communicative competence, we suspect, is that observations of communicative skill can rely on numerous units of analysis, of varying lengths and at varying levels of abstraction. The units that have been investigated range in length from a single-word or multiword utterance of one speaker to all of the utterances spoken within a single speaking turn, or to all of the utterances spoken by two or more speakers in a particular setting or during a particular time period. In addition to the great variation in length of units of analysis for pragmatics, there may also be vast differences in the number and abstractness of criteria used to identify them. For example, the recognition rule for a communicative event might be based on only one kind of information (e.g., if requests were to be identified strictly on the basis of syntactic form); alternatively, it might be necessary for the observer to use several kinds of information to identify the communicative event (e.g., if requests were to be identified on the basis of a constellation of syntactic, intonational, and listener response criteria).

Similarly, the abstractness of the phenomena to be identified may vary. At the extreme etic end of the inference continuum, a recognition rule might be written to classify utterances based strictly on their spectrographic characteristics (e.g., if a particular communicative event were defined solely according to utterance intonation contour or relative intensity). Toward the emic end of the continuum, the observer might be asked to identify a phenomenon based not just on an observable event but also on his or her own tacit social, cultural, and linguistic knowledge of the significance of the event (e.g., if the observer were to judge the "politeness" of an utterance, based not just on its syntactic or lexical characteristics but also on his or her knowledge of what makes it more or less polite given the context, participants, and preceding events).

That communicative events may be judged according to criteria at such widely varying levels of abstractness poses a challenge to the investigator of communicative competence, because a single utterance or behavior may be analyzed or classified in a number of different ways. This hierarchical organization leads to confusion if taxonomies and recognition rules fail to clearly distinguish among the various levels of analysis. For example, a single utterance identified on the basis of a fairly etic criterion (e.g., "A stretch of speech by a speaker that is bounded by 2-second silent intervals") may subsequently be analyzed with more abstract recognition rules that identify it as having a particular propositional structure, syntactic structure, illocutionary force, perlocutionary effect, relationship to antecedent and subsequent utterances, and so on (Chapman, 1981). A multilevel analysis is likely to present the most valid picture of communicative competence, but the various levels and their hierarchical relationships must be distinguished in order to write recognition rules that observers can use accurately and reliably.

Evaluating the adequacy of recognition rules, whether implicit or explicit, is a matter of empirical test. The investigator must determine whether the observers using the recognition rules agree in their decisions about the number and kind of events occurring (interobserver reliability) and whether a single observer agrees with his or her own decisions on different occasions or in different conditions (intraobserver reliability). The investigator decides what levels of reliability are acceptable, but confidence in observational data is strengthened to the extent that findings can be shown to be independent of any single observer's subjective judgment.

Step 4: Select a Data Recording System

Writing adequate recognition rules is only part of the process of ensuring adequate reliability. As noted previously, human information processing constraints limit the number and complexity of judgments that can be made at any one time in an observational session, regardless of how well the recognition rules are specified. Information processing demands may be severe if the events of interest are frequent or fleeting, if the implementation of recognition rules requires active thought, or if the manner of recording the information requires a significant amount of the observer's attention.

If the phenomena to be observed are discrete events toward the etic end of the continuum that occur fairly infrequently, and the recording system requires little active thought, observers may be able to record the desired information on-line. However, in studying complex communicative phenomena it is more often the case that the events must be preserved on videotape or audiotape for subsequent coding or analysis. For example, if recognition rules are based on a number of rapid, transitory types of information such as eye gaze, gestures, proximity, and so on, on-line data collection will probably not be possible. Even videotaping and audiotaping may fail to capture all of the information needed to make some coding decisions; for some questions it may be necessary to integrate video, audio, and on-line ethnographical methods to obtain an adequate base of observational data (Cherry Wilkinson, Clevenger, and Dollaghen, 1981).

On-line collection of observational data by a single observer is also unlikely to succeed if recognition rules require simultaneous attention to events at different levels of abstraction. Observers tend to have a great deal of difficulty making reliable, accurate judgments about more than one level of analysis at a time. For example, observers would likely find it impossible to classify utterances simultaneously with respect to both intonation contour and communicative intent. Thus, if multiple levels of analysis are to be conducted, it will usually be necessary to record the data, enabling observers to make repeated scans through it, with a single level of analysis being undertaken per scan. *The Language Assessment, Remediation and Screening Procedure* (Crystal, Fletcher, and Garman, 1977) exemplifies such a tactic in the analysis of the syntactic features of a language sample; word-, phrase-, and clause-, and sentence-level phenomena are identified on different scans through the transcript.

Ensuring that the mechanics of the recording system require as little of the observer's attention as possible is a relatively easy way to increase the amount of observational data that can be obtained on-line. Paper-and-pencil coding systems may be adequate for some purposes, but only if they are designed so that observers can use them rapidly and easily without having to search through columns or complicated codes. Technical developments have resulted in a number of electronic alternatives to paper-and-pencil coding that increase the number of judgments that can be made reliably by an observer on-line. For example, the SSR system (Stephenson and Dickson, 1978), which has been used successfully in live ethnological observations, is a portable, computerized keyboard worn by the observer, who merely keys in the necessary codes for events as he or she identifies them. This system provides a printout of coded data along with temporal information about the various coded events. The increasing availability of microcomputers likewise offers numerous possibilities for on-line coding of observational data. Ultimately, of course, the nature and purposes of the observation, along with the cost-effectiveness of various systems for recording it, will determine which methods are chosen. There will always be limits to the number of judgments that an observer can make at any one time, but a well-developed coding system that allows the observer to focus all of his or her attention on the events of interest rather than on the mechanics of recording the decisions about them will maximize the efficiency of observational data collection.

Step 5: Structure the Observational Context

At this step, the investigator makes a number of decisions about the characteristics of the situation in which the observation will occur, bearing in mind the extent to which she or he wishes to generalize from the data obtained in this context. Context specificity is one of the most consistent findings in the study of pragmatics, and numerous contextual factors can influence the picture of an individual's communicative competence that emerges from an observation.

The notion of "context" subsumes a number of variables, including the location, materials, and participants in a situation along with the degree to which the participants' behaviors are constrained by the investigator's task or response demands. Describing these contextual features is crucial when data from different contexts are to be pooled for analysis as well as when a direct comparison between individual data points is planned. Failure to replicate observational contexts across experimental sessions may present serious problems of external validity if the data are to be generalized; discrepancies in the findings from different observational investigations can often be attributed to undescribed contextual variations.

One contextual factor that deserves special mention is the effect, or "intrusiveness," of the observational process itself. The phrase "observer intrusiveness" can refer to a variety of influences, including such disparate factors as the physical presence of a camera, microphone, or observer within view of the participants and the comments or instructions provided to the subjects. Masling and Stern (1969) found that subjects adjusted to the presence of an observer (either human or mechanical) with relatively little difficulty, provided they were given sufficient exposure to the observer prior to the actual period of data collection. The investigator can estimate whether a subject has made this adjustment by documenting a decrease in the number of overt reactions to the observer or camera (e.g., utterances referring to the observer, glances at the camera) over the course of the acclimatization period.

Another important contextual decision is whether or not to involve a human observer as a participant in the situation observed. Should the observer be isolated as much as possible from the activities under observation and refrain from speaking or responding to overtures from another participant in the setting, or should he or she behave somewhat more "naturally?" The obvious tradeoff here is between the confounding effects of a completely silent human observer behaving in a very unusual way and the possibility that an observer who interacts with the participants will significantly alter the course of events in the situation. The investigator must decide which of the potential observer roles is least likely to significantly distort the data; ideally, pilot data would be collected prior to the observation itself, in order to empirically determine the impact of the various possibilities.

The effect of instructions given or comments made to the subjects prior to the observation must also be considered as a contextual variable. Ethical considerations dictate that subjects be informed when they are under observation, and the investigator can usually describe the aims of the observation in terms that are accurate yet sufficiently general to minimize their impact on the subject's behavior. If the goal of the observation is a record of behaviors in a "natural" situation, other instructions and comments will be kept to a minimum beyond attempts to put the subject at ease in the setting. However, if the goal is to observe a large number of occurrences of a particular event, the investigator may choose to provide instructions that increase the probability that it will occur. Both approaches can be valid, but when results from one kind of situation are unthinkingly generalized to the other, a significant risk of invalid or inaccurate conclusions exists. For example, if the focus of the observation is on a contingent phenomenon such as "answering," an investigator might instruct a mother to query her child frequently about his or her activities. The child's language would certainly be significantly constrained by these instructions, however, and the resulting language sample could not be taken to be a valid representation of the child's skills in a more spontaneous conversational situation.

Similar issues arise when confederates are used by the investigator to guide the events in the situation in some manner. Such a strategy is valid as long as the intervention is acknowledged from the start to be a major feature of the observational context and as long as results are not generalized to situations in which no such intervention occurred. Again, the aims and potential generalizability of the observation will dictate the approach taken; the important point is that observations should not be undertaken, or interpreted, without prior, conscious decision-making about these issues.

Another contextual decision to be made in planning an observation concerns the degree to which the subject's responses are to be restricted or controlled. Investigators may choose to influence subject responses directly, through instructions or commands, or indirectly, through manipulation of the other events in the context. An observational context may be termed more or less "contrived" depending on the degree to which its events are deliberately controlled by the investigator. Contrived contexts can be contrasted with naturalistic ones, in which there is no attempt by the investigator to influence the events that occur.

Both naturalistic and contrived contexts can provide valuable data on communicative competence. The main advantage of a maximally naturalistic study, in which the investigator attempts to avoid influencing the subject's responses in any way, is the increased likelihood that the behaviors observed will be representative of the subject's typical behavior in the context. For this reason, naturalistic observational contexts can be useful in the exploratory stages of an investigation or in an attempt to derive valid taxonomies for subsequent study. By restricting the subject's behavior as little as possible, the investigator ensures that the events observed are not just artifacts of the observational situation.

Once valid behavioral taxonomies have been derived, however, it is often more efficient to study communicative skills by structuring the observational context to increase the frequency of occurrence of particular kinds of events. By arranging a more contrived context, the investigator can often increase the amount of data obtained without directly controlling the subject's responses (unlike elicitation procedures of the "Say *X*–Do *X*" variety). A more contrived context can similarly be extremely informative when certain behaviors have not been observed to occur in a more naturalistic context. If a context is contrived to bias a subject toward producing certain behaviors, the investigator can more confidently interpret their absence as an indication of a true inability to produce them rather than as an apparent inability resulting from sampling limitations. Thus, data on frequency of occurrence of behaviors can only be validly interpreted in relation to the sampling context.

Although these steps in the observational process are presented as discrete stages, a great deal of interaction will typically be among them, and decisions about any one step will often have implications for both preceding and subsequent steps. For example, an investigator might select a taxonomy based on his or her observational objectives, but subsequently discover that it is not possible to write adequate recognition rules for its categories. The investigator would be forced to revise his or her objectives or select another taxonomy before proceeding with the observational process. It is probably most accurate to think of the observational process as a cycle; observations may be "recycled" through these steps a number of times in the course of obtaining useful information about a subject's communicative skills.

OBSERVATIONS OF COMMUNICATIVE COMPETENCE

How do these interdependent stages of the observational process relate to the study of communicative competence? As mentioned already, the first step in the observational process is that of specifying the objectives of the observation; clarity and specificity of goals are two fundamental factors predisposing an observational endeavor to success. Because of this, an attempt to use observational methods to study a construct as broad and vaguely defined as "communicative competence" is not likely to be either efficient or successful. The notion of communicative competence falls at the very end of the emic pole of the inference continuum; the likelihood of obtaining acceptable levels of accuracy and reliability from attempts to observe this construct without further specifying and defining it is very small. Even if observers could use implicit recognition rules to make reliable judgments about whether individuals are "competent" communicators, such gross judgments are not likely to be particularly useful for either clinical or research purposes.

The construct of communicative competence itself must be made more explicit if it is to be the subject of successful, empirically adequate observations. For the purposes of this chapter this task is undertaken in a very preliminary way by dividing communicative competence into three subdomains, the suggestion being that phenomena within the clusters cohere more closely than do phenomena across clusters. This cluster framework illustrates one possible way to begin the task of reducing the unwieldy construct of communicative competence to a set of specific events that can be rigorously studied through observational methodology.

The first of the clusters to which we will refer concerns communicative intents, communicative functions, or speech acts: the reasons for which speakers communicate. This cluster contains many of the most frequently mentioned pragmatic phenomena, and numerous category systems for analyzing the functioning of utterances or other communicative behaviors have been proposed (see, for example, the summary in Chapman, 1981).

A second cluster of pragmatic phenomena concerns the rules for sequencing communicative acts, or for constructing and managing discourse. In distinguishing this cluster it is acknowledged that speakers and listeners use rules, which might be viewed as a "syntax" of discourse, to create orderly stretches of communicative interaction. This cluster includes rules for initiating and terminating conversational sequences, for exchanging speaker turns (Sacks, Schegloff, and Jefferson, 1974), for introducing and maintaining topics (Bloom, Rocissano, and Hood, 1976), and for identifying and repairing conversational breakdowns (Gallagher, 1977; Garvey, 1977).

A third cluster of pragmatic phenomena concerns the ways in which speakers and listeners integrate linguistic and nonlinguistic information and includes rules for presupposing and foregrounding information (Bates, 1976; Chafe, 1970; Maratsos, 1979), for selecting and maintaining a speech register (Sachs and Devin, 1976; Shatz and Gelman, 1973), and for using cohesion devices and deixis (Halliday and Hasan, 1976; Wales, 1979).

In distinguishing these clusters, the implication is not that they are always clearly separable or entirely distinct; it is obvious that there are numerous ways in which the phenomena with the clusters impinge on one another. The preliminary step of dividing the notion of communicative competence into somewhat more manageable pieces, however, provides a framework within which we can explore the use of observational methods to study it. And, in fact, each cluster presents its own unique challenges to the five steps in the observational process described previously. Thus, having made this initial distinction, let us now consider each of the steps in the observational process with specific reference to these three subdomains.

Specify Objectives for Each Pragmatic Cluster

There are numerous potential objectives for observations within the domain of communicative intents, including, for example, a determination of the number, type, and proportion of various communicative intents in a client's repertoire or the gestural, semantic, syntactic, and phonological alternatives that the client uses to convey a particular intent. Given that preschoolers are typically able to reformulate their unsuccessful requests for action (e.g., by repeating the request with an added politeness marker or by making the request more direct by changing it from a syntactic declarative such as "I need a cookie" to a syntactic imperative such as "Give me a cookie"), an observation might be planned with the objective of examining a child's ability to vary his or her language forms in such situations (Ervin-Tripp, 1977; Read and Cherry, 1978).

Communicative Intents. Information from an observation of communicative intents is most likely to be used to compare the client with other individuals, either to determine whether a significant problem exists or to determine which aspects of the communicative intent system appear to require some sort of intervention. So, for example, in planning an assessment of a 2 year old child with a suspected delay in communicative development, one observational objective might be to determine whether the child expresses the diversity of communicative intents typical of children at his or her developmental stage. This is a reasonably well-specified observational objective that is more likely to be achieved than a general plan to observe the child's "pragmatic skills."

Sequencing of Communicative Acts. There are numerous observable and quantifiable phenomena within the domain related to sequencing communicative acts; the number of potential observational objectives is equally large. Within this subdomain we might be interested in observing a subject's ability to produce communicative acts in the appropriate sequence, e.g., by asking questions such as: Does the subject appear to understand the basic contingent relationship between such communicative events as requests for information and answers? Between detection of a comprehension breakdown and production of a request for clarification? Does the subject possess an age-appropriate ability to introduce new topics, such that the listener can make the transition from old to new with a minimum of difficulty? Is the subject able to maintain a topic by adding new information about it? Does the subject control the stereotyped social routines that function to regulate the flow of discourse, such as greetings, filled pauses, interruption devices, and so on. Does the subject adequately signal his or her willingness to relinquish the role of speaker or his or her desire to occupy it? Are the latencies of the subject's communicative initiations or responses significantly faster or slower than normal? All of these questions could be starting points for specifying observational objectives within this pragmatic subdomain.

Integration of Language and Context. Specifying observational objectives is probably most difficult for the cluster involving the integration of language and context. In fact, it may be overly optimistic to consider this a cluster at all, given the large assortment of phenomena that have something to do with the interaction between linguistic and contextual features. The knowledge that presuppositions, Gricean maxims, discourse cohesion, deixis, and code switching all concern adaptations of language to context does not make it easy to unravel the relationships among them or to structure an investigation of a client's abilities in these areas. Unfortunately for the would-be investigator of this domain, one of the few things these phenomena do share is a lack of definition. Clearly stated definitions for many of these intuitively appealing constructs have been notable for their absence from the literature. Although this lack heightens the need for an investigator to formulate detailed observational objectives, it also guarantees that this will not be a simple task. As the remaining steps of the observational process hinge on this initial step, however, it is particularly crucial for investigators to carefully specify their objectives in planning observations of phenomena in this domain. As mentioned previously, observations undertaken with general goals are likely to be less efficient than those undertaken with more detailed objectives. An observation undertaken with a general goal such as, "To evaluate the child's control of deixis," is likely to result in less information than an observation that divides this goal into a series of more specific objectives (e.g., "To determine whether the child spontaneously disambiguates deitic terms when necessary," "To determine whether the child can disambiguate a deictic term on request," and so on). These more detailed objectives allow the investigator not only to complete the remaining steps in planning the observation with relative ease but also to obtain observational data that is sufficiently specific to be relevant to diagnostic and treatment decisions.

Specific observational objectives are equally important for other phenomena in this cluster, such as code switching and control of devices for producing cohesive discourse. For example, an observation might be planned with the goal of examining a subject's ability to change speech registers in talking to listeners of different ages or status. Such an objective might be warranted in planning an observation of a "pragmatically disordered" school-aged child. By observing and comparing the characteristics of the language he produces in talking to peers and to adults, it might be possible to determine whether he is unaware of the need to switch registers or does not possess the necessary stylistic variants in his linguistic repertoire that would allow him to do so. Similarly, an investigation of cohesion skills would yield much more useful data if observational goals were written to differentiate among the various cohesion devices (Halliday and Hasan, 1976). Rather than talking about a general "problem with cohesion," the investigator could pinpoint the particular cohesion devices that the client was unable to use adequately (e.g., rules for accompanying exophoric references or deictic words with gestures when necessary or rules governing the use of pronominal reference).

Select or Construct a Pragmatic Event Taxonomy

At this step the investigator decides which categories of events are relevant to the observational objectives. As noted previously, this step is somewhat dependent on the first, and generating a valid set of categories may in fact be the objective of an initial, exploratory observation. Even when the observation is to be confirmatory, however, the content validity of the observational taxonomy must be evaluated.

Communicative Intents. Numerous taxonomies have been proposed for the domain of communicative intents; often these are tied to particular developmental levels. For example, the taxonomy of communicative functions that Halliday (1975) derived from observation of his 9 month old son contains different categories than the one that best captured his son's intents from 16 to 35 months of age. Similarly, various taxonomies have been devised to apply only to a particular developmental level, ranging from Bates's (1976) description of proto-imperatives and proto-declaratives in the prelinguistic infant to the analyses of adult performative verbs by Austin (1962) and Searle (1969).

As mentioned, taxonomies derived from observations of subjects with certain characteristics (e.g., particular developmental levels, motoric skills) may not be valid for other types of subjects; the applicability of category systems across subject groups should be tested, not assumed. Disordered subjects may use elaborate, idiosyncratic gesture systems to convey a variety of communicative intents despite significant deficiencies in productive speech; if taxonomies from normal speakers are not modified, these complex communicative gestures cannot be documented. Similarly, many motorically impaired individuals develop alternative means of conveying communicative intents, using facial expressions or postural changes interpretable only by those who are very well acquainted with them. An attempt to study communicative intents in these individuals would require an initial period of exploratory observation in order to determine which behaviors to include in a taxonomy for subsequent confirmatory observations.

Sequencing of Communicative Acts. Far fewer taxonomies have been proposed for the domain of communicative sequencing than for the domain of communicative intents. The descriptions of contingent query sequences by Garvey (1977) represent some of the more elegant analyses of the relationship between successive communicative events. Garvey's contingent query cycle is particularly noteworthy because it is based not just on immediately adjacent utterances but on cycles of related utterances that may be multiply embedded.

Possibly because of the paucity of published taxonomies for this domain, beginning clinicians often approach observations of phenomena within this cluster with an overly simplistic, two-category distinction between "appropriate" and "inappropriate" communicative acts. Thus, a clinician may report that a subject "responds inappropriately to questions." When pressured to define an inappropriate response, the clinician is often unable to provide more information, beyond saying that the subject "gives the wrong answer in response to a question." Such a broad and poorly defined description of subject behavior is likely to lead to equally broad and poorly defined treatment goals. Alternatively, by spending more time and effort to specify what is meant by an "inappropriate" communicative act, a clinician can generate a much more informative taxonomy, which will in turn provide a much more accurate and comprehensive picture of the nature and source of the subject's sequencing difficulties. For example, one might construct a taxonomy that at least distinguished between answers to "wh"-questions, yes-no questions, tag questions, and choice questions, or the clinician might conduct an exploratory observation of the subject's question-answering skills by recording and examining a number of events preceding and following successful and unsuccessful responses to questions. This exploratory phase might lead the clinician to realize that the subject's question-answering skill actually varies depending on the degree to which the question refers to some aspect of the "here-and-now" or the degree to which the answer can be produced through use of a comprehension strategy. The clinician could then proceed to construct a taxonomy distinguishing among these events and to write recognition rules for its categories; subsequent observations would yield a much better picture of the specific kinds of questions to which treatment should be addressed.

Integration of Language and Context. The domain of phenomena concerning the integration of language and context is not characterized by a proliferation of taxonomies; this is predictable given the lack of clear definitions for many of its constructs. The notions of presupposition and foregrounding appear in many analyses under different names or slightly different guises, but there seem to be very few taxonomies that go beyond these two general categories to differentiate among the phenomena of which they are comprised. The situation is somewhat better for analyzing cohesion in discourse, thanks to Halliday and Hasan's (1976) system describing seven types of cohesion and the various linguistic devices by which cohesion can be marked.

Code switching taxonomies have generally been based either on the characteristics of the codes that can be distinguished (i.e., the lexical, syntactic, prosodic, or phonological alternatives that are contingent on particular contexts) or on the characteristics of the contexts that elicit these modifications (e.g., age, status, familiarity, affiliation of listeners, setting formality or familiarity). In any event, that many phenomena in this cluster are identified through a lengthy chain of inferences rather than directly, coupled with the lack of a widely accepted theory of the phenomena in this cluster, make the issue of content validity particularly significant in constructing observational taxonomies within this domain.

Write Adequate Recognition Rules for Pragmatic Events

Communicative Intent. How will the observer know when one of the events from the chosen taxonomy has occurred? This is the question recognition rules are designed to answer. For each event, the investigator specifies what observable phenomena will serve as its indicators. For the communicative intent cluster, this is rarely an easy task. The problem comes in trying to balance the dual requirements of reliability and validity. Let's assume that an investigator has decided to use a simple taxonomy with three categories of communicative intents: comments, requests for action, and requests for information. If the investigation is concerned with reliability, she or he might be tempted to write some very explicit, etic-level recognition rules for these categories, based on the syntactic characteristics of utterances; for example, "Utterances with declarative syntactic structure shall count as comments, utterances with interrogative syntactic form shall count as requests for information, and utterances with imperative syntactic form shall count as requests for action." Assuming that the subjects had both the inclination and linguistic skill to unambiguously mark each of their utterances as one of these three syntactic forms, these recognition rules would likely result in high levels of observer accuracy and agreement. Unfortunately, of course, the literature makes it clear that syntactic criteria alone are not valid indicators of these various communicative intents.

At the opposite extreme, recognition rules might be based on the observer's emic-level inferences about whether each utterance was intended as a comment, a request for information, or a request for action. Such recognition rules might result in subjectively valid identification of these events, but rules based entirely on subjective inferences would be unlikely to result in acceptable levels of inter-observer reliability.

The solution to the problem of writing recognition rules for communicative intents lies somewhere between these two extremes, and the literature contains numerous descriptions of recognition rules that are based on a combination of etic and emic information. Table 3–3 presents some sample recognition rules written to enable the identification of a general communicative intent category (''Demand-request'') and two of its subcategories (''Demand-request for attention,'' ''Demand-request for action''). These rules illustrate a combination of relatively more etic information, such as utterance intonation contour and syntactic form, with more emic information, such as utterance relationship to antecedent and subsequent events and observer inferences about speaker intent. Regardless of whether recognition rules for communicative intents are based on etic- or emic-level information, observers are likely to require a significant amount of training before they are able to accurately and reliably identify complex phenomena such as these.

Sequencing Communicative Acts. Writing recognition rules for communicative sequencing phenomena is often quite difficult, first because the events of interest may take place over an extended or discontinuous period of time and second because sequential analyses are often based on highly interential or emic-level analyses. For example, the criteria that make an event an ''answer'' would be difficult to write in strictly etic terms; answers can take a variety of forms and need not occur immediately following a request for information or clarification (to take two possible precursors to the ''answer'' event). Writing a recognition rule that explicitly distinguishes between, for example, a delayed answer and a comment introducing a related topic may require a significant investment of time and thought.

To continue with an example mentioned previously, how might an investigator write a recognition rule by which an observer could identify ''Questions referring to the 'here-and-now' '' in order to study the relation of those events to answers? An initial attempt at a recognition rule for these questions might be, ''Questions that contain words referring to

Table 3-3. Sample Recognition Rules for Some Communicative Intents

Demand-Request:

Any intelligible or unintelligible verbalization produced for the purpose of obtaining a service or eliciting information or an opinion (e.g., "Bring me the ball," "Where did daddy go?"). Demand-requests require compliance on the part of the listener. Such utterances may consist of a single word (e.g., "Stop," "Hungry?"), may be accompanied with rising inflection on the terminal syllable, or may be accompanied by motor behaviors (e.g., grabbing, repetitive pointing, or attempts to ambulate toward or obtain an object).

Demand-Request for Attention:

An utterance initiated by one member of a dyad who solicits visual gaze from another (e.g., "Look at this," "Watch me").

Demand-Request for Action:

An utterance initiated by one member of a dyad who solicits the other participant to perform an action or discontinue an ongoing action (e.g., "Bring me the doll," "Stop hitting your teddy bear," "Can you find the ball?"). Also included in this category are requests for permission in which the speaker attempts to obtain the right to do or say something from the respondent (e.g., "May I go to the store?").

objects or persons in the immediate environment." However, an effort to implement this preliminary recognition rule would reveal that it is inadequate. For one thing, as it stands it does not provide criteria for identifying questions. A more serious problem is that although it includes questions that refer to objects in the immediate context, it does not exclude queries about actions or attributes that are not visible. Thus, even if the rule was modified to define questions as utterances having interrogative syntactic form, the rule would identify as "Questions referring to the 'here-and-now' " such diverse exemplars as "What is that train doing?" How old is your brother?" and "Is that train like the one you got at Grandma's?" The first of these questions is likely to be the most interesting sort; even though the other questions contain words pertaining to present referents, they do not query information that is available through visual inspection of the environment. A modification of the recognition rule that would come closer to delimiting the range of anticipated phenomena might be, "Questions referring to the here-and-now are defined as utterances that have interrogative syntactic form, contain at least one deictic word, and are accompanied with a pointing gesture occurring either simultaneously or within two seconds." This more restrictive rule not only makes the observer's task easier by more clearly specifying the kinds of events to which she or he must attend but also contributes to the investigator's awareness of the "distinctive features" of such events; that is, although we began with a fairly vague notion ("Questions referring to the here-and-now"), the process of writing a recognition rule has greatly sharpened our understanding of the features of this event that make it relevant to our observational objectives, allowing us to write even more adequate recognition rules on subsequent attempts.

Integration of Language and Context. Because of the abstractness of many of the phenomena relating to the integration of language and context, it is difficult and time-consuming to write adequate recognition rules for them; this step is consequently slighted more often than not. It appears that many observational investigations of these phenomena have relied primarily on observer inferences, rather than on clearly specified recognition rules relating the observable events to the emic-level phenomena that they are believed to reflect. Definitions of presupposed and foregrounded information, for example, often appear to rely solely on the observer's subjective impressions of features such as utterance "focus"; the observational study that reports data on the reliability of such judgments is unfortunately the exception rather than the rule.

The situation is somewhat better for observations of code switching, in which there are some directly observable, etic-utterance characteristics that can be more easily separated from inferences about their roles in marking different speech registers. Likewise, in the study of cohesion devices, it is relatively easy to distinguish observable utterance characteristics from the emic system inferred to underlie them; adequate recognition rules are correspondingly easier to construct.

Select a Data Recording System

Communicative Intents. In selecting a system for recording data on any of the three clusters of pragmatic phenomena the investigator must consider the frequency, rate, and level of abstractness of the events to be coded as well as the complexity of the recognition rules. The frequency and rate of speech production of 12 month olds may well be low enough to allow on-line, orthographic recording of their utterances; however, if complex recognition rules are being used to categorize these events, alternate methods of recording will likely be necessary. Similarly, if recognition rules require the observer to note a variety of events at a variety of levels of abstractness, on-line coding of information will be impossible, regardless of event frequency and rate. This would be the case in the domain of communicative intents, for example, if observers were attempting to identify several different intents on the basis of gestural, intonational, and syntactic information along with information about their contingent relationships with other events. If the observer's task is simplified by reducing the number of different phenomena to be identified and simplifying their recognition rules, on-line data collection would be a more viable option. However, the loss of information resulting from such tactics may outweigh the advantages of an on-line format.

If the data are to be recorded on-line, it is also critical that the recording system be designed to require as little of the observer's conscious attention as possible, in order to maximize his or her ability to monitor the events of interest in the communicative situation itself. For example, if the goal of the on-line observation were to obtain data on the frequency of three types of intents, checking off one of three columns on a data sheet would be easier than recording abbreviations or codes for the events. A paper-and-pencil system that could provide information not just on absolute frequencies of these intents but also on their sequence might consist of a one-letter symbol for each intent and a continuous "chain" of symbols recorded in the order observed.

In addition to well-designed coding formats, sampling decisions can often be made to enable on-line coding of pragmatic phenomena for portions of the data collection period. For example, several authors (Miller, 1981; Sackett, 1978) have suggested a strategy in which the stream of behavior is sampled at 30 second to 2 minute intervals, increasing the observer's ability to cope with rapidly occurring events and complex recognition rules.

Sequencing Communicative Acts. In contrast to the communicative intent cluster for which well-designed, "low-technology" recording methods as well as time-sampling strategies can often be used quite successfully, one of the distinguishing features of the cluster of sequential communicative phenomena is that its units of analysis are often based on sequences of events rather than on discrete behaviors or occurrences. As mentioned previously, human information processing constraints make it extremely difficult to obtain accurate, reliable on-line judgments about complex constellations of events, particularly when observations must be summed over time (Duncan and Fiske, 1977). Likewise, a time-sampling strategy is not applicable to the coding of sequential contingent relationships among communicative events, since the sampling periods might cut across the relevant set of contingent events, destroying their structure. Thus, on-line methods are of doubtful value for recording most observations in the sequencing domain.

Integration of Language and Context. In addition to their abstractness, phenomena related to the integration of language and context are often reflected in simultaneous clusters of semantic, syntactic, phonological, prosodic, and nonlinguistic events. Because of this, observations of most phenomena in this domain are likely to require recording of data for subsequent analysis. The kinds of events that can be coded on-line by a human observer are likely to provide only a small part of the data relevant to an evaluation of this cluster of pragmatic skills.

Structure the Observational Context

Communicative Intents. In planning an observation of communicative intents, contextual decisions are particularly important, for such factors as the number of persons present, their ages, status, and familiarity to the subject can have a significant impact on the number and kind of communicative intents observed, for communicators at all developmental levels.

Similarly, the degree of structure imposed by the investigator on the subject's behavior is likely to significantly influence the communicative intent data obtained. More naturalistic contexts, such as free play for young children and conversation for adults, are likely to be chosen if the investigator wants an overall picture of the subject's intentional communicative behaviors. However, the investigator may set up a more contrived situation in order to elicit a specific kind of communicative intent. For example, to observe a subject's ability to manipulate a variety of linguistic forms in producing requests for action, the investigator might contrive a situation in which the client's initial request for action is unsuccessful (e.g., Read and Cherry, 1978). Snyder (1975) structured a context to facilitate production of imperative and declarative intents by children at the earliest stages of language development.

Sequencing Communicative Acts. Similar issues arise in planning observations of the sequencing domain. There are numerous ways in which the observational context can be manipulated to facilitate the occurrence of particular sequences of communicative events or to facilitate observation of events that might otherwise occur infrequently. To return to a previous example, if our objective were to observe the subject's responses to questions referring to the immediate environment, the context could be structured by having a confederate ask the child a predetermined set of questions constructed to vary on this dimension (however, it had been defined in the recognition rule). The process of constructing a set of such questions might suggest other potentially revealing contrasts, such as their syntactic or lexical characteristics. A decision to explore these additional contrasts would entail returning to the beginning of the observational cycle to rewrite the observational objectives, taxonomy, and recognition rules.

Integration of Language and Context. Phenomena involving the integration of language and context are by definition contextual, which makes it imperative that the features of the observational context be consciously selected by the investigator. Because of the context dependence of many observational goals in this domain, the investigator can often contrive the observational context to facilitate the occurrence of the events of interest, making the observation both more efficient and more revealing. For example, an observation of a subject's ability to manipulate the presuppositional structure of his or her utterances could be designed in such a way that the speaker would be required to describe the same event to two listeners, only one of whom had been present when the event occurred. Contriving the context in this manner would provide more interpretable evidence on the speaker's control of presuppositional devices than if the investigator had simply attempted to discern presuppositional phenomena in a spontaneous conversation. Similarly, observations of code switching require that data be collected in the presence of different listeners or in different settings; the investigator who contrives contexts to facilitate the occurrence of just these kinds of events will obtain the relevant data much more rapidly and efficiently. Finally, such phenomena as narrative cohesion skills can be much more confidently compared across speakers if they have all engaged in identical narrative tasks; for example, if all speakers are exposed to an identical story that they must then retell to a new listener.

CONCLUSION

The preceding discussion has highlighted a myriad of considerations facing the investigator who would conduct even a minimally adequate observation of pragmatic phenomena. The adequacy of published data on pragmatics, of pragmatic assessment and intervention procedures, and of data used clinically to diagnose or treat communicatively impaired individuals should be evaluated with respect to these same considerations. Some of the available data concerning the pragmatic domain have been characterized by a less than impeccable record in relation to the dual demands of validity and reliability, which can probably be attributed to the eclectic nature of the construct of communicative competence, its relatively recent emergence on the empirical scene, and its position at the confluence of a number of disparate aspects of communicative skill. However, there is nothing inherent in the pragmatic domain that exempts it from the demands of scientific respectability; claims that communicative competence is somehow less amenable to the techniques of careful observational methodology are indefensible as well as counterproductive. It is unavoidable that a significant amount of time and effort is necessary to plan and conduct valid, reliable observations of communicative competence, but these are the only kinds of observations that will be useful for either clinical or research purposes. It is hoped that this chapter, by emphasizing the need for better observations in this area and presenting some suggestions for meeting this need, will assist readers in scrutinizing the observational methods used by themselves and others to obtain data on communicative competence. The sooner the notion that communicative competence can be evaluated through some sort of subjective, "gut-level" intuitions is abandoned, the sooner a truly useful base of information on the pragmatic abilities of children and adults will develop.

ACKNOWLEDGMENTS

Thanks to Anne van Kleeck for a number of valuable suggestions on this chapter.

REFERENCES

Austin, J. L. (1962). *How to do things with words.* Cambridge, MA: Harvard University Press.

Bates, E. (1976). *Language and context: the acquisition of pragmatics.* New York: Academic Press.

Bloom, L., Rocissano, L., and Hood, L. (1976). Adult-child discourse: developmental interaction between information processing and linguistic knowledge. *Cognitive Psychology, 8,* 521–552.

Boehm, A., and Weinberg, R. (1977). *The classroom observer.* New York: Teachers College Press.

Chafe, W. L. (1970). *Meaning and the structure of language.* Chicago: University of Chicago Press.

Chapman, R. S. (1981). Exploring children's communicative intents. In J. F. Miller (Ed.), *Assessing language production in children: experimental procedures.* Baltimore: University Park Press.

Cherry Wilkinson, L., Clevenger, M., and Dollaghan, C. (1981). Communication in small instructional groups: a sociolinguistic approach. In W. P. Dickson (Ed.), *Children's oral communication skills.* New York: Academic Press.

Crystal, D. (1980). *A first dictionary of linguistics and phonetics.* Boulder, CO: Westview Press.

Crystal, D., Fletcher, P., and Garman, M. (1977). *The grammatical analysis of language disability.* London: Edward Arnold.

Duncan, S., and Fiske, D. (1977). *Face-to-face interaction: research, methods, and theory.* Hillsdale, NJ: Lawrence Erlbaum Associates.

Ervin-Tripp, S. (1977). "Wait for me, rollerskate!" In S. Ervin-Tripp and C. Mitchell-Kernan (Eds.), *Child discourse.* New York: Academic Press.

Gallagher, T. M. (1977). Revision behaviors in the speech of normal children developing language. *Journal of Speech and Hearing Research, 20,* 303–318.

Garvey, C. (1977). The contingent query: A dependent act in conversation. In M. Lewis and L. Rosenblum (Eds.), *Interaction, conversation and the development of language.* New York: John Wiley and Sons.

Halliday, M. A. K. (1975). *Learning how to mean: Explorations in the development of language.* New York: Elsevier.

Halliday, M. A. K., and Hasan, R. (1976). *Cohesion in English.* London: Longman.

Hymes, D. (1974). *Foundations in sociolinguistics.* Philadelphia: University of Pennsylvania Press.

Kerlinger, F. N. (1973). *Foundations of behavioural research.* New York: Holt, Rinehart and Winston.

Maratsos, M. P. (1979). Learning how and when to use pronouns and determiners. In P. Fletcher and M. Garman (Eds.), *Language acquisition.* Cambridge: Cambridge University Press.

Masling, J., and Stern, G. (1969). The effect of the observer in the classroom. *Journal of Educational Psychology, 60,* 351-354.

Miller, J. F. (1981). *Assessing language production in children: experimental procedures.* Baltimore: University Park Press.

Read, B., and Cherry, L. J. (1978). Preschool children's production of directive forms. *Discourse Processes, 1,* 233-245.

Rist, R. C. (1977). On the relations among educational research paradigms: From disdain to detente. *Anthropology and Education Quarterly, 8,* 42-49.

Rosenblum, L. A. (1978). The creation of a behavioral taxonomy. In G. P. Sackett (Ed.), *Observing behaviour, Vol. 2.* Baltimore: University Park Press.

Sachs, J., and Devlin, J. (1976). Young children's use of age-appropriate speech styles in social interaction and role-playing. *Journal of Child Language. 3,* 81-98.

Sackett, G. P. (1978). *Observing behaviour, Vol. 2.* Baltimore: University Park Press.

Sacks, H., Schegloff, E., and Jefferson, G. (1974). A simplest systematics for the organization of turn-taking in conversation. *Language, 50,* 696-735.

Searle, J. R. (1969). *Speech acts.* London: Cambridge University Press.

Shatz, M., and Gelman, R. (1973). The development of communication skills: Modifications in the speech of young children as a function of listener. *Monographs of the Society for Research in Child Development, 38* (Serial No. 152).

Shriberg, L., and Kent, R. (1982). *Clinical phonetics.* New York: John Wiley and Sons.

Snyder, L. (1975). *Pragmatics in language disabled children: their prelinguistic and early verbal performatives and presuppositions.* Doctoral dissertation, University of Colorado, Boulder.

Stephenson, G., and Dickson, W. P. (1978). *SSR keyboard users' manual.* Working paper No. 232, The Wisconsin Research and Development Center for Individualized Schooling.

Tukey, J. W. (1977). *Exploratory data analysis.* Reading, MA: Addison-Wesley.

Wales, R. (1979). Deixis. In P. Fletcher and M. Garman (Eds.), *Language acquisition.* Cambridge: Cambridge University Press.

Chapter 4

Sequential Analysis of Naturalistic Communication

Howard M. Rosenfeld

The ability of a person to exchange information with other members of a culture is the product of a long and complicated learning history. For example, the development and usage of a child's verbal repertoire depends on the responses his utterances evoke over repeated opportunities. Thus, to understand the acquisition of communicative competence or incompetence, it is necessary to assess and analyze the developing child's interactions with his social and physical environment.

The child's verbal interchanges can be assessed in natural or experimental settings. The more natural the setting, the greater the opportunity to discover the range of behavioral and environmental variables involved in the communication process. The more experimental the setting, the greater the opportunity to determine if the relationships between a smaller number of variables are causal. Natural research emphasizes discovery and representativeness. Experimental research emphasizes certainty. The two approaches are complementary.

Natural and experimental approaches can be productively combined. The researcher may select settings that are conducive to expression of natural behavior yet are controlled enough to gain accurate conclusions. Although many variables in natural situations can be measured unobtrusively, often it is useful to introduce observers, recording equipment, and some constraints on permissible behavior. If these modifications of the natural environment are done carefully, subjects are likely to provide reasonably representative behavior. Another way to compromise is to build simulated features of the natural environment into experimental settings (Rosenfeld, 1972). The combination of natural and experimental approaches, or "naturalistic" research, will be emphasized in the present chapter.

In experimental studies, the researcher may control the setting (e.g., the presence or absence of playmates or playthings) or the occurrences of antecedent behaviors (e.g., the frequency or content of mother's utterances) to determine their effects on behaviors (e.g., the infant's vocalizations). In contrast, in natural studies the antecedents are allowed to occur as they may. Thus, in natural studies, it is more difficult to assure a sufficiently high rate of occurrence of antecedent behaviors to meet sampling requisites for statistical significance. Consequently, the researcher may need to devise ways of assuring sufficient samples of data. For example, in this chapter it is illustrated how imposed variations in the availability of toys and maternal attention in a naturalistic setting affect rates of several infant behaviors (see the section on complementary experimental analysis).

Another problem with natural studies is that the uncontrolled pattern of occurrence of behaviors makes it more difficult for the researcher to make accurate causal inferences about variables that are temporally related. The social effects of behaviors may be immediate, delayed, cumulative, or interactive. Thus, the researcher may need to invent statistical methods to help distinguish between competing causal interpretations of results. In this chapter statistical techniques developed for this purpose by Rosenfeld and Remmers (1981) as well as more recent improvements are discussed.

The communicative process may be broadly defined as the effects that interacting individuals have on each other over time (Altman, 1965, 1967). Statistical procedures for detecting these effects are known as methods of temporal or sequential analysis. Different methods serve as different kinds of "filters," each method sifting the data and allowing only selected features to fall through. By varying the filters and comparing the results, an increasingly accurate model of the communication process and how it changes can be developed. The filtering process begins when investigators decide which aspects of the natural flow of behavior they will record and which of the recorded variables will be analyzed. If no further assessments are made of variations in the pattern of distribution of each such variable over time, as is usually the case, this is referred to as conventional statistical analysis (or Type I analysis in Rosenfeld and Remmers, 1981). Analysis of the effects of temporal clustering of variables requires additional filtering techniques (see Fig. 4-4 for an example).

The literature on communicative development has paid little attention to the temporal distribution of behaviors and how variations are involved in causal relationships. Most researchers simply determine that rates of occurrence of certain classes of behavior by one category of person are nonrandomly associated with certain rates of behavior in another type of person. The researcher then offers an interpretation of the causal processes underlying these associations. But in such correlational studies of average rates of behavioral events, the absence of specific evidence about sequential connections between the events usually allows alternative causal interpretations. Sequential analysis can help determine directions of causality in correlated data and the effects of clustering of events.

For example, much is known about the utterances that children and adults perform during their social interactions, but little is known about how the acts of the participants influence each other. Considerable normative evidence indicates that children increase in linguistic competence with age. There is evidence that the utterances of mothers and other linguistically competent persons are similar in complexity to the utterances of infants and young children with whom they interact (Snow and Ferguson, 1977). However, from the correlation coefficients between the forms of utterance of mother and of child, it is not clear whether the mother's adjustments are a cause or a consequence of the child's performance. Conventional correlational evidence indicates that the levels of verbal complexity of mother and child tend to be similar, but sequential statistics are needed to reveal the direction of effect and the nature of the temporal or sequential connections.

Another limitation of most studies of communication is that the potential contributions of a variety of subcategories or features of behavioral variables are ignored. To what degree is the child responsive to the linguistic aspects of the mother's behavior versus to her voice quality and other nonverbal accompaniments? Among the nonverbal features, what is the contribution of gaze direction, facial muscle movements, and skeletal action? What are the effective temporal properties for any single feature or combination? Does the child respond to the mother's initiation of an utterance, to its termination, to segments within it, or to its repetition? These questions require a comprehensive multivariate classification system.

Sequential statistical methods in studies of human communication rarely are included in methodology books in the human behavioral sciences. Many sequential methods were initially developed for the physical sciences. In the behavioral realm, they have been used primarily by students of animal social behavior. Yet a variety of sequential analytic methods are applicable to the study of human communicative behavior (Fagen and Young, 1978; Gottman, 1980; Gottman and Notarius, 1978; Sackett, 1978; van Hooff, 1982). Individual investigators may need to adapt available procedures for their own purposes. Applications relevant to students of human communication include studies of peer and child-parent interaction (Patterson and Cobb, 1971), marital communication (Gottman, 1979), interviews (Hawes and Foley, 1973), and psychotherapeutic sessions (Lichtenberg and Hummel, 1976).

This chapter discusses major requisites and options for conducting sequential analysis of human social interaction. In particular, two widely divergent types of sequential method adapted for the purpose of analyzing interactions between infants and their mothers—holistic automaton analysis and bivariate lag analysis—will be reviewed. The methods will be illustrated on available data from the author's own research and their relative advantages and disadvantages evaluated. In addition, recent variations in the author's methods that make them capable of more precise interpretations, easier to use, and more broadly applicable will be noted.

BASIC METHODOLOGICAL CONSIDERATIONS

Many students of human social interaction are motivated by the broad and rather vague goal of finding out, "what is going on?" They want to explore the details of communicative interchanges to determine what variables are consequential and examine the nature of the relationships among variables rather than to formally test preconceived hypotheses. Such researchers face a fundamental problem. To extract all relevant information from their observations, they need to assess all potentially relevant acts and to check for all possible interrelationships. Yet most human interchanges are so complex that they could be coded in an indefinitely large variety of ways, and the coded behaviors could be interrelated in terms of a large number of alternative models.

Given sufficient time and resources, exploring such data might benefit the researcher in many different ways. But more often, the only practical solution is to make choices among the possibilities. The following sections set forth options in the selection of methods for sequential analysis of communication, starting with decisions relating to the coding of individual behaviors. (For more general issues regarding observational methods see the chapter by Dollaghan and Miller in this volume.)

Classifying and Encoding Variables

Some coding decisions pertain to substantive distinctions between categories and subcategories. Other decisions refer to temporal distinctions, including coding by order versus time interval of occurrence, size of time interval, and coding all intervals versus only those in which changes occur. Decisions also need to be made regarding use of observational and automated methods of recording.

Comprehensiveness of Classification System. Comprehensiveness of coding has implications for both the choice of analytic models and the results they produce. No single coding scheme is appropriate for all research purposes. This problem is complicated because communicative behavior may operate at a variety of levels, each with a different set of substantive distinctions (see the subsequent section on molarity of coding).

Current research indicates the importance of assessing not only verbalizations but also associated nonverbal accompaniments (Siegman and Feldstein, 1978) and orientations to physical and social objects (Sugarman, in press). The functional communicative element in an act of greeting, for example, may range from a full-body configuration such as a curtsy to a brief vocalization or lift of the eyebrow or head (Rosenfeld, 1982). Objective methods are now available for recording and categorizing nonverbal observable behavior, including vocal features, skeletal movements, and facial muscular movements (Scherer and Ekman, 1982).

Continuous Versus Discrete Measures. Many behaviors can be coded as either continuous or discrete. For example, the intensity or loudness of an utterance can be characterized on a continuous scale, or it can simply be noted whether or not it exceeded a given level of intensity or audibility. Most research on human communication has used discrete measures. One practical reason for the general preference for discrete measures is that they tend to be easier to assess. For a fuller discussion of reasons for and of differences in analytic procedures for discrete and continuous data, see Hewes (1980). The present chapter emphasizes discrete measures and corresponding analytic models. For examples of modeling of relationships involving continuous variables, see Gottman (1981), Martin (1981), and Thomas and Martin (1976).

Molarity of Event Categories. It is possible to categorize behavior at different levels of generality. Categories for describing behavior may range from relatively broad, summary characterizations of behavior (molar level) to the notation of detailed features and movements (molecular level). It is important to code the events at a level that reflects their actual use in communicative exchanges.

For example, persons who nod their heads more often during a social event tend to create a more positive social impression (Rosenfeld, 1966, 1967). However, overt behavioral reactions to head nods during the communicative process depend on variations in the features of each head nod, such as its vertical range and rate of up-down cycles (Birdwhistell, 1970; Rosenfeld and Hancks, 1980; Rosenfeld and McRoberts, 1979).

Thus, different levels of molarity are appropriate for different research purposes. Extremely detailed coding may be necessary for the analysis and training of skills requiring precise coordination of specified muscle groupings or for the basic study of perception of movement. Less detailed coding (and less complex statistical modeling) may be sufficient for testing theoretical propositions about rates of occurrence of commonly perceived gestalt configurations of behavior.

One strategy is to code behavior at the most elementary level (e.g., each momentary change in head position). An example is the preliminary discovery of the communicative significance of several different levels of eyebrow raise (Birdwhistell, 1970). The primitive properties of behavior then can be combined into more complex configurations whose communicative significance can be assessed. For example, there is evidence that larger units of utterance tend to be marked by correspondingly larger configurations of kinesic activities (Kendon, 1972).

Although improved methods for coding and summarizing details of movement are becoming available (e.g., Hirsbrunner and Frey, in press), research at the microscopic level can be expensive and time consuming. It also may become bogged down in so much detail that larger configurations having communicative significance are missed by the investigator. The researcher must guess at the likely payoff for the extra costs of assessing details. For example, some things can be learned about communication simply by assessing the pattern of occurrence and nonoccurrence of vocalization (Jaffe and Feldstein, 1970). Other kinds of information may require substantive distinctions between forms of vocalizations (see Figs. 4–2 and 4–3 for examples).

Size of Time Units. Molarity of behavior categories involve the consideration of substantive components and their temporal properties. Many researchers segment time into a sequence of 10 second intervals and then record whether or not various components or classes of behavior by each participant occur within each interval. But selection of size of coding interval should be guided by available information about the durations and rates of occurrence of events of interest rather than by arbitrary conventions.

Some events occur infrequently, such as major switches between speaker and listener roles in conversations. In studies of speaker switching it may be sufficient to include large time units that are capable of capturing changes in phrases rather than smaller time units that are necessary to include changes in more rapidly occurring events such as syllables (Duncan and Fiske, 1977). In contrast, some investigators of interpersonal synchronization of body parts between speakers and listeners have observed that change points in synchronization of small movements occur in conjunction with phoneme changes (Condon and Sander, 1974). To capture these changes it may be necessary to code vocal and other behavioral changes in intervals as small as 0.001 second (Rosenfeld, 1981).

Decisions about how to segment the temporal dimension are important for sequential analysis of communication because variations in the size of the chosen interval affect the conclusions. For example, in conversational situations, when using smaller-sized intervals, statistical methods for assessing sequential dependencies reveal relationships within one person's response pattern (e.g., word-to-word sequences). In contrast, with larger intervals the effects of one person on another are more likely to be detected (Hayes, Meltzer, and Wolf, 1970).

If intervals are large with respect to the frequency of occurrence of events, the effects of single occurrences and repetitive bursts will likely be confounded when both are identically scored as simply occurring in an interval. Thus, for statistical analysis, some investigators use an interval small enough to encompass only one occurrence of an event of interest (Sackett, 1978; Rosenfeld and Remmers, 1981).

Observational Versus Automated Coding. In sequential studies there is an increasing use of technical apparatus either as a supplement to or a substitute for observers. For sequential analysis, the selection of coding methods depends on the size of the time interval and the reliability of coding. If small time intervals are needed, manually or automatically operated digital event recorders can consult an internal clock to record the times of occurrence to the nearest fraction of a second. If the substantive categories are difficult to observe quickly or to record automatically, it may be necessary to record events on film or tape. These records then can be repeatedly scrutinized at desired rates with or without additional technical aids.

Automated aids can code detailed aspects of live action as well as synthesize the details into higher-order properties. For example, automatic voice transaction analyzers can detect vocalizations of individual conversants down to small fractions of a second and then compute temporal patterns of speaking and turn-taking (Jaffe and Feldstein, 1970). Other devices identify the boundaries of phonemes and locate them with respect to corresponding body movements on videotapes (Hirsbrunner and Frey, in press). An example of automated coding and analysis of movement patterns is the use of photoelectronic devices to record the exact three-dimensional position in space of each major body part involved within each small fraction of a second during ongoing behavior, along with the use of an associated computer to integrate the data into higher-order action patterns (Gustafsson and Lanshammar, 1977). The relative advantages of observers and automated coding devices, particularly in the assessment of nonverbal actions, are discussed more extensively by Rosenfeld (1982).

Change Point Versus Interval Coding. Coding observations for sequential analysis is a matter of assessing the intersection of two dimensions: content and time. The most common form of coding sheet consists of a matrix in which rows represent categories of content and columns represent time intervals (or vice versa). The coder marks the presence or absence of each event class in each time interval.

An alternative is to code only the time intervals in which particular events start and stop and to ignore intervals in which the events continue or in which no events occur. The data consist of a string of event labels, with each event marked by a start time or a stop time. This alternative saves coding time and space relative to the fixed-interval coding methods, particularly when a given event persists over a number of intervals.

Yet it also permits later reconstruction of all information that could have been obtained by coding continuations of an event repeatedly across adjacent fixed-time intervals. It permits segmentation of continuing events into sizes of time interval preferred by the investigator, down to the smallest reliable time unit that was used for making start-stop notations. Given these advantages, the change-point method of coding is highly recommended.

Interval Versus Ordinal Time Units. In some cases the effect of one person's behavior on another person is a function of the time between the behaviors, whereas in other cases the effect is a function of the sequence of occurrence of behaviors. Sequential analysis can be performed on events identified by their times of occurrence (clock-time intervals) or by their order of occurrence, but the conclusions may differ.

For example, according to one theory of conversational structure, a pair of conversants is expected not to leave noticeable temporal gaps in the exchange of utterances, and furthermore, the right to the speaking turn alternates between participants (Sacks, Schegloff, and Jefferson, 1974). Thus, if one person fails to take his turn at speaking within a brief time interval following an opportunity point, the other person immediately regains the right. Tests of this hypothesis would require coding the initiations and terminations of utterances by time interval, as recommended in the preceding section, so the temporal lengths of interutterance intervals can be assessed and related to who takes the floor.

Other kinds of interpersonal events, such as giving compliments or invitations, may depend on which person offered one last—regardless of the size of the interval. The exchange process may be detectable only if the sequence of the event, classes rather than their exact times of occurrence, is coded. Coding event start and stop times, as recommended previously, permit recoding for either interval or ordinal forms of analysis.

Multivariate Versus Univariate Events. Some events overlap. They are referred to as "*n*-tuples," with *n* referring to the number of categories simultaneously coded. Suppose we recorded when each participant in a conversation spoke and when each looked at the other. Within any arbitrarily defined time unit, at least four combinations of the two variables (2-tuple) could be recorded for each participant: the interval could contain neither looking nor talking, both looking and talking, only looking, or only talking. An example of this type of coding is the study by Jaffe, Stern, and Peery (1973) of the mother-infant relationship.

The number of possible states of an *n* multiply as one adds additional variables. For example, the addition of gesturing to looking and talking (a 3-tuple) would increase the number of possible combinations per interval to eight (two to the third power), and any additional binary category would double the possibilities again.

Some combinations may not make sense. For example, it may be irrelevant whether a person is gesturing or not while looking. Thus, separating looking into two types of 2-tuple subcategories may add noise or random error to the analysis of interpersonal effects. One might opt to instead code only meaningful combinations and ignore other combinations or collapse them into the most similar meaningful category.

Reclassifying Variables. The formation of *n*-tuples from coded event-time data is one of many ways that elementary event-time codes can be manipulated to construct more complex or more abstract variables. Reformulations may be done on on the basis of theoretical preferences or empirical evidence. Suppose we have coded a set of behaviors in terms of recommended start and stop times. Some investigators might recode the data into extended units consisting of all adjacent time units containing behavior of the same or similar type. For example, a series of discrete cries by a child might be collapsed into a single crying episode. Furthermore, a crying episode following by maternal soothing might be collapsed into a longer caregiving episode. Each level of complexity might be included as a separate variable if it seemed likely to have different social causes and effects.

The communicative functions of variations in length of extended units can be explored if the units are subclassified into multiple variables reflecting duration. Short and long crying episodes can be separate binary variables. This incorporates the advantages of continuous measures into a system of discrete measures.

Decisions about how to combine variables over time units can be based on consensual distinctions made by observers (e.g., Newtson, Engquist, and Bois, 1977) or by the application of statistical methods to coded data. One useful statistical basis is the log survivor function, which assesses discontinuities in the frequency distribution of interval sizes between sequential events (Fagen and Young, 1978; van Hooff, 1982). Such discontinuities indicate the presence of functionally different variables differentiated by timing rather than substance. For example, short intervals between cries may indicate breathing patterns, whereas larger intervals may reflect repetitions of unsatisfied efforts to gain attention.

Another statistical basis for segmenting temporally coded behavior is to test for significant repetitions, or runs, of the same class of event. Similarly, one can search for significant strings of behavior containing multiple classes of events within the same person. An example of a statistically detected string is the LEN response among monkey families (Bobbitt, Gourevitch, Miller, and Jenson, 1969) in which a particular combination of lip, eyebrow, and neck extensions occurred in sequence significantly more frequently than expected by random combinations. When this sequence was related to its social context it was found to occur in mothers when their infants had ventured beyond a safe distance. The LEN response increased the probability that the babies would return to close proximity.

There are many other possible bases for forming higher-order behavior categories from elementary ones. Differently named elementary behavior categories can be recorded into a single commonly named set on the basis of their theoretical connectedness or on evidence that they occur in similar contexts. One can define the higher-order units by applying logical operators such as "and" and "or" to the categories. The LEN response is an example of empirically derived "anding." An example of a combination of conceptually and empirically based "oring" is the category of coercive episodes studied by Patterson and Cobb (1971), containing whining, hitting, and other classes of "noxious" behavior that tended to have similar social antecedents and consequences.

The use of logical operators to redefine variables may affect sampling distributions (see the section on sampling issues further on). In recoding a limited body of elementary event data into complex configurations by "anding," data may run out quickly, resulting in too few events in the new category to permit reliable statistical analysis. On the other hand, the use of "oring" can increase the frequency of an event type that might otherwise occur too infrequently for analysis.

Reliability of Sequential Coding. In sequential studies, the computation of reliability of coding a variable should take account of the temporal level at which the variable is to be analyzed. If the effects of a behavior on what happens the next second are the area of interest, then it is important for the researcher to assess reliability within each 1 second interval. If the coding is reliable only within intervals of 5 seconds' duration, then the investigator could not determine the direction of relationships among variables separated by smaller time intervals.

Similarly, in relationships involving start and stop times of behaviors, reliability should be established for those features. If instead reliability is computed for occurrence of the behaviors within each time interval, it would be confounded with continuations between start and stop. The resulting reliability coefficient would be inflated in proportion of the average length of the behaviors.

Observer reliability on event occurrence tends to decrease with smaller time units. For example, in an analysis of adult conversations, agreement on duration (number of adjacent time units) of head nods by untrained observers was only 10 per cent if units of agreement were based on the same 0.1 second intervals, but agreement increased to 81 per cent as coding intervals were increased to 0.7 second (Rosenfeld, 1982, p. 223). With additional training, the range of percentages of agreement was raised to 21 to 98 per cent over the same increase in interval size. Similar results for the assessment of movements of various other body parts from filmed conversations were obtained by McDowall (1979).

Assessment of interobserver reliability for sequential data requires special attention to lining up multiple observational records so unintended displacements of temporal intervals can be adjusted. For suggested ways of dealing with this problem, and for recommended formulas for computing interobserver reliability for sequential data, such as the Kappa statistic, see Hollenbeck (1978), Gottmann (1979, 1980), and Reid (1970).

Selection of Analytic Model

After selection and sequential coding of a set of behaviors of interest, the problem becomes how to analyze interrelationships among them, both within and between participants in social settings. A variety of analytic alternatives is available. An ideal model would summarize the structure and dynamics of the system of relationships that our data represent.

Until the data have been analyzed, the best way to approach this ideal will remain unknown. For example, is it better to seek a complete but complex model of the data sequence or a simpler but incomplete model? Underlying these two extremes are two sets of choices. They are deterministic versus probabilistic relationships, and holistic versus piecemeal (e.g., bivariate) analysis.

Deterministic Versus Probabilistic Models. To accurately assess virtually all potentially relevant determinants of behaviors that must be explained the application of a "deterministic" model to the data—a model that specifies the conditions under which particular behavioral outcomes occur—becomes necessary. If all the relevant determinants cannot be assessed, a "probabilistic" model—one that specifies the degree of likelihood, ranging from 0.0 to 1.0, that an outcome would occur—can be used. The more comprehensive the assessment of relevant antecedents, the more the probabilistic model approaches a deterministic one; that is, the more the probabilities would approach the values of either 0 (no event will occur) or 1 (event will occur). However, considering the large number of overt and covert variables that affect communication, and the imprecision of the methods of measuring most of these variables, most statistics in the behavioral sciences assume a probabilistic model (see Hewes, 1980, and Remmers, 1985).

Holistic Versus Bivariate Models. A decision related to the choice of deterministic or probabilistic model is whether to attempt to analyze a whole communicative system at once or to study it piecemeal and then put the parts back together. The author prefers the holistic approach because of its greater likelihood of producing a representative model. But if many variables in the system exist, a comprehensive holistic analysis may result in a structure so complicated that it does not make sense.

At the other extreme, little difficulty is usually encountered in making sense of relationships between a pair of variables. But there is the risk that the relationship of the given pair is dependent on one or more additional variables. For example, a mother's reaction to her infant's vocalization may depend on whether or not the mother notices that the infant is oriented toward a particular object. If there are numerous complicated interrelationships within a network of variables analyzed as pairs, then it may be difficult to put them together in a comprehensible output model.

Although there is no way for a researcher to know in advance that he or she has selected the best method, each approach may offer insights complementary to the other. Intermediate approaches might also be selected. For example, sequential relationships between two variables can be compared when a third variable occurs in close proximity versus when the third variable is absent. More elaborate compromises include the search for longer chains of sequentially related behaviors (Altmann, 1965; Sackett, 1978), and the construction of holistic models that are probabilistic (Jaffe, 1970).

Sampling Issues

Statistical reliability increases as a function of size of sample. However, researchers accustomed to evoking high rates of a particular response category in an experimental setting may be surprised to find that many behaviors do not occur at high rates in naturalistic settings.

One way to deal with the problem of rarely occurring events is to extend the observation period. In a naturalistic study of intrafamiliar interactions, it was found that certain aggressive behaviors occurred about 1 per cent of the time; consequently, the investigators assessed behavior over more than ten thousand time intervals, averaging 6 seconds each, to obtain a sample sufficient for statistical analysis (Patterson and Cobb, 1971).

If researchers are more concerned with identifying the consequences than the antecedents of a particular class of behavior, they might choose to observe only those situations in which the given behavior has high probabilities of occurring. For example, children's aggression is more likely to occur in playgrounds than classrooms. However, the antecedents may differ in the two settings, which may in turn affect the consequences. See Figure 4–5 for an example of how rates of a variety of infant behaviors were affected by the intentional removal of toys and restriction of the mother's attention in research by the author.

Ethologically oriented researchers, who seek naturalistic evidence of evolutionary mechanisms, are often interested in compiling a complete list of behavior categories—an ethogram of the repertoire—for a particular species, including humans (e.g., see McGrew, 1972, for an ethological study of children at play). They provide formulas for estimating the probability than an increase in the number of observations will result in the appearance of additional categories of behavior (Fagen, 1978).

Another way to boost the rate of a category is to use the logical operator "or" to collapse different categories into one defined as containing Event Type A, Event Type B, or both. For example, brief vocalizations of the "mm-hmm" type and brief head nods tend to occur separately or together on the part of listeners during emphatic breaks in a speaker's utterance and to indicate attention (Rosenfeld, 1978). Thus the separate and combined occurrences might be combined into a larger category. On the other hand, the two kinds of response have also been found to communicate subtly different messages of approval and interest (Rosenfeld and McRoberts, 1979) that would not have been detected if premature collapsing of data had occurred.

To determine representative communicative habits of individuals, behaviors need to be sampled extensively within the same persons over time. Researchers who are accustomed to nonsequential research, in which they assess small amounts of behavior in each of many subjects, commonly fail to collect enough data within a communicative episode to permit reliable statistical analysis of behavior sequences. To test the generality of sequential relationships that characterize particular persons or dyads, data collection can be extended to additional sets of subjects and to other circumstances, and group statistics can be applied across the sets.

Measurement of Sequential Relationships

Sequential relationships between kinds of behavior can be measured in a variety of ways. If behavioral variables are continuous, a lag correlation coefficient is an informative measure. It describes the average strength of relationship between variables over the period sampled for any time lag of interest between occurrences of the variables (see Box and Jenkins, 1970; Gottman, 1981). If the variables are binary, a fundamental measure is the information statistic (see Losey, 1978; van Hooff, 1982). It describes, in terms of bits, the amount of uncertainty about the occurrence of one type of event that is reduced by knowledge of another type of event.

These measures of sequential relationships between behaviors should not be confused with other measures that summarize sequential patterns of behavior without directly assessing their interactive dynamics. Examples of the latter are the assessment of average differences in some behavior (e.g., conversational or physical dominance) between participants over their total interaction and trend functions reflecting change in a difference between participants over the period, (e.g., Hirsbrunner and Frey, in press). Such patterns can be used as dependent variables. For example, two cultures could be compared for the degree that they are organized by dominance hierarchies. Sequential analysis, in contrast, focuses on detection of dynamic effects within the temporal process. It models causal processes within social interaction rather than views the social interaction process itself as the outcome of other variables.

The most popular measure of sequential relationship between two categories of events is the "transitional probability." It refers to the probability that one type of event will occur given the prior occurrence of another. Thus, it is also referred to as a "conditional probability." Transitional probability is the basic relational measure in Markov chain analysis (see Breiman, 1969; Fagen and Young, 1978; Jaffe and Feldstein, 1970). Transitional probability also may be used in the closely related method of lag analysis (e.g., Sackett, 1978), in which the emphasis is on determining the time lag at which a given pair of discrete variables is related (whereas Markov chain analysis emphasizes the time lag that characterizes the relationships between all variables in a data set).

In the author's research on lag relationships (Rosenfeld and Remmers, 1981) relative frequency instead of transitional probability was used as a descriptive statistic. Relative frequency is the number of times that one type of event follows another. Relative frequency is an easier measure to visualize than transitional probability, and it is immediately informative about the number of replications of the lagged occurrences of paired events (see Fig. 4–2). The choice is a matter of preference. The measures are related to each other, and each has associated significance tests.

A transitional probability may be defined as the probability, on a scale of 0.0 to 1.0, that the occurrence of one type of event (A) will be followed by the occurrence of another type of event (B) at a specified time lag (k). Both events could be type A or B, but considering the focus on communication the A to B relationship will be emphasized, referring to the behaviors of two different persons.

Let us assume that events have been coded over a sequence of intervals and that the sequence represents a consistent underlying system—a stationary or steady state—in which particular probabilities remain the same throughout the entire sequence of data. (This assumption can be tested by comparing the given probabilities across different portions of the data sequence.) The probability of event A (pA) occurring in any interval is the frequency, or number of As (NA), divided by the number of intervals (NI); thus $pA = NA/NI$. Similarly, the probability of event B per interval is computed as $pB = NB/NI$. This measure may be thought of as the nontransitional or unconditional probability of the given event (A or B): its probability of occurrence without regard to what events precede it.

The transitional probability of B following A at a given lag of k intervals may be designated $p(B/A,k)$; see Remmers (1985). It may be defined as the number of AB pairs separated by the given lag of k time units (i.e., the lag frequency) divided by the number of As (the number of opportunities for an AB sequence to occur). Thus, the transitional probability of B following A in the next interval (lag $k = 1$) is $p(B/A, 1) = NAB/NA$. By comparing the transitional probability of B, i.e., $p(B/A,k)$, with its unconditional probability, pB, it can be seen how much the predictability of a B occurring is changed by having knowledge of whether or not it was preceded by an A.

Similarly, the obtained frequency of Bs at a given lag from A can be compared with the expected frequency of Bs at any lag from A, based on the assumption of no lag relationship (see Fig. 4–2). This expected frequency (FBe) can be computed by multiplying the probability of B per interval (NB/NI) by the number of As (NA) in the distribution: Thus $FBe = NA \times pB$.

Statistical Significance of Relationships. Assuming that a set of data consists of a randomly drawn sample of a population, the difference between the expected and observed probabilities (or frequencies) is evaluated in terms of the likelihood that a difference that large could have been due to variations in sampling from the same population. This is accomplished by computing the ratio of the difference to an estimate of sampling error.

Conventional parametric tests of the significance of differences in probabilities for nonsequential data are available in virtually all statistics books in the social sciences. But the assessment of significance for transitional probabilities requires some special adjustments, many of which have only recently been recognized. These adjustments are more thoroughly reviewed by Remmers (1985).

For example, adjustments must be made for the possibility that a sequential sample ends before the last occurring event A has an opportunity to be followed by an event B at some lag of interest (Remmers, 1985; Sackett, 1978). When As have no opportunity to be followed by Bs because of truncation of samples, their inclusion inflates the estimate of possible *AB* pairs. This problem can be resolved by reducing the number of *A*s in the formula for expected probabilities or frequencies of *B*s for lags at the truncated end of the distribution (Sackett, 1978), or if the data sample is long enough to permit the sacrificing of some data, the occurrence of events that happen less than the specified lag distance from the end of the distribution could simply be ignored (Rosenfeld and Remmers, 1981; Remmers, 1985).

It also has not always been recognized that expected (unconditional) probabilities of *B*s assessed from samples are not population probabilities. This requires the inclusion of an additional sampling error term in the formula for variance estimates (Allison and Liker, 1982). Such an error term was not included in most earlier formulas used for lag analysis (e.g., Bakeman and Dabbs, 1976; Sackett, 1978), but it was incorporated in the recent work of Gottman (1980).

Thus, Remmers (1985) recommends that the standard deviation of an expected lag frequency should be changed from the conventional formula

$$\mathrm{SD} = \sqrt{\mathrm{NA} \times \mathrm{pB} \times (1 - \mathrm{pB})}$$

to one that includes Sackett's (1978) suggested reduction of NA by the quantity $k \times pA$, and Allison and Liker's (1982) multiplication of pB by its error term, $1 - pA$. The resulting error term for testing the significance of the difference between an observed and an expected lag frequency as stated by Remmers is then

$$SD = \sqrt{(NA - k \times pA) \times pB \times (1 - pB) \times (1 - pA)}$$

Another issue is that transitional probabilities, being bound by 0 and 1, are not normally distributed. Thus, when sample probabilities are close to either of these limits the assumptions of normality underlying conventional parametric statistical tests may be violated. Allison and Liker (1982) offer a transformation of the probabilities that normalizes them.

Adjustments can also be made for small event samples that may result from rare occurrences or from construction of complex categories out of more elementary categories. Minimal event frequencies have been suggested for the appropriate use of the above normal-curve-based approximations of population parameters. For example, Hays (1963) suggests that the product of $NA \times pB$ and also $NA \times (1 - pB)$ should each be at least 10.

Otherwise, exact nonparametric tests based on the binomial distribution are more appropriate. Remmers (1985) offers the following form of the binomial formula to determine the probability that a frequency of

*B*s at least as large as that observed, $p(f \geq fo)$, at a given lag from *A*s could have occurred by chance:

$$p(f \geq fo) = 1 - \sum_{i=0}^{fo-1} \binom{NA}{i} \times (1 - pB)^{NA-i} \times pB^{i}$$

He also suggests that additional adjustments be made to this formula to deal with the issue of the sampling error of *pB* raised by Allison and Liker (1982) with regard to parametric tests.

In addition, Allison and Liker (1982) offer a useful statistical test that determines whether the difference between a transitional and non-transitional probability in one sample is significantly different from a comparable difference score in another sample. This test can answer questions such as, Do the effects of mothers on infants differ between cultures? Between developmental levels of the infants?

Other ways of computing the significance of sequential statistics are offered by Wampold and Margolin (1982). Their tests permit assessment of the significance of more complex transitions than were tested by the formulas just reviewed. For example, they can assess the significance of bidirectionality of relationship between event classes *A* and *B*, and they can simultaneously test for unidirectional significance of multiple transitional probabilities derived from a data sequence.

Many of the formulas given here are more complicated than conventional statistical tests. If they are to be applied frequently, and to large data sets, it would be wise to use computers. Some violations of assumptions might be tolerated in exploratory stages of research; in any case, the reader should be informed of the formulas that are used.

Order of Relationship. The number of time intervals (or the number of event intervals if ordinal coding is used) that characteristically separate sequentially related behaviors is referred to as the "order" of relationship. If the predictability of event *B* is greatest when it is the next event (or in the next coded interval) following event *A*, the relationship is designated first order. If event *B* usually occurs two intervals or events after event *A*, the relationship is second order, and so on.

In the application of Markov chain analysis to social interactional data, it has become conventional to summarize a network of sequentially related behaviors in terms of the highest order that significantly characterizes the relationships. Statistical techniques are available to determine if higher orders provide improved predictions over lower orders (e.g., see Jaffe and Feldstein, 1970). If the probabilities of next events are dependent on present events, then the relationship is at least first order. Then the first-order transitional probabilities can be multiplied over each two adjacent pairs of time intervals to determine the transitional probabilities at lag 2. The resulting probabilities can then be compared with the direct assessment of second-order (lag 2) transitional probabilities. If the latter provide significantly improved predictability, then the system of interrelationships is characterized as at least second order, and so on.

Many researchers who do transitional probability analyses of human social behavior assume that relationships are first order. Some do so on the basis of empirical evidence. Jaffe and Feldstein (1970) found that patterns of vocalization in conversations fit a first-order model and not second- through sixth-order models. Others hold to a first-order hypothesis in that they do not test for higher orders.

Many contemporary theories of human behavior emphasize immediate effects. For example, ethologists search for the immediate antecedent "causes" of behavior (McGrew, 1972), learning theorists look for immediate "reinforcers" as well as for antecedent stimulus control (Gewirtz, 1969), and pragmatically oriented linguists search for immediate "perlocutionary" consequences of utterances (Austin, 1962).

But higher-order relationships are likely to be found in these research domains, particularly as they come to deal with increasingly complex behavior sequences (Remmers, 1985; Rosenfeld and Remmers, 1981). For example, ethologists also look for more complex chains of behavior units within individuals that form characteristic "action patterns" and for future adaptive effects of these patterns. Indeed, Altmann (1965) found evidence for some third-order relationships among some behaviors in his study of primate communication.

In the application of learning principles to naturalistic observations of humans, Patterson and Cobb (1974; Patterson and Cobb, 1971) did not test for order, but they did report that the behavior-reinforcer sequence increased the probability of repetition of the behavior, which is potentially a second-order effect (see also Rosenfeld and Gunnell, in press). Cognitive learning theorists report evidence of delays in performance of new behaviors by observers of models until appropriate occasions for performance occur (Bandura, 1977), again implicating higher orders. Direct evidence of second-order question-answer-response sequences in natural conversations among adults was obtained by Brent and Sykes (1979).

Thus, it can be limiting to describe a set of interrelationships only in terms of the most characteristic order, although that be one useful summary statistic. A much more reasonable perspective is to anticipate relationships of different order between different variables as well as of multiple orders in relationships between the same variables. This is the perspective emphasized by lag analysis, in contrast to Markov analysis. For each pair of event classes, the order of relationship is assessed. It may be more difficult to integrate and interpret relationships among a set of variables that are interrelated at different orders, but it is also more informative. For examples of how different behaviors are related at different lags, see Figures 4–2, 4–3, and 4–4.

Filtering of Confounded Distributional Properties. A weakness in the methods reviewed for detecting lagged relationships between *A* and *B* is that they fail to consider that unassessed variations in the distribution of each of these variables can affect the meaning of the obtained relationships. In some cases an apparently meaningful causal relationship may be based on statistical artifacts. In other cases, more specific underlying causal processes are involved.

It has been noted that behaviors may cluster sequentially into repetitive episodes (bursts or clusters) of different lengths. One way to prevent hidden bursts in the data is to use a time unit small enough so only one event can occur within it. Significant bursting can then be detected by assessing the autolags of behaviors: the transitional probabilities of *A* to *A* and of *B* to *B*. When bursting occurs it is not clear from the conventional lag statistics if the effective determinant of a significant lagged relationship is due to the first occurrence, the last occurrence, the length, or some other structural property.

The possibility of redefining bursts into single extended units was noted. If the extended units are the actual causes of sequential relationships, then the inclusion of the separate components as separate events in a statistical analysis would inflate the frequencies of the variables. This could result in erroneous interpretations.

As a first step toward assessing differential effects of distributional properties of *A*s and *B*s, Remmers prepared a set of "filtering" statistics to be applied initially to Rosenfeld's mother-infant data sequences (Rosenfeld and Remmers, 1981). These statistical filters attend to various features of the distributions of *A*s and of *B*s in lag relationships.

To illustrate distributional problems that require disambiguation, Rosenfeld and Remmers (1981) invited comparison of the following three types of mother and infant behaviors:

1. M---I-M---I---M---I
2. M-M-I-M---I---M-MMI
3. MMM-III--MM--IIM--I

time: 123 . . . . *k*

Let us assume that each M and I entry represents the start of some class of behavior, that each start occurs in a separate interval, and that each series is representative of an indefinitely large population of sequential events. All three distributions suggest an effect of mother upon infant at a lag of four intervals. Yet very different processes are involved in the three series that would not be differentiated by the conventional lag analysis.

The first sequence is a straightforward example of the infant responding to individual mother events. In the second sequence, the infant responded to the first occurrences of repeated mother events but not to the intervening ones. In the third sequence the infant imitated the rhythm of repetition of the mother.

The conventional form of lag analysis is an unfiltered form in that any combinations of *A*s and *B*s can occur in the intervening intervals between a given *A* and a given *B* separated by a particular lag. The filtered forms described by Rosenfeld and Remmers (1981) place restrictions on the intervening behaviors. For example, their Type II analysis (illustrated in Fig. 4–4b) includes only those *AB* pairs at each lag in which *B* is the first *B*-event following *A*; thus, for example, in a lag 2 analysis of the string *ABB*, the second of the *AB* pairs would be excluded owing to the intervening *B*.

To compute the expected frequencies of *B*s at each lag by the filtering method, it is necessary to take account of the required nonoccurrences of specified events in the intervening intervals between *A* and *B* at each lag. In the example of a Type II filter applied at lag 2, it is necessary for the event "not *B*" to occur in the interval between *A* and *B* for these data to be included in the analysis. In the filter formulas the expected probabilities of *B*s decrease multiplicatively with greater lags from *A*, in contrast to the uniform expectancies per lag that characterized the conventional, unfiltered analysis (or Type I analysis) already reviewed.

For the Type II analysis the expected frequency of *B* is calculated by the following formula (Rosenfeld and Remmers, 1981):

$$f\,(Be) = NA \times (1 - pB)^{k-1} \times pB$$

where $(1 - pB)^{k-1} \times pB$ is the expected transitional probability of *B* given *A* at lag *k* (i.e., $p[B/A,k]$).

The statistical significance of the observed frequency of *B* at each lag may be tested by the same formulas used for the conventional lag analysis (the author's Type I) but with the substitution, for *pB*, of the transitional probability, $p(B/A,k)$, expected at each lag *k* under the null hypothesis. For example, the formula (1985) for the calculation from the binomial becomes

$$p(f \geq fo) = 1 - \sum_{i=0}^{fo-1} \binom{NA}{i} \times [1-(1-pB)^{k-1} \times pB]^{NA-i} \times [(1-pB)^{k-1} \times pB]^{i}$$

An additional filter (Type III) described by Rosenfeld and Remmers (1981) excludes the occurrence of additional *A*s between any *AB* pair; the filter Type IV excludes both extra *A*s and *B*s between an *AB*. An example is given later in this chapter of the use of Type II and IV filters (see Figs. 4–4b and 4–4c respectively) to disambiguate the interpretability of a relationship between behaviors of a mother and her infant for which multiply significant lags were detected by a conventional Type I lag analysis (see Fig. 4–4a). A formula for the Type IV analysis is given by Rosenfeld and Remmers (1981) and Remmers (1985). For Type II analysis the formula given in this chapter should be used.

Integrating and Presenting Results. In Markov chain analysis the transitional probabilities at a given lag are arranged in matrices in which the rows represent the first behavior and the columns the second behavior. These matrices can be rearranged into state transition diagrams, which are directed graphs indicating direction and strength of connection between event classes. For lag analysis the diagrams would further indicate the order at which each pair of variables was related.

The results of a deterministic sequential machine model, illustrated in the following section, are best comprehended when displayed in a state transition diagram (see Fig. 4–1), but in this case a "state" refers to a hypothetical variable that underlies changes in the relationship between *A* and *B* at different times rather than to the classes of behavior. Other measures are displayed in other formats. For example, the information statistic commonly is represented as a Venn diagram (van Hooff, 1982).

ILLUSTRATIVE DATA

This section illustrates the application of the methodological principles, using examples from the author's research on communication between mothers and infants (Rosenfeld, 1971, 1973; Young-Browne, 1972). A review of the application of two different sequential analytic methods to the coded data, a holistic "automaton" model and a bivariate "lag" model is included. Although enough systematic variations in the uses of the two models to permit a formal analysis of their relative merits were not performed in the study, a sense of the methodological usefulness of alternative choices in the application of each model can be obtained.

Basic Design, Sampling, and Coding Decisions

The primary purpose of the study (Rosenfeld and Remmers, 1981) was to determine the ability of different sequential analytic methods to elucidate the development of communication between mothers and infants. These goals affected the choice of research design, sampling strategies, and data coding procedures. To construct a causal model of the natural social interaction process, it was necessary to assess the natural sequence of infant and mother behaviors. A naturalistic study in which the mother and infant were free to initiate behavior and respond to each other, was chosen. The setting stimulated and supported behaviors representative of those in the participants' home environment; it permitted reliable assessment of behaviors that are likely to be involved in communicative development; and sufficient quantities of behavior were assessed to permit analysis of short-term and longer-term functions of a variety of behaviors.

The naturalistic setting was a laboratory simulation of a living room and nursery—a carpeted, furnished, well-lighted room including sofa and chairs, magazines, television set, pictures, mirror, infant seat, mobile, and manipulable toys. Unobtrusive observation of the participants' behavior was made from an adjacent room through a half-silvered mirror-window.

The developmental period selected for exploring communication within mother-infant pairs (dyads) was the second quarter of the infant's first year, during which evidence of specific "social attachments" most commonly appears (see Schaffer and Emerson, 1964; Bowlby, 1969). Through birth notices in a local newspaper, prospective mothers were contacted and asked to participate in a study of the development of infants. Of the five dyads who initially participated, two were able to attend with reasonable regularity throughout the requested 3 month period of the study. These two, referred to here as Dyad A and Dyad B, provided the data for most of our applications of sequential statistical methods.

Without knowing ahead of time what behaviors would occur at what rates during the course of the study, the determination of an adequate length and frequency of sessions for sequential analysis was a matter of guesswork. Practice sessions indicated that the optimal length was about 45 minutes. Dyads A and B each participated in a minimum of nine naturalistic sessions, which was thought to be enough to provide sufficient rates of a variety of interesting behaviors. We assumed that some communicative analyses could be done within single sessions, and that others that involved lower rate behaviors might be done by combining the data of adjacent sessions.

While the researchers observed practice sessions they also developed concerns about relying totally on naturalistic methods. Mothers would often use the available toys in the setting as a substitute for their own stimulation of the infants thereby limiting the proportion of time that social interaction occurred. Thus curiousity arose about how the kinds and rates of social behaviors observed reflected the behavioral capacities of the infant rather than limitations imposed by the social and physical environment. It was also noticed that infants sometimes seemed to induce the mothers to provide objects the infants might otherwise reach and manipulate themselves. Consequently, it was decided to add experimental probes to the naturalistic design to determine the effects of toys and the availability of the mother on the infant's social and solitary behaviors.

The final design was a mixture of naturalistic and experimental methods, with an emphasis on the former. It consisted of naturalistic (or baseline) sessions between which were interspersed additional sessions in which toys were absent or the mother was requested not to participate except in emergencies or in which both limitations were imposed. The resulting series of sessions for Dyads A and B are listed in Table 4-1.

Most of the sampling effort went into maximizing the likelihood of obtaining large samples of behavior within sessions to permit reliable assessment of communicative relationships within sessions. Secondarily, repetition of sessions at relatively short intervals to allow assessment of the emergence of changes in communicative relationships as well as longer-term stabilities was emphasized and sampling of individual or group differences was minimized. Thus the problem of determining the generality of application of any substantive results across social groups (e.g., socioeconomic and cultural), personalities, and other individual differences, was left for future studies.

The methods of collecting data were a combination of automated and observational. All sessions were videotaped, providing an automated audiovisual record. Most of the time a wide-angle lens and an omnidirectional microphone were used. These assured that the entire range of potential stimuli was recorded. However, it also meant that some detail was sacrificed. For example, the infant's orientation toward objects had to be based more on observations of videotaped head orientation than direction of gaze. More expensive alternative methods might have been to use multiple cameras to get higher-resolution closeups of focused mother-infant interaction or to get a three-dimensional rather than a two-dimensional record of the sphere of action (see Rosenfeld, 1982).

Observers of the videotaped records coded the behavior of participants for computer analysis of sequential relationships. Coding decisions were made on the basis of successive approximations and emerging consensus. Several observers reviewed practice tapes and recorded events likely to function as social stimuli. The researchers looked for categories of events that were meaningful on the basis of both prior research and personal experience and tried to define them in terms of the smallest size of unit that was likely to have an effect and that could be communicated clearly to other coders.

The code category system that emerged was comprehensive and molecular. It contained a large number of behavior categories, particularly nonverbal categories. The latter emphasis reflected biases of the principal investigator regarding the limited verbal capacities of the infant participants and the importance of nonverbal behavior in human com-

Table 4–1. Coded Mother-Infant Video Tapes

	Session	Age (in weeks, w, and days, d)	Condition*
Dyad A	1	12w–4d	Baseline
	2	14w–4d	Baseline
	3	15w–4d	Baseline
	4	17w–4d	Baseline
	5	19w–6d	No toys
	6	21w–4d	Baseline
	7	24w–4d	M ignores
	8	27w–5d	Baseline
	9	28w–3d	M ignores
	10	29w–2d	Baseline
	11	29w–4d	No toys, M ignores
	12	31w–3d	Baseline
	13	33w–3d	No toys
	14	34w–3d	Baseline
Dyad B	1	9w–4d	Baseline
	2	10w–4d	Baseline
	3	11w–4d	Baseline
	4	13w–1d	Baseline
	5	14w–4d	No toys
	6	16w–1d	Baseline
	7	17w–4d	M ignores
	8	18w–1d	Baseline
	9	18w–3d	No toys, M ignores
	10	24w–4d	Baseline
	11	26w–1d	M ignores
	12	26w–4d	Baseline
	13	27w–3d	No toys, M ignores
	14	28w–4d	Baseline
	15	29w–4d	No toys
	16	31w–4d	Baseline

*Sessions were approximately 45 minutes long and were naturalistic (Baseline) except when toys were absent (No toys) or mother (M) was asked not to respond to infant (M ignores).

munication in general. Other investigators might reasonably put greater emphasis on verbal contents.

The coding system was hierarchical, with the most general feature of behavior notated first and subcategories notated subsequently. The first symbol referred to the actor (mother or infant). The next symbols referred to basic categories (seven were included) and subcategories (26 included) of action in the visual, vocal, and kinesic realm (e.g., visually orienting toward objects; talking in animated or soothing tones; moving relative to objects by approaching, reaching, touching, and manipulating). The next symbol referred to objects of behavior, 26 included (e.g., a specific person, toy, or body part). Coding was discrete (versus continuous), with only the occurrence and nonoccurrence of each behavior noted. When assessments of variations in quantity or quality of a behavior seemed desirable, additional discrete categories were included; for example, gentle stimulation and rough stimulation were assessed as separate variables.

The other feature of each event was its time of occurrence. A half-second time interval was selected as a compromise between a time interval small enough to reveal meaningful changes in action and one large enough to permit reliable observational coding. A visible digital clock image was superimposed on duplicate copies of the videotapes, with time noted in half-second increments. Observers recorded the time intervals during which changes in behavior occurred. If an event lasted longer than one interval, the time at which it started was marked (with a +) and the time it stopped was marked (with a −). Momentary or single interval events were unmarked and were considered to represent both starts and stops.

Each event change was coded by time and category using brief alphabetical and numerical symbols that a computer could be programmed to analyze. For example the code "25 I1.E+" meant that in the 25th half-second time interval (i.e., 12.5 seconds into the session) the infant (I) started to look (1) at its mother (.E). As noted in the first part of this chapter, univariate events coded at this elementary level could later be combined in a variety of ways.

Table 4–2 lists several categories of events used in the statistical analyses along with the average number of times they occurred (started) per naturalistic session. Some of the examples refer to elementary coding; for example, mother looks at infant (M1)—the only object of her gaze that we included—and mother's vocal qualities, such as animated (M4A) and soothing (M4B). Other examples refer to combinations of elementary categories. For each category, a mnemonically based, four-letter acronym that is more communicative than the original codes was constructed; for instance, for mother looks (at infant) MVIS was used as an alternative to M1. Examples of higher-order categories are M4, or MVOC, a superordinate category that includes all vocalizations regardless of their quality, and M, or MANY, which includes any of the mother's actions regardless of content. Other higher-order categories were based on combinations of selected subcategories; for example, M4F-J, or MODD, combines a set of vocal oddities such as whistling or clicking sounds, and I4A,H, or IPOS, includes coos (I4A) or laughs (I4H), both of which may be hypothesized to represent a positive state. Note that as the "or" combinatorial categories become more inclusive, the frequencies of behavior increase, sometimes dramatically.

Although the small elementary time interval has the potential for highlighting quick and fleeting social effects as well as for assessing the effects of interval length, it also makes reliable coding more difficult. It is often difficult to detect the moment a bodily organ starts to move, even

Table 4–2. Mean Frequencies Per Session of Selected Behavioral Categories

Actor-Behavior	Code	Acronym	Mean Starts Per Session *Dyad A*	*Dyad B*
Mother (any act)[b]	M	MANY	512	200
Look at infant[a]	M1	MVIS	67	44
Vocalize[b]	M4	MVOC	283	91
Animated[a]	M4A	MANI	84	7
Soothing[a]	M4B	MSTH	12	2
Questioning[a]	M4E	MQST	98	52
Misc. Noise[c]	M4F–J	MODD	29	5
Move[b]	M3,5–7	MKIN	212	63
Move object[b]	M3	MSTM	86	21
Relocate Infant[b]	M5	MRLC	60	17
Touch infant[b]	M6	MTCH	86	21
Move self[b]	M7	MMOV	15	6
Infant (any act)[b]	I	IANY	345	260
Look at mother[a]	I1.E	IVIS	109	10
Look at toy[c]	I1.A, . . .	ITOY	38	39
Vocalize[b]	I4	IVOC	182	112
Positive[c]	I4A, H	IPOS	71	29
Ambiguous[c]	I4B,E	IAMB	79	75
Negative[c]	I4F,G	INEG	15	8
Move self[b]	I2	IMOV	23	9
Manipulate Object[b]	I3	IMNP	98	67

Note: Bases of categorization: a = elementary; b = superordinate; c = combinational "or." Entries are based on nonexperimental (Baseline) sessions: 9 for Dyad A, 10 for Dyad B (see Table 4–1). Other categories referred to in Chapter 4: MNON (absence of codable behavior by mother), ISLF (infant looks at own body), and MGTL and MRUF (gentle and rough subcategories of MSTM).

though observers agree that a discrete movement has occurred. Table 4–3 reveals some of the problems of reliability encountered in attempting to code behaviors at half-second intervals. For example, for the category MVIS (or M1: mother looks at infant), the first two coders had an 89 per cent agreement (Table 4–3, Column 1) on occurrences of the mother looking at her infant during the same half-second intervals. But when these coders attempted to determine the interval during which the mother initiated her gaze the agreement was only 47 per cent (Table 4–3, Column 4). It was difficult for coders to determine exactly when a gaze was initiated, but they had little problem recognizing its continuation.

If, however, a two-interval "window" was allowed, in which the start of a gaze was considered the same if the coders were within a one-interval lag of each other, the agreement on starts was raised to a creditable 84 per cent (Column 5 of Table 4–3). Although analyses of the start and stop data were based on half-second intervals, any effects might be sharpened if the interval size were increased.

It was noted earlier that percent agreement between coders is not a sufficient method of assessing reliability relative to more complex alter-

Table 4–3. Intercoder Reliability (% Agreement) on Occurrences of Temporal Features of Selected Mother and Infant Behaviors per Coding Condition

Feature:	**Interval Content**			**Start Interval**		
Interval Lag:	**0 (same 1/2 sec)**			**0**	**1**	**2**
Condition:	**Original**	**Transfer**	**Feedback**		**Original**	
Coders:	**1, 2**	**2, 3**			**1, 2**	
Categories:						
MVIS	89	97	—	47	84	84
$MSTM_j$	82	32	70	27	61	73
$MTCH_j$	70	86	—	30	67	85
$MMOV_j$	95	50	82	36	70	70
$MVOC_j$	83	35	80	36	79	86
IVIS	89	86	91	—	—	—
$IVOC_j$	83	40	75	—	—	—
MEAN:	84	61	80	35	72	80

Note: Interval lag refers to temporal lag in 1/2 second units permitted between coders for the same codes to be considered agreements; e.g., Lag 2 permits discrepancy up to 1 second. Category labels, identified in Table 4–2, are subscripted "j" here if agreement was based on subcategory contents (not shown here) as well as general category shown. Per cent agreement entries are based on the formula Number of occurrence-intervals agreed upon ÷ Number of occurrence intervals scored by either coder, × 100. Reliabilities of Coders 1 (author) and 2 (Virginia Stark) were computed after substantial collaboration in developing original written code definitions from practice videotapes. Subsequent Coder 3 (Margaret Hancks) initially used original written code (transfer condition) and then her revision of the code based on inspection of videotapes of discrepancies from Coder 2 (feedback condition).

natives such as the Kappa statistic. The major source of bias in the percentage agreement statistic is the inclusion of agreements on nonoccurrences as well as occurrences. For rarely occurring events, such as most of those assessed at the half-second level in this study, agreements on nonoccurrences tend to give an inflated estimate of reliability. However, the reliability statistics reported in Table 4–3 refer to agreements on occurrences; thus they should be free of this bias.

An additional problem of intercoder reliability is apparent in a comparison of the first two data columns of Table 4–3. When the coding system was used by a new coder, with only the written definitions provided by the original coders, there was poorer agreement with the original coders than the original coders had had with each other. Some variables such as the mother's looking at the infant (MVIS), and her subcategories (i) of touching the infant (MTCHi), retained high reliability with new coders. But other subcategories, such as the mother's ways of stimulating the infant (MSTMi), decreased in reliability.

When specific discrepancies between initial and later coders were reviewed on videotape, it was clear that the original coders had unknowingly shared some unwritten definitions with each other. When previously unwritten defining properties were then used explicitly by the new coder, reliability improved. For example, agreement on MSTMi increased from 32 to 70 per cent (Table 4–3, Column 3). This is another case of how an emerging consensus can contribute to the development of a coding system. It also demonstrates the advantage of analyzing data from a single trained coder.

Analytic Methods

A variety of analytic methods were tried on the same data set. This allowed the researchers to determine their relative abilities to generate interesting results, at least on their own data. Some analyses were applications to sequential data of conventional statistical methods used in nonsequential analyses. For example, data was factor analyzed (and the discovery was made that the thing an infant initiates most often in an elementary time interval is nothing). A nonparametric analysis of variance model was applied (and some interesting observations about the ways mothers unwittingly contribute to their infants' crying episodes were noted; see Young-Browne, 1972). An attempt was also made to determine how molecular coding of specific behaviors relates to the molar environmental force units coded by ecological psychologists (see Barker, 1963), but it was unsuccessful.

Extensions of methods specifically designed to reveal sequential relationships were most interesting. Allusions to the application of two very different analytic approaches to the analysis of the elementary data strings described have been made. The uses of the two approaches, referred to as "automaton" and "lag" models, can be differentiated in terms of methodological taxonomy. The essential difference between the models is that the automaton model is based on a holistic analysis of an entire data string, whereas the lag model is based upon bivariate relationships (two variables at a time).

Other differences were a matter of preference, guided by the researchers' desire to make the two approaches as different as possible. Thus, the version of the automaton model is deterministic, providing as full an historical account of events as the data set permits, whereas the lag analysis describes sequential relationships between pairs of behaviors probabilistically. Other differences involved the recoding of the elementary data string. The data set for the automaton analysis, compared with that for the lag analysis, included multivalued or n-tupled variables versus single-valued variables, extended units of behavior versus elementary units, and ordinal time (behavioral clock) versus interval time (mechanical clock).

Automaton Model. From a systems perspective, a human communicative act can be fully understood only in terms of the entire context that affects its occurrence. Adaptation of holistic field–theoretical concepts from physics to account for social-psychological events has had considerable appeal at the theoretical level but little effect at the empirical level. For example, the field theory of Lewin (1951) has been popular among social psychologists, yet Lewin's disciples tested his hypotheses by traditional experimental investigations of probabilistic relationships between two or three variables at a time (see studies in Cartwright and Zander, 1953). Another popular holistic perspective in contemporary research is the ethnolinguistic approach (e.g., Sacks, Schegloff, and Jefferson, 1974). It is more sophisticated in contextual comprehensiveness than in scientific methodology. Similar holistic approaches to the study of nonlinguistic aspects of communication have been proposed by Birdwhistell (1970) and Hall (1968).

Automaton theory offers sophisticated mathematical models for holistic-systems analysis of sequential events (e.g., Booth, 1967). With the encouragement of colleagues in the engineering sciences, Rosenfeld and Remmers (1981) decided to subject a lengthy string of comprehensively coded mother-infant data to an automaton analysis in the hope that the application of the model would reduce a complicated data set into a reasonably coherent systematic representation of the communication process. (The researchers did this with some trepidation, at one point considering that Einstein is reputed to have selected physics in preference to biological science as his area of study because he considered the latter to be too complicated (Clark, 1972, p. 34).

Automaton theory is a part of systems theory that deals with relationships between inputs, outputs, and states. At a psychological level we might view these terms as corresponding to the familiar concepts of stimuli, responses, and states of mind. Thus, when an infant is in a particular state of mind, a particular behavioral input from the mother results in a particular behavioral output from the input. For example, if the infant is in a rested state, animated talk by the mother may result in cooing by the infant; whereas if the infant is in a tired state the same input might result in crying. The automaton model adapted for analysis has the formidable-sounding title of a deterministic finite chain sequential machine (Booth, 1967). A brief mention of its use is reviewed here (see also Rosenfeld and Remmers, 1981).

Inasmuch as the researcher's dominant substantive goal was to understand the contribution of the mother to the social development of the infant, the initial task was to construct an infant machine. (It also is possible to construct a mother machine or even a dyad machine.) Thus the behaviors of mother were viewed as inputs, those of the infant as outputs, and the logically required internal processes of the infant that mediate the input-output relationships as states. A basic requisite for the analysis was that the behaviors of mother and infant be segmented into a chain of discrete acts: a sequence of input-output pairs. Initially, each of these input-output sequences is considered to represent a corresponding state. The task of the automaton program is to generate a simpler model of the data, one that contains the minimum number of states that allows an exact reproduction of the original input-output string.

To construct the requisite input-output sequence, the researchers first chose a set of mother and infant variables that seemed to represent a wide range of behaviors of communicative importance. Some of the behaviors were primitives in our coding system (such as mother looks at infant, and infant looks at mother); others were higher-order constructions. Most of the examples of variables shown in Table 4–2 were included. Altogether 22 mother behaviors (1 visual, 5 vocal, and 16 kinesic) and 23 infant behaviors (8 visual, 6 vocal, and 9 kinesic) were selected. Initial analysis was limited to the data from the first session of Dyad A.

Inasmuch as each of the variables was coded by start and stop times to the nearest half second, it was possible for multiple behaviors to occur by each participant during any given time interval. For example, the mother could simultaneously be looking at the infant, talking in a soothing voice, and jiggling a toy. But the automaton program required a single string of discrete events as the starting data. Thus co-occurring behaviors of mother and of infant in each interval were converted into multivariate events or *n*-tuples. If all mother behaviors occurred simultaneously, a 23-tuple would result; the infant could have up to a 22-tuple; and the dyad could have up to a 45-tuple. Fortunately, an interval containing larger than a 3-tuple per person, such as in the example just given, was rare.

To further simplify the data all adjacent dyadic *n*-tuples that had identical content were collapsed into single extended-unit *n*-tuples; that is, a multivariate act by either participant was considered to have continued until there was a change in action by either participant. Thus the initial fixed-interval sequence of approximately 5,000 half-second units in the session was reduced to a sequence of 1,197 extended units of variable length. In terms of a conceptual system clock time was transformed into behavioral time (without the researchers knowing whether or not this would contribute to the resulting model or detract from it). The resulting chain of extended-unit *n*-tupled behaviors contained 61 varieties of mother acts and 27 varieties of infant acts. These were distributed in a string of 1,197 mother-infant input-output sequences.

This string constituted the data to be processed by the automaton program. As noted earlier, each input-output pair in the data string initially was considered to correspond to a particular state. From a social-psychological perspective, it was initially assumed that each time the mother acted the infant was in a particular state, that the mother's act resulted in the subsequent infant act, and that the infant proceeded to the next state.

Figure 4–1a displays a simplified representation of an initial sequence of inputs, outputs, and states. In the figure, when the infant was in presumed State 1, the mother's failure to engage in any codable activity in the first extended unit (input of MNON, for nonactive) was followed by the infant's ambiguous vocalization (an output of IAMB) and by the infant's change to State 2. While the infant was in State 2, the mother's questioning voice (MQST) resulted in another instance of IAMB. By the time the infant reached State 4, physical stimulation by the mother (MSTM) resulted in crying by the infant (INEG). The entire original sequence met the requisites for the deterministic automaton in that when the infant was in any state, a given input resulted in only one kind of output. Otherwise the input-output relationship would have been probabilistic.

The automaton program reduced the number of states that were necessary to account for the original seuqence of input-output relationships. This required that the program search for strings of input-output relationships that did not violate the requirement that in a given state a particular input cannot lead to more than one kind of output. If a contradictory input-output relationship occurred, then a different state had to be presumed to precede it.

After trying out various alternative ways of collapsing input-output sequences into substrings that were compatible with single states, the researchers succeeded in reducing the original set of 1,197 states to 215 states. Using percentage of reduction of states as a summary statistic to reflect the amount of organization in the data that was detectable by the automaton program, an 82 per cent reduction in the complexity of the original data string was achieved. This reduction, however, could have been due to two sources of redundancy: that contained in the mother-infant relationship, which was of interest, and that contained within the data strings of each of the participants, which was not of any particular interest.

To estimate the amount of data reduction that was due to the within-participant redundancies, the automaton programs were rerun after removal of the opportunity for relational effects to occur. The mother-infant behavior sequence was halved, and within each half the order of either the mother or the infant behaviors was reversed. This procedure provided four sets of data in each of which the interpersonal structure had been removed while most of the within-person structure was retained. The average result of the automaton analysis of these four data sets was the reduction of the initial 1,197 states to 600 states. Thus, about 50 per cent of the total initial redundancy was attributable to the

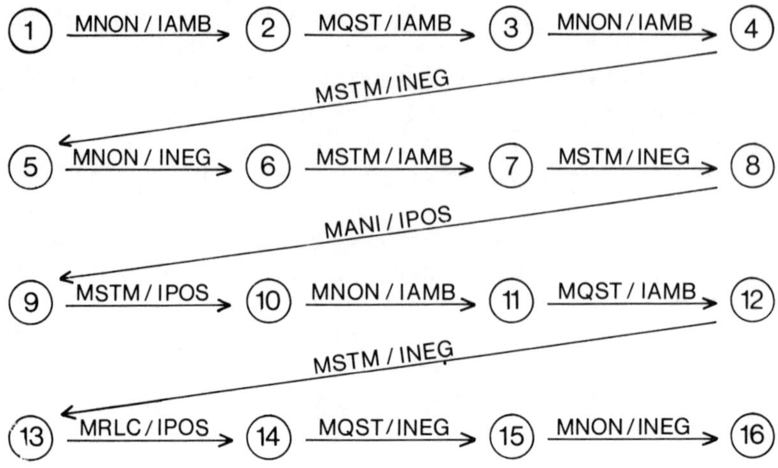

a Original sequence of inputs/outputs (mother-infant behaviors) and inferred states (numbered)

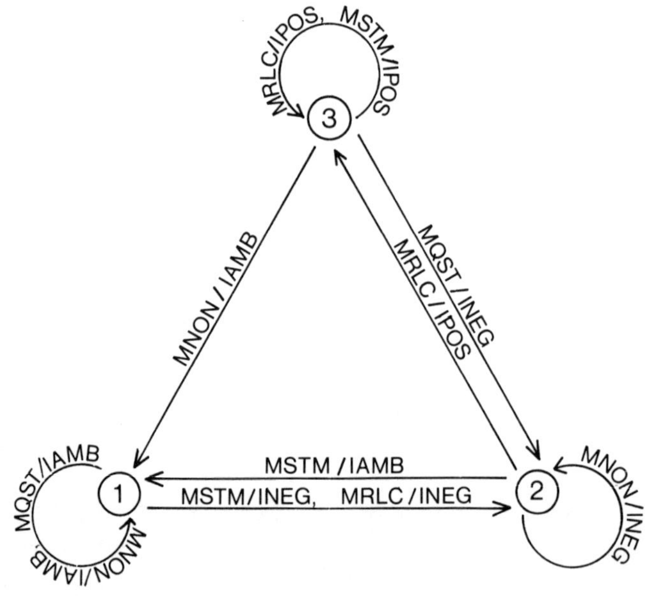

b Minimization of original sequence

Figure 4–1. Automaton representation of mother-infant interaction. (Fictitious simplification of deterministic chain sequential machine model reported by Rosenfeld and Remmers, 1981. Variables are identified in Table 4–2). From Rosenfeld, H. M., and Remmers, W. W. (1981). Searching for temporal relationships in mother-infant interactions. In B. L. Hoffer and R. N. St. Clair (Eds.), *Developmental kinesics: The emerging paradigm.* Baltimore: University Park Press.

structure within the sequences of behavior of each individual. Comparing this 600 state model with the original 215 state model, the amount of data reduction due to interpersonal structure would then be estimated to be about 64 per cent.

The amount of simplification of the original mother-infant data string by the automaton program was impressive, but the resulting data structure was still too complex to be interpreted. The minimized model, containing a network of 215 complexly connected states, each associated with a variety of input-output relationships, can be represented in two ways: matrix form and directed graph form. The graphic form tends to be easier to comprehend intuitively, although in the case at hand neither form made much sense. This does not make the model impractical. Major business organizations have been run profitably on models that nobody understands. Perhaps analogous practical applications could be made in interpersonal relationships. Yet one traditional criterion of a good theory is that in addition to allowing prediction and control it also must make good sense. An example of a comprehensible model is presented in Figure 4–1b, where a ficticious string of 16 mother-infant behavior sets is minimized into a three-state model.

Changes in research procedures should result in more interpretable automaton models of the mother-infant relationship. One recommended change would be to rely less on the computer and more on our own intuition in selecting variables for the input string. It is likely that many of the *n*-tuples that emerged from sequential segmentation of the multivariate behaviors coded were not functional. For example, a mother may sooth an upset infant by picking it up regardless of whether or not the mother simultaneously is speaking, is making odd vocal sounds, or is silent. If each of these pairs (2-tuples) is a separate type of behavior, their separation may add unnecessary complexity to the analysis.

Other sources of error may be attributable to the original data set. Many observable behavior categories that were involved in mother-infant interactions were not included. Also, few researchers would argue that all of the relevant determinants of an individual's behavior in a social setting are located in observable actions. Physiological and cognitive variables, not to mention potentially communicative variables such as olfactory stimulation, also contribute. In addition, much error undoubtedly remains in systems of measurement, as shown by imperfect reliability coefficients within and between observers. Measurement error also occurs within automated measuring devices (see Rosenfeld, 1982). Thus, efforts at comprehensive measurement fall short of the completeness and accuracy of assessment that is required for a deterministic model.

One solution is to use an automaton with probabilistic connections between inputs and outputs per state, between state transitions, or both. A smaller variety of behaviors may also help simplify a probabilistic automaton model. For an example of a probabilistic automaton model applied to sequences of vocalization and silence in adult dyads, see Jaffe (1970). For a Markov chain (probabilistic, nonsystems) model of the same kind of data also see Jaffe and Feldstein (1970).

Although the author and co-worker Remmers discontinued automaton models in favor of the bivariate lag model to be described next, their potential advantages should not be overlooked. Most analyses of interpersonal behavior sequences assume that relationships between behaviors reflect a "steady state" over the course of an observation period; thus, an assessment is usually made of the average probability or strength of relationship. Greater attention to possible shorter-term changes in state that affect the probability or strength of a social effect may lead to more accurate models.

Lag Model. In contrast to the automaton analysis, bivariate lag analysis allows a breakdown of the complexity of interpersonal relationships into subparts that tend to be much easier to comprehend. Thus bivariate methods have been the dominant form for social and behavioral scientists. In this section some of Rosenfeld and Remmers' more informative experiences (1981) in the use of bivariate lag analysis are reviewed. In addition to considering relationships between only two variables at at time, the bivariate approach was further simplified in contrast to the aforementioned automaton approach by considering the relationships to be probabilistic rather than deterministic.

Initially, preliminary evidence indicating which of the many variables assessed were most likely to be involved in lag relationships was sought. Chi-square statistics were used to see which pairs of behaviors tended to occur mutually beyond randomly expected levels within 4 second intervals. This is referred to as an approximate co-occurrence analysis in that it did not allow identification of the precise ways the behaviors were related within or between intervals. Contrary to expectations, the approximate co-occurrence analysis did not consistently identify variables that proved to be of communicative significance in subsequent precise lag analyses. A review of the approximate analysis will highlight the advantages of the lag analysis.

The data were segmented by computer into a series of 4 second time intervals. Using a 4 second interval resulted in 675 intervals to be analyzed in a 45 minute session (15 per minute times 45 minutes). Each behavior of interest was said to "occur" if it was present during the interval and to "not occur" if it was not present. An occurrence of an event within an interval could be a start, a stop, a continuation, or any combination of these. For a pair of variables, the frequency distribution of all possible simultaneous combinations in intervals could be set up in a two-by-two matrix. Occurrence and nonoccurrence of one variable are the column categories, and occurrence and nonoccurrence of the other variable are the row categories. Thus, in any interval of the data string, four combinations of two variables were possible: Both occur, neither occurs, only the one occurs, and only the other occurs.

The frequencies in each of these four cells were compared with the frequencies expected if the variables were unrelated (using the marginals in the conventional chi-square formula). If the co-occurrence was significantly greater than expected, the pair of variables were candidates for sequential analysis. The researchers' interests at this point were heuristic—to seek promising variables—rather than confirmatory. Likely violations of the chi-square statistic resulting from lack of independence of events across intervals, were ignored (e.g., continuation of the same event across intervals).

Table 4–4 summarizes the co-occurrence analysis for relationships between nine mother and six infant behavior categories that occurred enough in multiple sessions in Dyad A and Dyad B to permit application of the chi-square statistic. Entries in the cells of Table 4–4 show the number of baseline (nonmanipulated) sessions in which a pair of behavior categories was related. The criterion of relationship was a chi-square value of 3.8 or greater, which is significant at the $p < .05$ level (two tails, one degree of freedom). In addition, the entries show whether the relationships were positive (designated by a plus sign), reflecting co-occurrence significantly above chance, or negative (designated by a minus sign), indicating that when one variable was present the other tended to be absent.

Some general inferences about mother-infant relationships can be drawn from Table 4–4. For example, mother and infant regularly gazed at each other within the 4 second interval framework. The infant's gaze (IVIS) usually was associated with the mother's use of animated and odd voices, less so with her questioning, and not at all with her soothing voice. The mother's gaze usually was positively associated with the infant's attention to toys but less often with the infant's voice. Few associations occurred between mother and infant vocalization categories, an exception being the positive association of mother's soothing voice with infant's negative voice (crying, fussing) in Dyad A and with infant's ambivalent voice in Dyad B.

Let us assume that the "significant" positive associations between mother and infant behaviors detected by the heuristic procedures were indicative of real relationships. A variety of patterns of connections between the behaviors could underlie the associations, allowing a corresponding variety of alternative causal inferences. Did the mother's behavior cause (or at least precede) the infant's behavior? Or was the infant the cause the mother's behavior? Or did they alternatively effect each other? Or did they simultaneously occur, perhaps as the result of some

Table 4–4. Number of Baseline Sessions With Significant Associations Between Mother and Infant Behaviors within 4 Second Intervals

Mother's Behavior		Dyad	Infant's Behavior					
			Visual			*Vocal*		*Kinesic*
			IVIS	*ITOY*	*IPOS*	*IAMB*	*INEG*	*IMNP*
Visual	MVIS	A	8+	7(+)	3(+)	0	3(+)	4
		B	7+	6(+)	3+	5(+)	3(+)	3+
Vocal	MQST	A	3+	5−	2+	2−	2+	4−
		B	5+	3+	1−	1−	2	4(−)
	MANI	A	6+	4(−)	2+	2−	2−	3(−)
		B	6+	3(+)	1+	1−	1+	1+
	MODD	A	9+	5−	3+	0	1−	5−
		B	5+	2−	4−	5+	1−	0
	MSTH	A	1+	3−	1−	0	6+	2−
		B	1+	0	0	6+	1−	0
Kinesic	MSTM	A	6(−)	4+	5(−)	1−	4(−)	2−
		B	2+	7+	1−	3−	1−	1+
	MGTL	A	4(+)	8(−)	3(+)	2−	3+	4
		B	1−	5(+)	1+	0	1+	1+
	MRUF	A	8+	5−	3+	0	0	3−
		B	2−	1+	1−	2	1−	3+
	MRLC	A	1−	6(−)	2−	1+	6+	6−
		B	1+	3+	1+	1+	0	1−

Note: Entries are the numbers of baseline sessions for Dyad A and Dyad B in which occurrences of the paired behaviors were associated at a chi-square value of ≥ 3.8 (p = .05 for 1 degrees of freedom). Signs indicate "direction" of association in the combination "M occurs and I occurs": + indicates mutual occurrence was consistently above expected level, and − indicates it was consistently below expected level in all the significant sessions. ( ) indicates the dominant direction of inconsistent results across sessions. Behavior categories are defined in Table 4–2.

other event? If any of these causal possibilities were true, were the relationships based upon starts of the behavior? Upon stops? Were relationships dependent on particular time lags within the 4 second periods? Were there effective lags greater than 4 seconds, which might have resulted in negative associations or no associations between the behaviors when using the 4 second intervals?

It was noted in the earlier section on analysis of sequential relationships that lag statistics are capable of discriminating between a variety of causal interpretations that may be confounded in nonsequential methods, such as the aforementioned co-occurrence analysis. Most fundamentally, lag statistics have the capacity to reveal direction of relationship. Lag analysis also has some advantages over the most popular sequential statistic, Markov chain analysis. The latter emphasizes first-order (lag 1) relationships in particular and fixed-order relationships in a network of variables otherwise. Lag analysis, in contrast, is oriented toward finding the orders or lags that best characterize relationships between each pair of variables in a network. Even conventional uses of lag statistics can be improved upon. In particular, a new set of improved lag statistics that filter out selected distributional properties, thereby permitting tests of alternative explanations of a given lag relationship, have been offered.

The conventional statistic used to describe the strength of sequential relationship between a pair of variables is the transitional probability $p(B/A)$. This is the statistic used in Markov chain analysis, which emphasizes lag 1. For lag analysis of mother-infant communication, the statistic is more properly written $p(M/I,k)$ or $p(I/M,k)$ indicating directional effects at each of k lag intervals of infant on mother and of mother on infant, respectively.

The set of k lagged relationships between a pair of behaviors was described in the form of a histogram of relative frequencies rather than as probabilities. Frequencies are more informative of the number of replications of a lagged event that are involved in a relationship, and they are easier to visualize than are probabilities.

The researchers also chose to separate the variables by clock time rather than by behavior time, in contrast to the automaton analysis. The time unit selected was the elementary one-half second interval at which the data initially were coded. This choice lent assurance that in any time interval only one occurrence of a type of behavior could occur, thereby preventing different numbers of sequential repetitions of one participant's behavior from having confounded effects on the occurrence of the other participant's behavior. The behaviors analyzed were only in the form of starts or stops (not continuations). This choice assured that the same event could not be represented in more than one interval, thereby preventing the inflation of frequencies in statistical analysis.

The number of temporal intervals, k, between a pair of variables for which lag relationships were computed was set at 30 in the examples. One practical reason was that description of lag frequencies over 30 intervals happened to fit conveniently on computer output sheets. In addition, it was believed that enough relationships of interest were likely to occur within 15 seconds (30 half-second intervals) to justify that selection.

A bivariate lag analysis on data from mother-infant Dyad A—our more active pair of subjects—was performed. By limiting the definitions of behaviors to starts and stops and ignoring continuations between them, the researchers found that the number of behaviors per session was substantially lower than was the case for the prior analysis of approximate co-occurrences. To maximize the frequency distributions of behaviors for statistical purposes, data from the eight baseline sessions were combined. This resulted in a total of 35,229 elementary time units.

For the initial lag analysis relationships between mother and infant behaviors at three hierarchical levels were inspected. First each participant's behaviors were collapsed into one general category—mother behaves (M or MANY) and infant behaves (I or IANY)—and these two high frequency categories were tested for lag relationships. Then each participant's behaviors were subdivided into three major categories of visual orientation to the other participant (MVIS and IVIS), vocal activity (MVOC and IVOC), and kinesic activity (MKIN and IKIN). These too were tested for lag relationships. Note that the vocal categories and the mother's kinesic category were combinations of the subcategories used in the approximate co-occurrence analysis summarized in Table 4–3. Finally, relationships among those vocal subcategories that had sufficient frequency distributions for statistical analysis were studied. These were the mother's questioning (MQST), animated (MANI) and soothing (MSTH) voices, and the infant's positive (IPOS), ambivalent (IAMB), and negative (INEG) voices.

For each ordered pair of behaviors, the computer printed out a frequency histogram of occurrences of the second category of behavior across the first 30 half-second intervals following occurrences of the first category of behavior. A conventional type (Type I) of lag analysis was performed initially, allowing all occurrences of each category of behavior to be included in the analysis (including runs or clusters of starts of the same behavior.) For current purposes (the efficient production of illustrative data) the significance between expected and obtained lag frequencies using the normal curve approximation statistics rather than exact statistics was tested. In addition, the uncorrected variance term $NA \times p(B) \times p(1 - B)$ was used rather than the more elaborate corrected version that further accounts for truncation of the B distribution and sampling variation of $p(B)$. However, more recent computer programs incorporate the statistical corrections and automatically switch to exact statistics when needed to meet assumptions (Remmers, 1985).

Examples of the output of the lag program are presented in Figure 4–2. Three of the four possible interpersonal relationships between starts and stops of the behaviors IVOC and MVOC are shown (not included is the effect of mother stops on infant stops, for which no significant results were obtained). In the illustrations starts are inferred, unless stops are explicitly identified.

First, note the distribution of effects of IVOC on MVOC. The histogram is elevated above the .05 significance level at lags 2, 3, and 4 only, with the largest effect at lag 3 ($p < .0001$). This is an ideal distribution for interpretation in that the elevations on both sides of the most significant lag indicate some random error in the effective size of lag. If only lag 3 were elevated, suspicions might be raised on the assumption that the mother is unlikely to have an internal clock that counts lags to the exact half second. Some error is particularly likely in that the boundaries of the half-second intervals are arbitrarily located in time (see Rosenfeld,

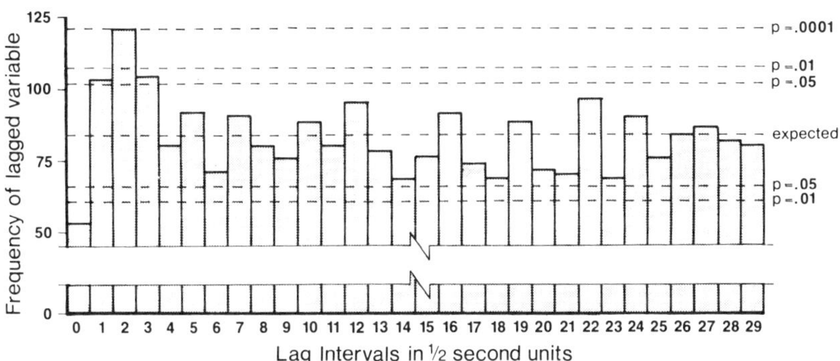

a Infant vocalizing followed by mother vocalizing (IVOC→MVOC)

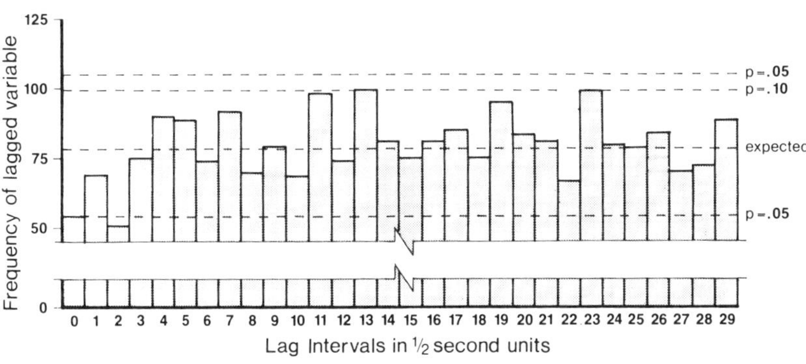

b Mother vocalizing followed by infant vocalizing (MVOC→IVOC)

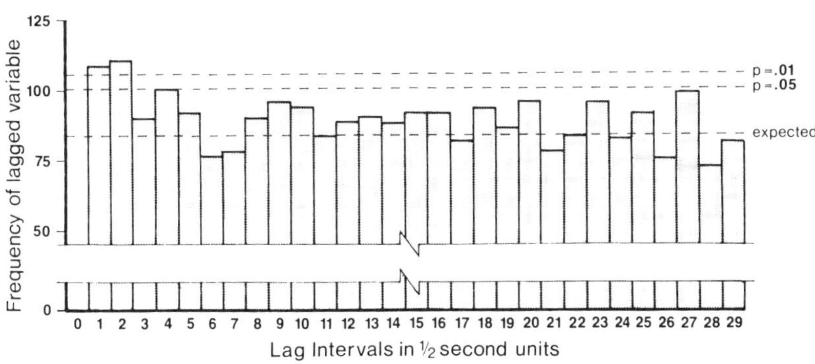

c Mother stops vocalizing followed by infant vocalizing (MVOC, stop → IVOC)

Figure 4–2. Lag histograms showing significant temporal relationships between vocalizations of mother and infant in Dyad A (first interval shows co-occurrence or zero lag).

1981). It would be even more suspicious given the relatively high errors of measurement found when using such a small interval. Thus this first histogram can reasonably be interpreted to indicate that when the infant initiates vocalization, the mother typically replies vocally an average of 1.0 second later and within the range of 0.5 to 1.5 second.

The next histogram in Figure 4–2 shows the reverse relationship: the effect of MVOC on IVOC. In this case none of the lag frequencies is elevated beyond the .10 level of significance. No other general pattern is evident, other than a possible tendency toward suppression of simultaneous responding. This tendency occurs in all of the vocal histograms and might be due to difficulties, and thus errors, in separating two voices from a monophonic recording. Thus, the relationship between vocalizations is unidirectional; mother replies to infant, but infant does not reply to mother—at least within the 15 second lag period we inspected.

The final histogram in Figure 4–2 assesses the effect of the mother's termination of speech (MVOC stop) on the initiation of infant speech (IVOC). Here, the most significant elevations are found at lags 1 and 2 ($p < .01$). Two other lags, lag 4 and lag 28, reach the .05 level, but given their isolation the researchers are reluctant to consider them as representing more than random error. Certainly the most justified interpretation of this histogram is that when the mother stops talking, the infant replies from 0.5 to 1.5 seconds later.

Considered as a whole, the set of histograms in Figure 4–2 supports a simple model of the relationship between vocalizations of mother and infant. They tend to engage in a form of turn-taking but the mother responds to the initiation of the infant's utterance and the infant responds to the termination of the mother's utterance. From an adult perspective the infant engages in the more polite conversational behavior in that he waits for his mother to finish her utterance before replying, and additionally, he leaves only a minimal pause between speaking turns (see Rosenfeld, 1978, for a review of vocal turn-taking conventions).

There is speculation, however, that from an infant's perspective the mother's speech evokes an alerting response that temporarily inhibits his or her tendency to vocalize. Still, the infant's elevation of speech following mother's termination suggests the emergence of rudimentary turn-taking. If greater amounts of data had been collected by observation of longer or more frequent sessions, it would have been possible to search for developmental changes in the infant's vocal participation patterns by comparing the size of significant lags across samples. Whatever the answer to these additional questions, it is already clear that the lag analysis of vocalizations gives much more precise model of vocal interaction between the mother and infant than was provided by the earlier nonlag analysis.

By applying similar procedures and interpretations to the lag relationships between the full set of visual, vocal, and kinesic behaviors of mother and infant, the more elaborate model displayed at the top of Figure 4-3 was constructed. It includes both a graphic and linear representation of the vocal interchanges discussed above. Direction of significant effects is shown by arrows connecting behavior codes, and the first significant lag, or else the average of the first cluster of significant lags, is marked to the nearest half second.

In the earlier analysis of approximate co-occurrences consistent evidence that mother and infant gazed at the other sometime within a 4 second interval was found. The present lag analysis supports the conclusion that the infant returned the initiation of the mother's gaze at a 0.5 second lag but that the mother was nonresponsive to the initiation of the infant's gaze. Furthermore, the infant looked at the mother 1.0 second after she initiated vocalization.

Although it is possible that the infant detected the direction of the mother's gaze by peripheral vision, it is more likely that the mother's vocalization was the effective stimulus for his gazing toward her. Perhaps the mother followed her initiation of speech with gaze about a half second later, an hypothesis that could be tested by assessment of the lag relationship between the two mothers' behaviors. If so, the infant's visual response may have been stimulated by the mother's speech component at a 1 second lag rather than to the gaze at a half-second lag. The infant's visual reply to the mother's vocal-visual initiation is an additional indicator of the performance of a normative form of adult conversational participation (Rosenfeld, 1978); the first indicator was the infant's reply to the mother's termination of utterance.

The MVOC and IVIS behaviors were initiated enough in Dyad A (see average frequencies in Table 4-2) to permit statistical analysis of lag relationships in individual sessions. This allowed us to look for developmental trends. Significant lag effects of MVOC and IVIS were found in five of the nonexperimental sessions. A developmental trend appeared over the first three sessions, with the first significant lag appearing at 2.5, 2.0, and 1.5 seconds respectively. However, in the fourth session the significant lag was 4 seconds. The remaining significant lag, occurring in the seventh nonexperimental session, was at 1.0 second.

Finally, the skeletal actions of mother (MKIN) and infant (IKIN) tended to co-occur but showed no lag relationships. Thus, mother and infant tended to be physically active at the same time, but movements per se did not appear to serve as significant social stimuli to the participants.

At the bottom of Figure 4-3 a model is presented of the pattern of lag relationships among the vocal subcategories of infant and mother.

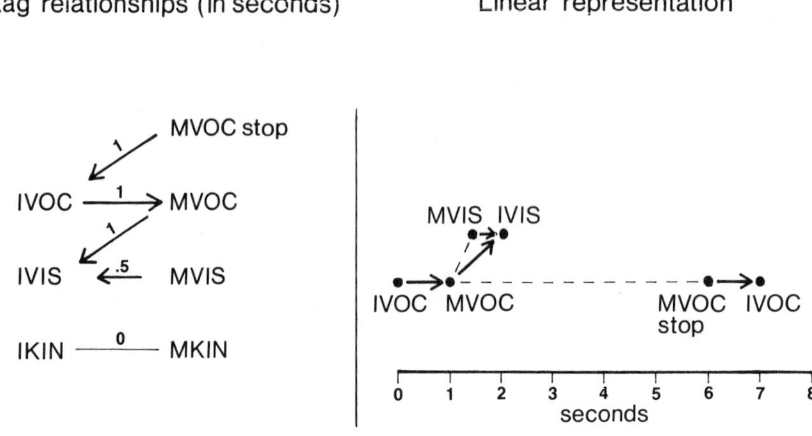

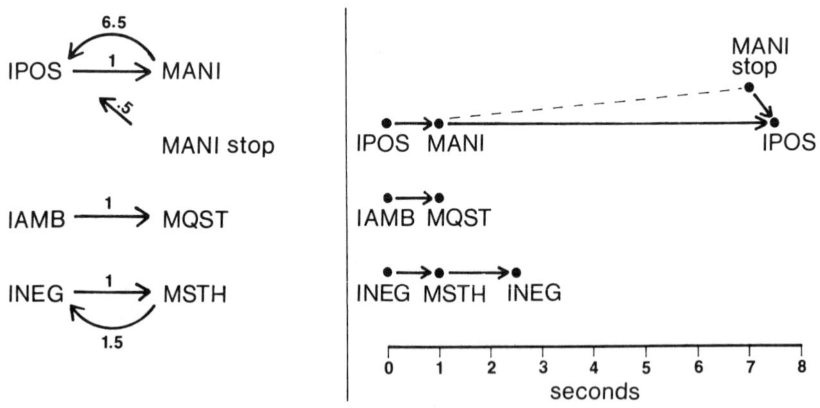

Figure 4–3. Graphic representations of significant lag relationships between mother and infant behaviors in Dyad A at two levels of specificity. (Solid lines show first lag significant at .01 level. Arrow shows direction of relationship. Dotted lines show implicit intrapersonal lags. Variables are identified in Table 4–2.)

This model provides refinements to the aforementioned lag analysis of undifferentiated vocalizations. Each of the three significantly related pairs of behaviors retained the 1 second lag from infant vocalization to mother vocalization. However, each of the three maternal vocal categories was related to a different infant vocal category.

Mother's animated voice only followed infant's positive voice. In addition, infant's positive voice followed mother's animated voice but at a 6.5 second lag. The latter effect was disambiguated by the further finding that the infant's positive voice followed termination of the mother's animated voice at a 0.5 second lag. The final piece of the puzzle fell into place when it was further found that the typical duration of mother's animated utterances was between 5 and 6 seconds. Thus, the infant waited for his mother to finish her vigorously inflected sentences (MANI stop) before cooing or babbling (IPOS) in reply.

Ambivalent-sounding infant vocalizations (IAMB: grunts or irritated-sounding coos) resulted in questions by the mother (MQST: the content usually indicating a concern or an hypothesis regarding the infant's welfare). But unlike the above reciprocal effect of MANI or IPOS, MQST did not result in IAMB.

Finally, negative infant vocalizations (INEG: fussing or crying) resulted in utterances by the mother that were soothing (MSTH) in both tone and content; and in addition MSTH was followed by INEG at a 1.5 second lag. The last result indicates that the mother's efforts at improving the infant's negative state were ineffective, at least in the short run (see Young-Browne, 1972, for a dedicated analysis of types of maternal determinants of infant crying in our two dyads, based on more conventional nonlag statistical methods). The lag analysis reported here was not complete enough to determine whether the mother's attempts at soothing actually exacerbated the infant's negative state or whether they temporarily interrupted an ongoing negative mood (see Bloom, 1977, and Kaye, 1977, for studies that have teased out evidence to distinguish between maternal interruptions and maternal effects on infant behavior).

This demonstration of the uses of bivariate lag analysis will conclude with an example of an application of Remmers' distributional filter statistics (Remmers, 1985; Rosenfeld and Remmers, 1981). Distributional filter statistics were developed for disambiguating the confounded contributions of isolated versus sequentially clustered occurrences of a type of behavior on the lag relationships detected by the conventional lag procedures such as those described before.

The filter programs were applied to the analysis of the previously discussed lag effect of MVOC on IVIS in Dyad A for the seventh nonexperimental session, at which time the infant was 29 weeks. The analysis was described by Rosenfeld and Remmers (1981). Earlier in the chapter a corrected version of the formula for the Type II filter was provided. The histograms in Figure 4–4, showing the results of the filter analysis, include some simplifications and other minor changes in format compared with those presented in the prior report.

The three kinds of analysis shown in Figure 4–4 are based on exact statistical tests, which are appropriate to the small samples representing a single session, rather than on the normal curve approximations used in the preceding analysis of combined sessions. The first interval shown in each histogram represents co-occurrence or no lag and the next 28 intervals show increments of 0.5 second. Figure 4–4a shows the conventional lag histogram (Type I) of the sequence MVOC preceding IVIS. Highly significant lag relationships ($p < .005$) were found at intervals 3 and 4 (1 and 1.5 second lags) and at interval 23 (11 seconds), with a weaker effect ($p = .035$) at interval 16 (7.5 seconds).

Our Type II and Type IV lag analyses were added to test the validity of several possible confounded interpretations of the significant lag relationships found in the conventional analysis. These additional filtering programs excluded pairs of behaviors if they contained certain intervening events. By comparing the results of the filtered analyses with those of the conventional (unfiltered) analysis, it is possible to assess the contribution of clustering of the variables to lag relationships. It should be recalled that in the filtered analyses, unlike the conventional analysis, the larger the lag the lower is the expected probability of occurrence. This is because increasing strings of nonoccurrences of an event are required in the calculations.

The first filtering program (Type II in Rosenfeld and Remmers, 1981) retained for analysis only the first occurrence of IVIS after any occurrence of MVOC. That is, in contrast to the conventional analysis, it excluded all repetitions of IVIS (subsequent occurrences of IVIS not preceded by a MVOC). The result, shown in Figure 4–4b, was that all four of the lag relationships that had been detected by the conventional analysis remained significant. Thus the significant lags could not be accounted for by clustering of IVIS behaviors.

The second filtering program, using the Type IV formula in Rosenfeld and Remmers (1981), eliminated not only repetitions of IVIS but also repetitions of MVOC. It retained for analysis only pairs in which neither variable was repeated in between. In the resulting histogram, shown in Figure 4–4c, the significant effects previously found at intervals 3 and 4 were upheld but there were no longer any significant effects at intervals 16 and 23. Thus the larger lags detected by the conventional analysis were attributable to repetitions of the MVOC variable.

On the basis of the results of the three kinds of lag analysis, the best supported conclusion regarding the relationship between the behaviors is that the mother's utterance typically evoked the infant's visual attention after about a 1 second lag. Further refinement of the description of the

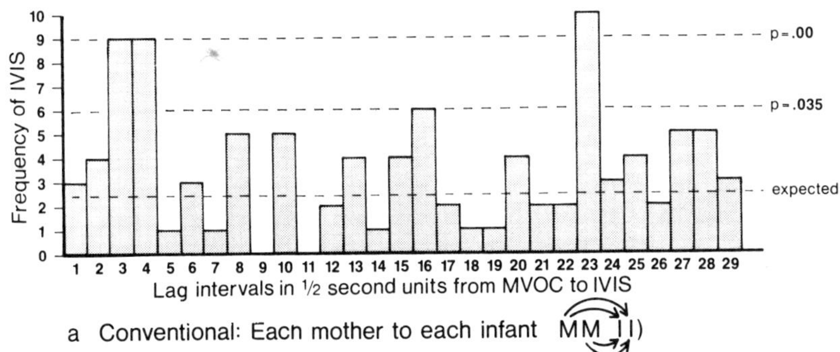

a Conventional: Each mother to each infant (MM II)

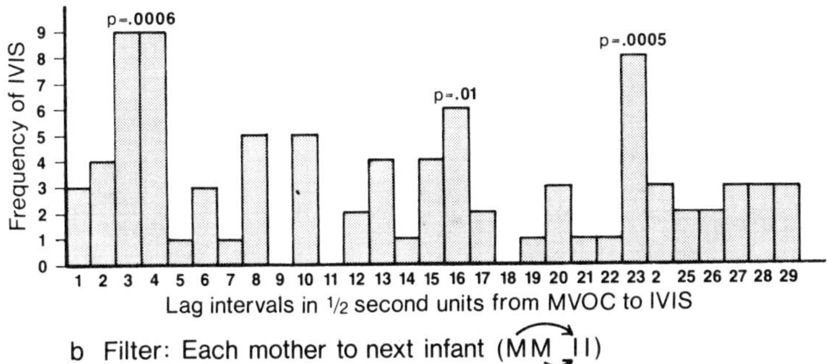

b Filter: Each mother to next infant (MM II)

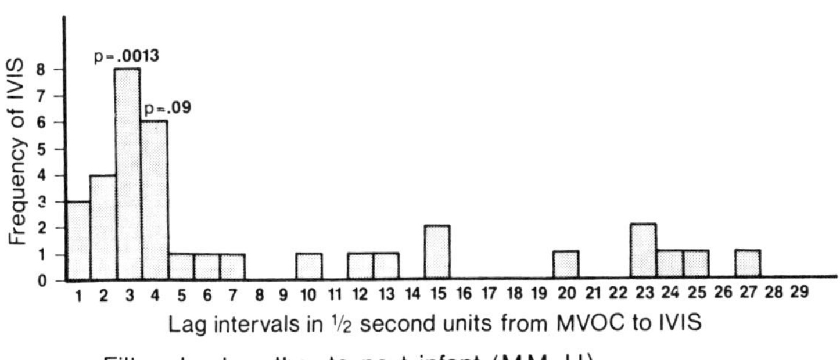

c Filter: Last mother to next infant (MM II)

Figure 4–4. Conventional and filtered lag histograms showing significant effects of mother's vocalization on infant looking at mother in Dyad A Session 10 (First interval indicates co-occurrence. Histogram *b* is based on Filter Formula Type II as given in Chapter 4 and Remmers (1985). Histogram *c* is based on Filter Formula IV as given in Rosenfeld and Remmers (1981).

relationship might be obtained by assessing histograms of the MVOC to MVOC relationship to see how this behavior is clustered. Then clusters of various sizes could be defined as variables, and the contributions of repetitions of MVOC to the occurrence of IVIS could be assessed. Analysis of the effects of stops as well as of starts might add even greater accuracy to the interpretation.

The various lag analyses of the mother-infant relationship demonstrate the value of a successive-approximations approach to causal modeling of the communication process. Each additional form of lag analysis tended to answer questions raised by prior forms of analysis. Some forms disambiguated previously confounded causal possibilities; others added detail about the contents and temporal-distributional properties of interrelated behaviors. Each new contribution of information tended to stimulate further questions, requiring additional forms of analysis for their answer.

If an investigator has the ability to ask good questions and to propose productive hypotheses about sequential relationships, then the availability of flexible methods for providing answers should be extremely valuable research tools. The tools of Rosenfeld and Remmers (1981) and of other investigators referred to only scratch the surface of what is possible. But if such tools are to be attractive to investigators, they must be made easy to use.

During the author's experience with lag analysis, he found several discouraging sources of inefficiency for which he is currently developing solutions. Searching through masses of batch computer output of lag histograms to find the few that are likely to answer a current hypothesis or empirical question breeds impatience, and the author has been frustrated by having to interrupt the excitement of zeroing in on more precise answers in order to redefine variables in computer analyzable form and to create filter programs that are more appropriate to the questions that have arisen.

Work on solutions to these problems continues. Remmers (1985) has written a computer program that will allow the investigator to interact with the computer so as to redefine variables in various ways and to perform only the specific lag analyses that are needed at the moment. It offers either parametric or nonparametric statistics. Only if the resulting histograms shown on screen are satisfactory to the user must they be saved on disk or printed. The program is written in BASIC for use on popular microcomputers. In addition to providing the conventional and filtered statistical tests with corrections, as described previously, the program also allows the user to test for the effects of any third variable *C* intervening between *A* and *B*.

Complementary Experimental Analysis

A variety of ways in which experimental analysis can complement naturalistic analysis was noted earlier. In the present study the author was interested in the degree to which the emergence of skillful behaviors by the infant was dependent on the availability of certain physical and social opportunities in the setting. To generate relevant evidence, sessions in which one or both of two constants of the surrounding naturalistic sessions were removed or restricted were included: Either the infant's toys were removed (two sessions), or the mother was instructed not to interact with the infant except in emergencies(two sessions),or both (one or two sessions).

Effects of the experimental manipulations could be assessed by comparing rates of particular behaviors in the replicated manipulated sessions with those of the surrounding nonmanipulated sessions. Although a formal statistical analysis of these differences has not been done, inspection of data from Dyad A indicates that the restriction of toys and of mother's availability had some strong effects on the infant's behavior rates. Several of the more interesting effects from Dyad A are shown in Figure 4–5.

The absence of toys seemed to be particularly effective in increasing the rate of certain infant behaviors. Two of the infant's behaviors, looking at mother (IVIS) and positive vocalizations (IPOS), had been shown earlier to be related to mother behaviors in the nonexperimental (baseline) sessions. As shown in Figure 4–5, both IVIS and IPOS increased when toys were unavailable. These results indicate that communication between mother and infant becomes more salient when alternative sources of attention for the infant are lacking.

Some complementary confirmatory evidence was available from the lag analyses. The same bivariate lag analyses were performed within the no-toys sessions as in the baseline sessions. One result was that in the no-toys sessions IVIS responded more quickly to both MVIS and MVOC than in the baseline sessions; both lag histograms had significant elevations within the first half second.

Particularly surprising were the effects of the unavailability of toys on the infant's direction of visual attention to parts of his own body (e.g., hands or feet) and on his initiation of locomotion (see Fig. 4–5). Neither behavior had been found to occur during the first four sessions in all of which toys had been present. Of course, it cannot be proved that the infant would not have initiated these behaviors in the fifth session even if it had contained toys. But their reduction in the subsequent baseline session and their increase in the much later replication of the no-toys

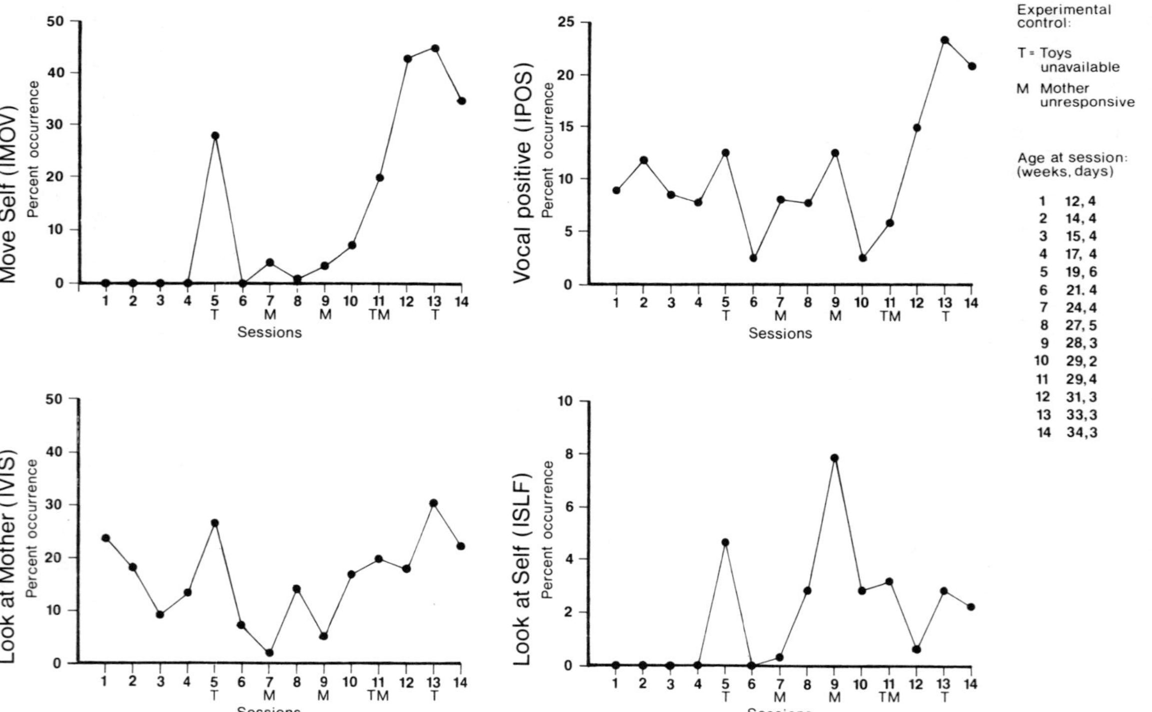

Figure 4–5. Effects of modifications of the physical and social environment (availability of toys and mother) on rates of occurrence of infant behaviors in Dyad A (Entries show per cent of 0.5 second intervals per session during which behavior was "on.")

session increases confidence that they were indeed initiated in response to the unavailability of toys.

Inspection of details of the sequentially coded data from the no-toys sessions revealed several instances in which the infant's locomotion resulted in manipulation of otherwise unreachable objects. These included the legs of both the mother and a table as well as an electrical outlet, the last of these resulting in a high transitional probability of mother uttering "No!" Without the addition of the experimental sessions, the investigator would have been susceptible to the erroneous inference that the infant was incapable of locomotion until at least the sixth baseline session. Furthermore, rare opportunities to observe the context of maternal scolding would have been missed.

SUMMARY AND CONCLUSIONS

Methodology for the study of communicative development has lagged far behind theory. A clear example is the body of research testing the popular hypothesis that mothers and other agents of socialization contribute to the development of language acquisition by means of social interchange. In particular children's verbal skills are thought to be facilitated by the mother's verbal reactions to the infant's verbal and nonverbal behavior. The correlational evidence that is consistent with this proposition also is consistent with other interpretations as well. There is a scarcity of evidence relating to direction of causality and to the effects of various temporal features of categories of behavior.

Thus a major limitation of methods that commonly are used for analyzing human communicative development is insufficient attention to temporal processes. Yet many methods for sequential analysis exist and have been applied with considerable success in other fields. It is rare to find such methods included within statistics texts in the social sciences. Fortunately, an increasing number of students of human communication are becoming familiar with these sequential methods.

In this chapter the experience that the author and his colleagues have had in delving into sequential relationships in mother-infant interaction has been reviewed, and a set of methodological prerequisites that need to be satisfied in conducting sequential studies has been proposed, with particular emphasis on the elementary coding of temporal properties of behavior. The wide range of methods for statistically analyzing sequential relationships and providing models of the results was pointed out. Holistic and piecemeal approaches to data analysis were contrasted; the applications of each to data sequences coded from observation of individual mother-infant dyads were reviewed. The results have been more valuable for demonstrating the relative usefulness of alternative methods for analyzing sequential relationships than for providing substantive generalizations about communicative development. But the methods demonstrated and others referred to in the chapter can be adapted for a variety of substantive uses.

One of the practical lessons learned in this study was that sequential studies require data strings that are substantially longer than do experimental studies. This is particularly true in exploratory studies in which the investigator proceeds in detective-story fashion to unravel a gradually unfolding mystery. As more specific forms of behavior become implicated, including both rarely occurring single behaviors and complex functionally connected sets of behaviors, the problem of finding sufficient replications for statistical analysis increases. But the potential for information that permits more accurate causal modeling may be worth the extra effort required to obtain sufficient samples.

It was suggested that more precise causal inferences may be derived from sequential data than some popular methods have permitted. In particular the importance was demonstrated of adding a process of comparative filtering to conventional lag methods so as to assess the contributions of different forms of sequential clustering to relationships between event classes. Finally, the complementary contributions of experimental methods were demonstrated.

In conclusion researchers are urged to use the increasingly available tools for sequential analysis in basic and applied research on human communicative development. However, the case for hardware and software must not be overstated to the neglect of the personal input of the researcher, who must also ask the right questions; there is no single all-purpose tool for answering all questions about communicative development. But intelligent selection of available tools and their sensitive application to good questions should allow researchers to optimize the wealth of information that can be provided by naturalistic studies.

ACKNOWLEDGMENTS

Preparation of this chapter was supported in part by funds from NICHHD Grant 002528, administered through the Bureau of Child Research, and by Biomedical Sciences Support Grant No. 4082–711 through the University of Kansas. The author wishes to acknowledge the invaluable contributions of Bill Remmers. He wrote the innovative automaton and lag-filter computer programs for analyzing social behavior and helped clarify many methodological issues. Other contributors to the methods and results reported here include Gail Young-Browne (videotaping), Virginia Stark (primary coding), Margaret Hancks (reliability coding), Jeff Bangert (data formatting for the computer), Robert

Haralick and Nimitra Kattiyakulwanich (formatting of data for automaton analysis), and Maxine Schoggen and Beverly Ayers-Nachamkin (comparison to ecological units).

REFERENCES

Allison, P. D., and Liker, J. K. (1982). Analyzing sequential categorical data on dyadic interaction: a comment on Gottman. *Psychological Bulletin, 91,* 393–403.

Altmann, S. A. (1967). The structure of primate social communication. In S. A. Altmann (Ed.), *Social communication among primates.* Chicago: University of Chicago Press.

Altmann, S. A. (1965). Sociobiology of rhesus monkeys. II. Stochastics of social communication. *Journal of Theoretical Biology, 8,* 490–522.

Austin, J. L. (1962). *How to do things with words.* Oxford: Oxford University Press.

Bakeman, R., and Dabbs, J. M. (1976). Social interaction observed: Some approaches to the analysis of behavior streams. *Personality & Social Psychology Bulletin, 2,* 335–345.

Bandura, A. (1966). Vicarious processes: A case of no-trial learning. In L. Berkowitz (Ed.), *Advances in experimental social psychology, Volume II.* New York: Academic Press.

Barker, R. G. (Ed.). (1963). The stream of behavior. New York: Appleton-Century-Crofts.

Birdwhistell, R. L. (1970). *Kinesics and context.* Philadelphia: University of Pennsylvania Press.

Bloom, K. (1977). Patterning of infant vocal behavior. *Journal of Experimental Child Psychology, 23,* 367–377.

Bobbitt, R. A., Gourevitch, V. P., Miller, L. E., and Jenson, G. D. (1969). The dynamics of social interactive behavior: A computerized procedure for analyzing trends, patterns, and sequences. *Psychological Bulletin, 71,* 110–121.

Booth, T. L. (1967). *Sequential machines and automata theory.* New York: Wiley.

Bowlby, J. (1969). *Attachment and loss. Volume 1: Attachment.* London: Hogarth.

Box, G. E. P., and Jenkins, G. M. (1970). *Time-series analysis: Forecasting and control.* San Francisco: Holden-Day.

Brent, E. E., Jr., and Sykes, R. E. (1979). A mathematical model of symbolic interaction between police and suspects. *Behavioral Science, 24,* 388–402.

Breiman, L. (1969). *Probability and stochastic processes.* Boston: Houghton-Mifflin Company.

Cartwright, D., and Zander, A. (1953). *Group dynamics: Research and theory.* Evanston, IL: Row, Peterson.

Clark, R. W. (1972). *Einstein: The life and times.* New York: Avon.

Condon, W. S., and Sander, L. W. (1974). Synchrony demonstrated between movements of the neonate and adult speech. *Child Development, 45,* 456–462.

Duncan, S. D., Jr., and Fiske, D. W. (1977). *Face-to-face interaction: Research, methods and theory.* Hillsdale, NJ: Erlbaum.

Fagen, R. M. (1978). Repertoire analysis. In P. W. Colgan (Ed.), *Quantitative ethology.* New York: Wiley.

Fagen, R. M., and Young, D. Y. (1978). Temporal patterns of behavior: Durations, intervals, latencies, and sequences. In P. W. Colgan (Ed.), *Quantitative ethology.* New York: Wiley.

Gewirtz, J. L. (1969). Mechanisms of social learning: Some roles of stimulation and behavior in early human development. In D. A. Goslin (Ed.), *Handbook of socialization theory and research.* Chicago: Rand McNally.

Gottman, J. M. (1979). *Marital interaction: Experimental investigations.* New York: Academic Press.

Gottman, J. M. (1980). Analyzing for sequential connection and assessing interobserver reliability for the sequential analysis of observational data. *Behavioral Assessment, 2,* 361–368.

Gottman, J. M., and Notarius, C. (1978). Sequential analysis of observational data using Markov chains. In T. Kratochwill (Ed.), *Strategies to evaluate change in single-subject research.* New York: Academic Press.

Gottman, J. M. (1981). *Time-series analysis: A comprehensive introduction for social scientists.* New York: Cambridge University Press.

Gustafsson, L., and Lanshammar, H. (1977). *ENOCH: An integrated system for measurement and analysis of human gait.* Uppsala, Sweden: Institute of Technology.

Hall, E. T. (1968). Proxemics. *Current Anthopology, 9,* 83–108.

Hawes, L. C. and Foley, J. M. (1973). A Markov analysis of interview communication. *Speech Monographs, 3, 40,* 208–219.

Hayes, D. P., Meltzer, L., and Wolf, G. (1970). Substantive conclusions are dependent upon techniques of measurement. *Behavioral Science, 15,* 265–268.

Hays, W. L. (1963). *Statistics for psychologists.* New York: Holt, Rinehart, and Winston.

Hewes, D. (1980). Stochastic modeling of communication processes. In P. R. Monge and J. N. Cappella (Eds.), *Multivariate techniques in human communication research.* New York: Academic Press.

Hirsbrunner, H. P., and Frey, S. (in press). Movement in human interaction: Description, parameter formation, and analysis. In A. W. Siegman and S. Feldstein (Eds.), *Nonverbal behavior and communication (2nd ed.).* Hillsdale, NJ: Lawrence Erlbaum Associates.

Hollenbeck, A. R. (1978). Problems of reliability in observational research. In G. P. Sackett (Ed.), *Observing behavior. Volume 2: Data collection and analysis methods.* Baltimore: University Park Press.

Jaffe J. (1970). Linked probabilistic finite automata: A model for the temporal interaction of speakers. *Mathematical Biosciences, 7,* 191–204.

Jaffe, J., and Feldstein, S. (1970). *Rhythms of dialogue.* New York: Academic Press.

Jaffe, J., Stern, D. N., and Peery, J. C. (1973). "Conversational" coupling of gaze behavior in prelinguistic human development. *Journal of Psycholinguistic Research, 2,* 321–329.

Kaye, K. (1977). Toward the origin of dialogue. In H. R. Schaffer (Ed.), *Studies in mother-infant interaction.* London: Academic Press.

Kendon, A. (1972). Some relationships between body motion and speech: An analysis of an example. In A. W. Siegman and B. Pope (Eds.), *Studies in dyadic communication.* New York: Pergamon Press.

Lewin, K. (1951). *Field theory in social science.* New York: Harper.

Lichtenberg, J. W., and Hummel, T. J. (1976). Counseling as stochastic process: Fitting a Markov chain model to initial counseling interviews. *Journal of Counseling Psychology, 23,* 310–315.

Losey, G. S. (1978). Information theory and communication. In P. W. Colgan (Ed.), *Quantitative ethology.* New York: Wiley.
Martin, J. A. (1981). A longitudinal study of the consequences of early mother-infant interaction: A microanalytic approach. *Monographs of the Society for Research in Child Development,* 46, Serial No. 190.
McDowall, J. J. (1979). Microanalysis of filmed movement: The reliability of boundary detection by observers. *Environmental Psychology and Nonverbal Behavior, 3,* 77–88.
McGrew, W. C. (1972). *An ethological study of children's behavior.* New York: Academic Press.
Newtson, D., Engquist, G., and Bois, J. (1977). The objective basis of behavior units. *Journal of Personality and Social Psychology, 35,* 847–862.
Patterson, G. R. (1974). A basis for identifying stimuli which control behaviors in natural settings. *Child Development, 45,* 900–911.
Patterson, G. R., and Cobb, J. A. (1971). A dyadic analysis of "aggressive" behaviors. In J. P. Hill (Ed.), *Minnesota Symposia on Child Psychology, 5,* 72–129.
Reid, J. B. (1970). Reliability assessment of observational data: A possible methodological problem. *Child Development, 41,* 1143–1150.
Remmers, W. W. (1985). An interactive microcomputer program for the disambiguated analysis of lag relationships between discrete behavioral events. Unpublished doctoral dissertation, University of Kansas, Lawrence.
Rosenfeld, H. M. (1966). Approval-seeking and approval-inducing functions of verbal and nonverbal responses in the dyad. *Journal of Personality and Social Psychology, 4,* 597–605.
Rosenfeld, H. M. (1978). Conversational control functions of nonverbal behavior. In A. W. Siegman and S. Feldstein (Eds.), *Nonverbal behavior and communication.* Hillsdale, NJ: Lawrence Erlbaum Associates.
Rosenfeld, H. M. (1971). Development of social competence (Project Report 1H0K01). Lawrence, KS: Center for Research in Early Childhood Education.
Rosenfeld, H. M. (1972). The experimental analysis of interpersonal influence processes. *Journal of Communication, 22,* 424–442.
Rosenfeld, H. M. (1982). Measuring body movement and orientation. In K. R. Scherer and P. Ekman (Eds.), *Handbook of methods in nonverbal behavior research.* New York: Cambridge University Press.
Rosenfeld, H. M. (1967). Nonverbal reciprocation of approval: An experimental analysis. *Journal of Experimental Social Psychology, 3,* 102–111.
Rosenfeld, H. M. (1973). *Time series analysis of mother-infant interaction.* Paper presented at the Symposium on the Analysis of Mother-Infant Interaction Sequences, Annual Meeting of the Society for Research in Child Development, Philadelphia.
Rosenfeld, H. M. (1981). Whither interactional synchrony? In K. Bloom (Ed.), *Prospective issues in infancy research.* Hillsdale, NJ: Lawrence Erlbaum Associates.
Rosenfeld, H. M., and Gunnell, P. K. (in press). Pragmatics versus reinforcers: An experimental analysis of verbal accommodation. In H. Giles and R. N. St. Clair (Eds.), *Recent advances in language, communication and social psychology.* London: Lawrence Erlbaum Associates.
Rosenfeld, H. M., and Hancks, M. (1980). The nonverbal context of verbal listener responses. In M. R. Key (Ed.), *The relationship of verbal and nonverbal communication.* The Hague: Mouton.

Rosenfeld, H. M., and McRoberts, R. (1979). *Relationship of topographical features, verbal and nonverbal context, and ratings of head nods.* Unpublished manuscript, University of Kansas, Lawrence.

Rosenfeld, H. M., and Remmers, W. W. (1981). Searching for temporal relationships in mother-infant interactions. In B. L. Hoffer and R. N. St. Clair (Eds.), *Developmental kinesics: The emerging paradigm.* Baltimore: University Park Press.

Sackett, G. P. (1978). The lag sequential analysis of contingency and cyclicity in behavioral interaction research. In J. D. Osofsky (Ed.), *Handbook of infant development.* New York: Wiley.

Sacks, H., Schegloff, E. A., and Jefferson, G. (1974). A simplest systematics for the organization of turn-taking in conversation. *Language, 50,* 696–735.

Schaffer, H. R., and Emerson, P. (1964). The development of social attachments in infancy. *Monographs of the Society for Research in Child Development, 29*(3).

Scherer, K. R., and Ekman, P. (Eds.). (1982). *Handbook of methods in nonverbal behavior research.* New York: Cambridge University Press.

Siegman, A. W., and Feldstein, S. (Eds.), (1978). *Nonverbal behavior and communication.* Hillsdale, NJ: Lawrence Erlbaum Associates.

Snow, C. E., and Ferguson, C. A. (Eds.). (1977). *Talking to children: Language input and organization.* Cambridge: Cambridge University Press.

Sugarman, S. (in press). The development of preverbal communication: Its contribution and limits in promoting the development of language. In R. L. Schiefelbusch and J. Pickar (Eds.), *Communicative competence: Acquisition and intervention.* Baltimore: University Park Press.

Thomas, A. C., and Martin, J. A. (1976). Analyses of parent-infant interaction. *Psychological Review. 83,* 141–156.

van Hooff, J. A. R. A. M. (1982). Categories and sequences of behavior: Methods of description and analysis. In K. R. Scherer and P. Ekman (Eds.), *Handbook of methods in nonverbal behavior research.* Cambridge: University of Cambridge Press.

Wampold, B. E., and Margolin, G. (1982). Nonparametric strategies to test the independence of behavioral states in sequential data. *Psychological Bulletin, 92,* 755–765.

Young-Browne, G. (1972). Infant crying: An exploratory analysis of maternal elicitors in naturally occurring mother-infant interactions. Unpublished master's thesis, University of Kansas.

SECTION III
INTERVENTION PROJECTS AND PROCEDURES

Chapter 5

Language Intervention Through Sensemaking and Fine Tuning

Judith Felson Duchan

Every decade has gaps between research and practice, gaps between old theory and new theory, or gaps between one discipline's discovery and another's incorporation of it. Usually we language clinicians identify our gaps by looking outside our own discipline. We spend our time trying to "keep up with the Joneses"—that is, with what is going on in neighboring disciplines such as linguistics or psychology—and trying to apply those findings to everyday dealings with the communicatively handicapped. This decade is going to be different. The gaps language clinicians will choose to bridge will be of our own making: the discrepancy between assessment and intervention techniques and the gap between the theories held about language and the approaches used to guide them in language intervention.

Unfortunately, successfully filled gaps of one decade create new ones for the next. In the 1960s and early 1970s the gap was bridged between linguistic theory and language assessment. It was done by developing language sample analysis, a set of techniques for discovering the linguistic structures undergirding the language of language impaired children (for examples see Miller, 1981, and Lund and Duchan, 1983). The new approach was called *informal assessment* to contrast it with formalized test procedures that had been used previously.

The gap between theory and therapy was felt in the later 1970s when language clinicians began to look at how various contexts influenced language interpretation. At first attention was paid to language use (Bloom and Lahey, 1978), and assessment and intervention approaches that focused on intentionality were devised. Since then the focus has broadened to include other aspects of the communicative interaction, such as the script (Johnston, 1982), turn-taking (Prutting and Kirchner, 1983), the topic (Hurtig, Ensrud, and Tomblin, 1982), and breakdowns and repairs (Gallagher and Darnton, 1978). Thus the original category of pragmatics is now expanded to include a variety of factors that come into play during communicative interactions.

The newly created gap between pragmatics theory and therapy indicates the need for a conceptual framework for evaluating what goes on during clinical interactions. This chapter attempts to develop such a framework and lay out principles of clinical intervention that would follow from it. The framework uses ideas from informal assessment and pragmatics, so it has its theoretical biases, but it is also critical of its own history. It is hoped that the principles can be used to evaluate and expand upon diverse clinical approaches, even those that derive from theories that have historically been viewed as incompatible.

The framework being proposed builds on two conceptual cornerstones: *sensemaking* and *fine tuning.* Briefly, sensemaking is what the participants in the interaction think is going on and what ideas structure that thinking; fine tuning involves the various ways partners adjust their part of the interaction to be in accord with their model of the person they are interacting with.

SENSEMAKING

Sensemaking pervades and underlies all interactions. It is done by whoever is participating in the interaction and even by whoever watches it. The sensemaker brings to bear theories and ideas about the world that seem pertinent for creating an interpretation of what is currently going on. Children who participate in the clinical interaction make sense of it from their orientations, clinicians make sense of that same interaction from their orientations, and those analyzing the interaction can bring yet another set of vantage points from which to interpret the event (Berger and Kellner, 1981).

Because the idea of sensemaking is derived from the pragmatics revolution, it can best be discussed in relation to some selected themes found in the pragmatics literature: script, turn-taking, intent, topic, breakdowns, and repairs (Gallagher and Darnton, 1978; Prutting and Kirchner, 1983; Irwin, 1982). Two new constructs—overall sense and agenda— will be added to round out the sensemaking framework. The discussion strives to bind these eight constructs together into a unified conceptualization that involves rendering some of the ideas as peripheral and others as more central to the process of sensemaking. It begins with a central construct: the overall sense of the event.

Overall Sense

One important component of the answer to "What's going on?" is an *overall sense* of the event, e.g., we are playing, we are eating, we are shopping, we are in speech class. Overall sense is close to what the words "gist" or "main idea" mean for written language. The overall sense can be about what people are doing, why they are doing it, or how a particular participant feels about it. Or it can even be about what the person wants to have happen. Thus, if we ask about a child's trip to the zoo and he talks about a hot dog, we must acknowledge the possibility that the animals were of secondary importance and the hot dog was more integral to the child's overall sense of the zoo event.

The overall sense of the event is often informed by the event's *script*. The script is the person's conceptualization of how events will unfold. Scripts contain a skeletal depiction of the main parts of the event, parts that the participants use to move from one part of the event to the next. A restaurant script, according to Shank and Abelson (1977), includes being seated, ordering from a menu, being served, eating, getting and paying the check, and leaving. Scripts can be idosyncratic. For example, the child's script may highlight dessert or eating Big Macs. Scripts can also vary from being highly specific (restaurant script = what you do at all McDonald's restaurants) or very schematic (restaurant script = what do you do at all eating establishments). Scripts do not contain all the knowledge needed for an enactment of an event. For example, they do not contain plans about unforseen circumstances such as what to do about a broken chair or what to say or do in response to a particular question. Scripts are general plans, something like guidelines that can be violated, but even in their violation they can offer meanings to the overall sense (e.g., "This is not the way things should have gone"). Some events are highly scripted, whereas others are not, and the degree of scripting contributes to our sense of whether the event is structure or nonstructured.

Turn-taking

In the actual enactment of an event, partners often take turns. Sometimes those turns are prescribed by the script. For example, a lesson script may involve each person reading a page and the turns proceeding in a prearranged order around the circle. Sometimes turn-taking must be negotiated, such as in situations in which specific bids must be made for getting a turn (Sacks, Shegloff, and Jefferson, 1974). The outcomes of these negotiated turns are not part of the script but follow from the negotiation.

The dynamics of turn-taking depend not only on whether or not they are clearly scripted but also on the participants overall sense of the event. For events that are not understood, are not liked, or are understood differently from other participants, interactants may show "turn-taking problems." The problems are not a result of their inability to take turns but are because they do not want to or they do not know the event well enough to know when it permits accepting or relinquishing a turn—or worse yet, they do not know what to do when the turn is theirs.

Intents

Turns contain *acts,* sometimes one, sometimes many. Acts may be verbal or nonverbal, and for oral speakers they are usually both. Nonverbal acts are actions such as reaches and gives; verbal acts have been called propositions. Acts are performed for many reasons. They can be prescribed by the script, the actor may want to accomplish something in particular, the actor may want to make a general impression on the listener, or any combination of these and others. These reasons are called *intents,* and the usual conceptualization of intents is that there is at least one per act. This one-intent-per-act idea has led to coding schemes for assessing what intents a child expresses (Coggins and Carpenter, 1981; Dore, 1975) and to remedial programs for teaching children to express a variety of intents (Watson and Lord, 1982; Cole, 1982).

Another way to conceptualize intents is to see that they are closely intertwined with the sensemaking enterprise; thus, an act can have an intended function that may contribute to sensemaking, such as carrying forward the event, taking an assigned turn, keeping to the topic, or receiving the right answer.

Agenda

Acts often conspire to achieve the same goal. A request, for example, can be set up in the first act, issued indirectly in the next, then reissued more directly (Garvey, 1979, calls this the request domain). Sometimes acts tie together in more indirect ways to achieve a more general goal. These overall goals are called *agendas* (Duchan, 1984a). Children may be performing all the acts in an event perhaps to please the teacher, to avoid embarrassment, or to earn tokens. Conspiracies and agendas are often closely related to sensemaking in that the main thing going on is the attempt to achieve a particular goal.

Topic

Verbal acts not only tie together by virtue of their goals but also cohere in content. In other words, they are topically related. Sentences in a sequence may be about the same topic. In fact, competent speakers are obliged to keep to the same topic unless they indicate otherwise (van-Dijk, 1979). Topics may or may not have to do with intents or agendas. Sometimes the topic is simply a vehicle for carrying out an agenda that has nothing to do with the vehicle. For example, *small talk* is seen as a way to continue the interaction with the topic of the talk being immaterial to the agenda. What is really going on is that the people are getting to know each other. Sometimes topics are highly congruent with the agenda of both parties as when one asks for directions and the other gives them. In these cases topic and agenda are one and the same, and they both are the main contributors to the participants' sense of that event.

An event may have many different topics or only one. In one sitting, a reading group can cover many stories. Going to the zoo can involve many conversations about many things, but getting directions has only one topic. Topics can be embedded, in that specific topics can tie together under an overriding topic. One person's discussion of a car breakdown can occur inside her discussion of a trip to Philadelphia, which can, in turn be followed by another person's description of his car problems or a joke about Philadelphia by W. C. Fields. Sometimes topics are controlled by the script: "Your turn to read." In those cases, the topics are often closely allied to the overall sense of the event.

Breakdowns and Repairs

Breakdowns in interactions can occur for as many reasons as there are components to the event. They can occur because the participants have a different overall sense of the event, because someone fails to take an expected turn, because the intent or agenda being worked on is not fulfilled, or because the topic is not maintained by the partner. Some breakdowns surface and interrupt the event; others are felt but do not surface to intrude on the ongoing event (Earle, 1983; Vuchinich, 1977). The covert breakdowns can, for example, be talked about later: "Remember when she made that off-the-wall comment?" When there are many breakdowns the inability to proceed in the event becomes paramount and the sense of the event can change from "a reading lesson," for example, to "I'm not getting anything right."

Sometimes people become aware that their participation in the event is not meeting the demands of the event, and they develop strategies for getting by. When the person sees the strategy as a way to pass, the strategy is deemed compensatory (Kirchner and Skarakis-Doyle, 1983). When the strategy is a short cut or plan for keeping the interaction going, without being a cover-up, we call it a repair (Gallagher and Darnton, 1978).

What the sensemaking framework offers the pragmatics framework, then, is a grounded overall organizational perspective in which scripts, acts, intents, agendas, topics, breakdowns, and repairs can vary in their influence and can be seen as related to one another in different ways, depending on the person's overall sense of what is going on.

FINE TUNING

Fine tuning, like sensemaking, allows us to stand outside the pragmatics constructs that have emerged from the literature and to look at them from a particular point of view: that of how adults and children adjust to one another in the course of an interaction. Fine tuning is observable when examining how children and adults make their adjustments. There are many diverse aspects to those adjustments. What is even more fundamental than detection of what adjustments are being made is what role the adjustments play in each partner's sense of the event and whether or not the tuning serves the interaction well.

The role fine tuning plays in influencing the overall sense of the interaction varies with the event and with the style of the interactant. Interactants who have a social bent incorporate the other person into their main sense of the event. ("This event is good because my interactant is doing well," or, for the more perverted fine tuners: "I got his goat that time!")

The particulars of fine tuning involve being sensitive to the partners' ideas about how the event is scripted. The more tightly prescribed the script, and the more familiar the adults and children are with it, the less they need to fine tune to one another. That is, when rituals are the order of business, it is not necessary for either partner to decide what vocabulary or syntactic level to use, nor do they need to determine the other's background knowledge except in terms of what is known of the script.

Similarly, when the event has the turns incorporated within its structure, neither partner must be concerned about taking turns—the turns are directed by a prearranged plan. It is only when events are less scripted that they require the participants to figure out what the turns are to be and when to assume them. It is likely that under circumstances in which adults are highly tuned to a child's knowledge and language system that the child will assume turns readily. Indeed, one indicator of fine tuning by an adult is when a child is able to assume a turn when it is offered and to relinquish readily it when it is time. If the adult directs a question or comment to a child that the child fails to understand, it is likely that the child will not respond, thereby not taking a turn. This lack of response is also likely if the adult underestimates the child's competence. What would be required in either overestimation or underestimation of the child's competence is a readjustment of the event, that is to say, a tuning. The readjustment may be either a scaling up to make it more difficult or a scaling down to make it easier. Scaling is done in order to match the input language to the child's cognitive and linguistic competence.

Fine tuning also pertains to the intent and agenda of the interactants. In finely tuned interactions, each partner assumes responsibility for helping the other fulfill his or her communicative intents. It is what might be called in common parlance "being sensitive" and entails fulfilling requests, commenting on comments, accepting offers, and supporting agendas. Typically, in events that are designed to teach the child something, the child has little opportunity to construct utterances with a variety of intents. Instead, he or she is in a nonreciprocal position of fulfilling the request of the teacher to say and do what the lessons entail. The child must fine tune to the teacher by contriving right answers. In interactions in which the agendas of the participants are at odds, fine tuning may entail an adjustment of one person's agenda to be compatible with the other's or an abandonment of the agenda if adjustments are not feasible.

Topic continuation across a turn involves fine tuning on the part of the new speaker. Lack of continuation, without warning, is interpreted as being "tuned out." Topic shifts are often the source of interaction breakdowns, in which the originator of the topic is faced with reestablishing it or going with the topic change. These rough spots in topic continuation often arise because partners neglect to tune into what the speaker was saying.

Finally, repairs, for whatever reason they are needed, also require that participants work with one another in interactions to get the event moving forward once again. The participants must, for example, hypothesize why the interaction broke down. Did the listener not understand the content? Was he preoccupied? Did he hear it? These hypotheses are more correct when the participants have a good model of the listener and represent yet another aspect of fine tuning.

Fine tuning adds to the sensemaking framework a perspective-taking component from which to evaluate the sensitivity of the interactants to one another. It, too, is grounded in a pragmatics conceptual network that includes scripts, acts, intents, agendas, topics, and breakdowns and repairs and works with the sensemaking network as a way to assess clinical interactions. This network will be discussed later. First, the current intervention practices and how they were influenced by the pragmatics revolution of the 1970s will be examined.

LANGUAGE INTERVENTION

Before the pragmatics revolution, teaching methods were evaluated primarily on whether an identified goal was obtained either in terms of a well-specified behavioral objective, or, more generally, on whether or not the lesson "worked" (Johnston, 1983). The pragmatics sensibility upset the "it works" criteria by adding more context-related questions such as: Where? For whom? Under what circumstances? And among the more radical pragmatists the even more difficult question arose: What difference does it make, even if he or she does learn it? How will it affect his or her everyday life?

In order to evaluate language intervention approaches, they must be typecast. The common categories used to describe intervention have been designated as either structured or unstructured in organizational plan; cognitive or behavioral in theory; naturalistic or clinical in style or setting. The particular dichotomy used depends on which of the many differences among the many therapy approaches the classifier wants to highlight.

Intervention programs differ not only in organization, theory, and style but also in whether they are directed toward working with teachers (Blank and Franklin, 1980), with families of the language impaired child (Bromwich, 1981; Clezy, 1979; Manolsen, 1983), or directly with the language impaired child (Cole, 1982). They also differ in what is being taught: language structure, conceptual understandings, or pragmatic competencies. The following discussion targets two general types of language intervention, pragmatics therapies and behavioral intervention. By pragmatics therapies is meant those that are loosely structured, are cognitive in theory, and are concerned with naturalistic simulation of everyday events. Behavioral interventions, in contrast, are usually tightly structured, are behavioristic in theory, and are usually conducted across the therapy or classroom table. Both pragmatics and behavioral interventions may target aspects of pragmatics such as what should be taught, so pragmatics lessons may be found in either type of intervention. The therapies differ in how they organize the pragmatics lessons, in the theoretical frameworks used to interpret pragmatics, and in the way the therapy is set up.

Sensemaking and Fine Tuning During Pragmatics Intervention

Pragmatics therapy is a recent development for language clinicians, and it comes in a variety of forms. The most conservative form is therapy whose format is in lessons, whose setting is in the therapy room, and whose content is on an aspect of pragmatics such as turn-taking or intentionality. Such therapy tends to have the traditional focus on right answers that are defined beforehand by the language clinician. This "teaching pragmatics skills" approach leads to clinician egocentricity in that the focus is not on the child's sensemaking nor does the approach require that the clinician fine tune to what the child is saying and doing.

A less conservative type of pragmatics therapy has three defining features. The clinician organizes the therapy around naturalistic interactions, assigns the child the interactive lead, and concentrates on modeling and expansion of what the child says and does (Duchan and Weitzner-Lin, 1984). Each of these three components can be evaluated within the sensemaking and fine tuning frameworks.

The naturalistic emphasis is dedicated to teaching communication in everyday contexts. The problem with this emphasis on everyday events is that there is an implication that such contexts can be talked about unidimensionally. Everyday events come in many varieties. Some are highly scripted, others are open. Some are arranged to be in keeping with children's agendas (e.g., playing); others are planned to ensure everyday things are accomplished (e.g., eating, bathing). Some involve considerable amounts of new knowledge; others are ritualized reenactments of familiar events. Most importantly for planning naturalistic interventions, some are regarded as similar by the child in that they are seen as versions of one another, whereas others are considered different events. Thus, the unidimensional view of everyday contexts carries with it the potential for our reverting back to prepragmatics ideas about language—a conceptualization that fails to acknowledge the importance of contexts.

Even if the view of everyday contexts were more multidimensional, conducting interventions to simulate everyday events may or may not be in keeping with those everyday events. Having the language interventionist at home may make the event so different that the "lesson" is not generalized. Lessons in the speech room or clinic that have to do with, for example, setting the table may be just that, setting the table during speech class, and may not be seen as relating to what goes on at home.

A concomitant aspect of naturalistic interactions is sometimes termed "unstructured." This approach allows the child to do what he or she wants, and the clinician follows the lead, *que sera sera*. The judgment that the lessons are unstructured seems to be based on the clinicians' egocentric idea that structure must originate with them. Thus, if the child initiates a ritualized event, such as the highly structured game of peekaboo, clinicians still typically regard the lesson as unstructured because it was not organized by them.

Approaches advocating that the clinician talk about what the child has said or done, that is, the "parallel talk," "modeling," and "expansion" techniques, also may lead to clinicians' egocentricity. These response procedures, which can be grouped together as procedures involving "semantic contingency" on the child's acts, carry no commitment for the clincian to be in accord with the children's overall sense of the event, their agenda, or intent. The assumption is that what the adult interprets as the child's semantic meaning also matches what the child intends. The neglect of the child's intent could be dangerous, as in the following:

Child: (asking for help to unbuckle his belt) Go bathroom.
Semantically contingent adult: Uh huh. You have to go to the bathroom.
Intent contingent adult: Come here, I'll help you with your belt.

Nor does the notion of semantic contingency acknowledge the impact of the event structure on the interaction. Modeling in a tightly scripted, recurring event such as peekaboo will have a different future impact on the child than modeling in a free-wheeling play event. Indeed, the modeling under tightly scripted conditions has been dubbed scaffolding by Bruner (1975) because it requires that the child rotely learn what is being modeled. Modeling under loosely scripted conditions is more abstract in that the child or the adult is likely to say something different the next time those conditions obtain.

When considering parallel talk, modeling, and expansion in light of event structure, it becomes apparent that what people do when they scaffold is to model the event structures that are tightly scripted. Thus, ideas about semantic contingency need to be refined to include not only responsiveness to the child's overall sense, intent, and agenda but also the acknowledgement that what is often being modeled is the adult's sense of the event as carried by the event structure.

In sum, the sensemaking and fine tuning frameworks ask that language clinicians broaden their thinking about what they are doing when they engage in naturalistic interactions and when they respond contingently to the language impaired child's interactive leads. The clinician's tuning is not so fine when responding to the children only in terms of what he or she takes them to mean without regard for why they acted or how their acts fit with their sense of the event.

Sensemaking and Fine Tuning During Behavioral Intervention

Language intervention programs employing applied behavior analysis are more widely used and written about than any other kind (Craig, 1983). Clinicians designing operant approaches, although confirmed behaviorists, have recently opened their doors to teaching mentalistic constructs such as "rules" and "intents." The behavioral approach to teaching rules and intents has been to determine the overt behavioral manifestation of the targeted rule or intent and to teach these behaviors in a highly structured way. As described by the most prolific of the behavior analysts, Guess, Sailor, and Baer (1978), the technique nearly always includes the following:

> . . . reinforcement of correct behavior; extinction and brief timeout from the opportunity to gain more of that positive reinforcement, contingent on incorrect, inappropriate, disruptive, or inattentive behaviors; careful detailed programming of small new increments to be learned; and repetitive modeling of those new responses, usually coupled with the fading and shaping techniques well known in operant technology. (p. 105)

In order to place these behavioral constructs into a sensemaking framework, clinicians are required to reorganize their thinking about them. For example, as the programs now stand, correct and incorrect or inappropriate behaviors are determined by the adults' sensemaking perspective. Thus, a child who calls stacking rings "bagels" in response to the question "What are these?" is wrong from the adult frame of reference. They are not bagels, they are rings. But the rings, in fact, do look like bagels, and the child's sense of the event is appropriate in that he understands that he was being asked to label the object and that he even offered a sensible label, when seen from his point of view. Behavioral programs are designed to model or correct the child when the answer is inappropriate; thus, they would have the teacher say "No, these are rings." The behavioral programs, just as the pragmatics lessons requiring right answers, house the potential for clinician egocentricity.

The sensemaking perspective suggests that the child when corrected may come to interpret the correction as a breakdown and a failure, thus changing his sense of the event to one that is going less well than before. The repair strategies under the behavioral paradigm require the child to correct his answer, that is to say, to recast it in terms of what the adult expects for an answer. The event therefore becomes a guessing game in which the child must guess what answer the adult wants, even when he thinks he knows another answer that seems to be sensible. In the future, he may learn to say rings in response to questions about those objects in order to receive positive reinforcement, but that may be the only sense he has for why he should say "rings" when he is asked to label what he thinks of as "bagels."

Besides modeling and correction, the behavioral clinician may use "shaping" to get the child to say "rings." The clinician takes whatever approximations the child is making of the correct response and adds new pieces bit by bit until the new response is achieved. To analyze a task into parts for shaping, a response is only understandable from the children's point of view if they know what the pieces are part of. Otherwise they are learning to perform a set of meaningless tasks that are all the more difficult to remember because they make no internal sense. A reach, a grasp, a lift, and a back-and-forth movement of the hand when learned as a meaningless sequence is more forgettable than learning that the sequence of movements are all part of a hair-brushing act. Bransford and McCarrell (1974) found this constructive aspect of memory in adults whom they asked to recall a set of sentences. When the adults knew what the sentences were about they remembered them much better. Thus, task analysis works best when children understand how these sequenced acts make overall sense.

Reinforcement also relates to sensemaking. Extrinsic reinforcement, in which the learner is rewarded with anything that is deemed reinforcing, does not tie to the sense of the act. You do something right and get praise for it, whereas intrinsic reinforcement is by definition related to the sense of what is going on. A child is learning to request and is reinforced by being given what he has just requested. In Guess and coworkers' (1978) program the teacher is directed to give the learners what they are requesting (if they ask in a clear, two-word sequence, that is). The reinforcement is thereby intrinsic.

Intrinsic reinforcers may or may not be congruent with the child's view of the event. That is, reinforcers are deemed intrinsic to the task by the adult's definition, not the child's. Once again bias leads away from asking what the child understands. Instead of choosing what is thought of as intrinsic to the event, clinicians should choose reinforcers that are congruent with the child's intent, agenda, and overall sense of the event.

When the child's response has been shaped and the child has learned to say "rings" in response to the stacking rings and the questions "What are these?" a response that satisfies the behavioral goal of teaching him or her a new correct response has been made. But the lesson may fall short of the sensemaking goal for the child: to understand why "rings" are what you call those bagel-shaped objects at school and "bagels" are what you call them at home.

The child's confusion about what objects to call "bagel" has been dubbed a problem of generalization. Behavioral approaches, like other intervention approaches, aim for the learner generalizing from what has been learned to new appropriate contexts. Behavioral approaches, unlike other intervention approaches, ask the important question; "What does the generalization entail?" It is presumed in the behaviorist framework that when the child gains some context specific knowledge, that is, when the response comes under stimulus control, children must then learn to generalize that knowledge to contexts that were not like the original. Perhaps the language is different in the new context; perhaps the task varies; perhaps the interaction partner changes; perhaps the setting is different. Stimulus generalization is the process by which the child can generalize from one context to another. Response generalization is the process by which that child changes the original learning to fit the new context.

The behavioral framework, then, offers the capability for talking about how original learning transfers to new situations. Ironically, the behavioral approach, unlike more mentalistic approaches, comes to grips with the question of what is significant to the child. It does this by trying to determine the discriminative stimuli (SD), or those parts of the context that control the child's responses. An autistic child who focuses on a table and chair present in the learning context may not generalize his learning to another context in which the table and chair are absent (Rincover and Koegel, 1975). Autistic children are thus described as having stimulus overselectivity: they pick aspects of the stimulus context that are not relevant to other members of the culture for a particular act of sensemaking. All that is needed to bring this behavioral view under the control of the sensemaking paradigm is to add an interpretive component that assigns meaning to the SD and to generalization constructs. Autistic children fail to generalize because their sense of the event is one in which they are asked to say something while sitting at that table and on that particular chair, and they do not interpret a second situation without that table and chair as the same event, so it does not occur to them that they should display their new learnings in that second situation.

INTERVENTION PRINCIPLES

Sensitive clinical interactions require that the clinician "fine tune" to the child's level of language structure and content, and, more importantly, successful interactions require that the clinician be tuned in to the child's intent, agenda, and sense of the event. The fine tuning has its effects at every step of the way of the intervention process. The appropriateness of the intervention goals and the quality of the lesson plans hinge on the accuracy of the clinician's model of what the child is thinking and wanting. The actual playing out of the lessons should involve on-the-spot tuning to the child and should not only provide the child with interesting lessons but allow that child the opportunity to take the interactive lead. Subsequent assessment of the interaction and of the ability of the child to generalize to new contexts offers insights for later finer tuning.

These various stages in conducting language intervention—establishing goals, planning lessons, executing the lessons, and evaluating the lessons—all require different sorts of fine tuning. A set of principles for each will be drawn up as guidelines for approaching language intervention.

Fine Tuning for Deciding What Goals to Work On

It is often the case that language impaired children have many communicative incompetencies. Children classified as retarded, autistic, or learning disabled or as having specific language disabilities often have communication problems in more than one area of language performance. This "multiple problem" phenomenon can be seen most clearly by looking back to see what happened when new areas of language and communication to examine were found. For example, in the last 20 years, the discovery of syntax has led to the realization that many language impaired children have syntax problems. When semantics was discovered, many children were found to be deficient in that area. Cognition offered the same results: Some language impaired children could not perform at age level on tasks designed to measure cognitive competence. Now, as the discipline looks at pragmatics, sure enough, children with problems in areas that fall under the rubric of pragmatics—turn-taking, expression of intentions, and so on—are found.

This multiplicity of problem areas has led to an unmanageable battery of assessment instruments and procedures and has placed language interventionists in the unhappy position of having to decide which of the many deficit areas to focus on as they move from assessment to remediation. Decisions are often made on the basis of the latest clinical interest of the language interventionist rather than derived from a set of principles that best fit the needs and knowledge gaps of the child and his or her interactants.

The sensemaking framework suggests that the interventionist work on teaching language impaired children things that are most compatible with the children's sensemaking and are most needed to build an overall sense of events. The sensemaking approach assigns priority to teaching children to understand event structure and to better express their intents and agendas, and it assigns secondary importance to work on language form unless it interferes with the sensemaking enterprise. In other words, if a child fails to understand what is going on because he has misinterpreted a lexical item, then work on the semantics of that item receives priority. Otherwise, clinical energies should be given to helping the child understand the themes of what goes on around him and to participate in culturally acceptable or interpretable ways.

What the sensemaking construct does is postpone work on structures that are not essential to the sensemaking of the child. If the child has trouble with basic sensemaking, work on phonological problems or on semantic or syntactic structures conveying nuance is delayed. These structures are saved until the child is in a position to make sense of what is going on and is able to convey that sense to others.

Even when work is restricted to those knowledges that are involved in basic sensemaking, a position of choice still exists. Which event structures are to be taught? How can children be encouraged to express their intents and how can their intent types be expanded upon? This choice of what to work on should be based on which knowledges the child finds most graspable. Vygotsky offers a construct that he called "zone of proximal development'' (Cole, John-Steiner, Scribner, Souberman, 1978), that makes this selection process more tangible:

> . . . the zone of proximal development is the distance between the actual developmental level as determined by independent problem solving and the level of potential development as determined through problem solving under adult guidance or in collaboration with more capable peers. (p. 86)

Vygotsky saw the zone of proximal development as marking off potential areas of learning that are in an embryonic state and will develop with a little assistance. The closest language interventionists have come to acknowledging proximal development is in the measure of ''stimulability'' which they employ by seeing which sounds are imitable upon request and are thereby judged as learnable. What language interventionists need are measures to detect which learnings are in the buddings stages for other areas of communication so that they can evaluate children not only on what they know but on what they can most readily learn.

Another avenue to explore when deciding on directions for intervention is to examine the breakdowns between the child and familiar interactants. The breakdowns most easily identified are those that are overt, such as obvious misunderstandings between interactants, failure to answer questions by one or the other partner, queries for clarification, and lack of response to requests (Lubinski, Duchan, and Weitzner-Lin, 1980; Weitzner-Lin, 1981). Covert breakdowns can be identified through a postsession interview that may include asking either the child or the adult to recollect aspects of the event that went poorly or by playing a video of the interaction and asking participants to identify significant places in the interaction (Campbell-Taylor, 1984; Frankel, 1982; Sonnenmeier, 1984).

Once breakdowns are identified, speculations can be made about their origins and strategies can be developed toward prevention of the same sorts of breakdowns in the future. These strategies can become the goal of intervention, either for helping the child understand and make himself understood or for helping the interactant understand and be understood. This could be dubbed the ''fix the breakdown'' approach and differs from the usual ''fix the deficit'' approach in that it places the emphasis for treatment on the interaction rather than on remediating a deficit located within the child. (See Chapman, 1983, for a discussion of this event-oriented approach.)

Finally, there are things that children and adults need to know how to do together to make everyday life more livable. For example, all children need to learn the meaning of ''no'' as a command to stop, adults of echolalic children need to recognize the difference between an echo that means ''yes'' and one that means, ''I'm thinking about it'' (Prizant and

Duchan, 1981). Clinicians must help children and adults communicate about everyday needs.

These priorities can be formulated into a set of principles and accompanying implications:

Principle 1: Help the child make sense of what is going on.
- Implication A: Work on event structure before teaching turn-taking.
- Implication B: Work on intent before (or along with) form and content.
- Implication C: Work on pragmatic knowledge before linguistic knowledge and on linguistic knowledge before metalinguistic knowledge.

Principle 2: Work within the child's zone of proximal development.
- Implication A: Find which structures are most stimulable through imitation, hints, and scaffolding, and work on those.

Principle 3: Fix the interaction.
- Implication A: Work on strategies for enhancing communication between the child and familiar interactants.
- Implication B: Work on having significant others be fine tuned to the child as well as on the child's taking the listener's perspective.

Principle 4: Work on those categories significant and functional for the child and the categories significant to those people responsible for that child.

Fine Tuning for Planning Lessons

Written lesson plans can be viewed as overt scripts that are designed to carry out the clinician's agendas. They may be written to inform an onlooker such as a parent or supervisor about what will be happening, or they may be written as a plan for the clinician's eyes only. In either case, they are likely to be only the explicit part of the clinician's more elaborated covert plan. For example, the clinician may write ''map activity'' on his or her overt script as a mnemonic for a covert script explicating needed materials, what the players are supposed to say, procedure for turn-taking, and how the activity begins and ends. Overt and covert plans vary in detail. Some are scripted for most eventualities and may even include a verbal script detailing what the clinician and the child are supposed to say (Englemann and Osborne, 1976). Others are more loosely scripted, perhaps including simply a listing of possible activities. Some are in between, with the event outlined but the enactment subject to negotiation.

Tightly scripted plans are likely to be called "structured" and dydactic," although in actuality, loosely scripted events can also be carried out in structured and dydactic ways. For example, it is often the case that clinicians ask many questions whenever they are with children, regardless of whether they make explicit overt or covert plans ahead of time. These on-the-spot procedures have been called local formats (Jones, Rogerson, Weitzner-Lin, Duchan, 1983). In these ways unplanned lessons can easily become dydactic in quality.

The lessons appearing most unstructured are those called "play," in which the clinician allows the child the lead (Shriberg and Kwiatkowski, 1982). The child initiates and the clinician responds accordingly. However, even these play lessons may be scripted in that the clinician decides beforehand that he or she will use explicated techniques such as parallel play, modeling, or elaboration.

There are benefits to highly scripted plans. They work well to foreground new information against a background of familiar and formatted information. For lessons depending on formats such as "What's that?" or "Point to . . ." or "It's a . . .," the child does not have to attend to how to display that knowledge and can instead concentrate on the new information. All the children must do is think about what to put into the blanks.

A second advantage to highly scripted plans is that some scripts, once they are learned, can be transported as whole units elsewhere. For example, practicing steps for assembling a bicycle brake can be used later to assemble a bicycle brake (Gold, 1972). Scripts that recur in whole packages in everyday life have been taught under the rubric of *task analysis* and most often involve motor tasks or vocational tasks, such as dressing or sorting items and putting them in a container.

Problems occur with tight scripts. The most serious problem is that the new learning that takes place in them may not generalize to highly scripted events. "It's a . . ." and "Point to . . ." lessons may not teach names of things but rather what to say in that lesson frame.

A second problem with scripts is that even if they were generalized, performance is likely to be inflexible, with little capability for constructing detours when parts of the script do not work. This inflexibility is due to a lack of understanding of how and why the parts of the script go together. When children (and adults) fail to grasp the *sense* of the script, they must memorize each part. Thus, task analysis must be accompanied by the child's understanding of what is going on and how the parts logically relate to one another and to the whole.

A third problem for tightly scripted lessons is that they disallow children to take initiative and to act in behalf of their own agendas and intents. Thus, although pieces of everyday life may be learned, the child also learns to play a passive role in them. Weisz (1979) has called this "learned helplessness."

Loosely scripted lesson plans point the clinicians in the direction of paying more attention to the child's thoughts and actions. This finer tuning results from the removal of a comfortable script that provides a way of interacting on the basis of a right or wrong response. In unstructured events clinicians must work harder to keep the interaction going and still move toward the stipulated goals. Another positive quality of loosely scripted lessons is that they allow for more initiative from the child, militating against learned helplessness.

Children may not have the requisite knowledge of event structures or enough interest in exploring the world around them to benefit from the lack of structure in loose scripts. Also, the targeted structures may not occur in the child's initiated events. If a clinician wants to teach someone to keep to the topic but the child chooses well-defined games to play, the work on topic maintenance cannot commence.

Because tight and loose scripts serve different functions and serve a child differently depending on how those scripts fit with everyday realities, the choice of which type of teaching is appropriate should depend not only on the preferences of the clinician but on the learning style of the child, on what is being taught, and on the type of scripts that that knowledge appears in the child's everyday life. The following principles can serve as points of departure for designing overt as well as covert lesson plans:

Principle 1: Teach new structures to generalize into scripts found in everyday situations.

Principle 2: Teach new structures in familiar formats.

Principle 3: Perform task analyses by dividing tasks into units that are in keeping with the child's sensemaking.

Principle 4: Teach structures in naturally occurring contexts.

Principle 5: Use teaching styles compatible with the child's learning styles.

Principle 6: Teach the child to be assertive and to require that he or she be treated by others as legitimate. (Guard against learned helplessness.)

Implication A: When possible use open-ended scripts that require child initiative.

Implication B: For tight scripts, allow children power for negotiation, such as choice of activity, who is leader, and when turns begin and end.

Fine Tuning for Carrying Out Lessons

There are several viewpoints about how adults fine tune to children in the course of an interaction. The most familiar view is to focus on the input language to the child for adult-initiated sequences. This can be done in many areas (e.g., linguistic or cognitive) and at levels within each (e.g., phonological, syntactic, and semantic). The fine tuning would involve a match of the adult-input language with the child's level of competence.

Other studies in a separate literature in pragmatics that look to the other side of the adult-child exchange—not to how the adult begins the exchange but to how they respond to what the child says (Cross, 1978; Duchan and Weitzner-Lin, 1984). Adults have been found to imitate children, to expand on the content of the child's comment, and to model new content, and adults who operate under principles of behavior modification reinforce the child's desired responses through social means (e.g., "good talking") or more tangible reinforcers (Guess, Sailor, and Baer, 1978).

There is yet a third, more recent literature in pragmatics on adult-child interaction that describes the whole event structure, tracing the adult-child talk throughout the event. Bruner (Ratner and Bruner, 1978) is the spokesman of this research effort, and his interest is in studying infants and mothers engaged in circumscribed ritualized interactions, such as give and take and peekaboo. Bruner has found that (1) the mother first demonstrates all the parts of the interaction, (2) she scaffolds them, (3) the child begins assuming one of the roles, and (4) the child assumes any of the roles in the interchange.

All three literatures, the first one adult input, the second on adult response, and the third on scaffolding, neglect to ask about how the adult's actions fit with the child's intent and sense of the event and about the ways the adult and child fine tune to one another as the interaction is played out.

I would like to call for a fourth type of fine tuning, in which clinicians look to see how adults adjust to the child's intent as well as sense-making. For example, modeling or reinforcing may or may not be in keeping with the child's intent. A case in point is found in a recent language program explicated by Guess and co-workers (1978). The lesson is "designed to teach the student to request things using a two word response, *Want (object).*"

	Trainer	Student
Trial 1		
	(Holds up cookie)	
	Want what?	"cookie"
	That's close, Dick. Let's try again.	
	Say, want cookie.	"wa cookie"
Trial 2		
	(Holds up Coke)	
	Want what?	"wa Coke"
	Good! You want Coke.	
Trail 3		
	(Holds up piece of candy)	
	Want what?	"want candy"
	Very good talking, Dick.	
Trail 4		
	(Holds up toy car)	
	Want what?	"car"
	No Dick, you want car.	
	Want what?	"want car"
	That's right. Want car.	

When judging how well the clinician's response matches the child's intent, consistent potential mismatches can be found. They all emanate from the clinician's placing the child in an intentional state of wanting an object and then treating the child's verbalization as good talking rather than as a request for something. The clinician's evaluation of the quality of the act diverts the child's sense of the act from one intended to obtain objects to another involving talking competence. One could argue that being praised for something you do not feel at the time to be significant makes for a covert breakdown in the interaction. The classic example is to have the disconcerting experience of being told, "You're so cute when you're angry."

As for sensemaking, clinicians must ask: How well does the adult respond when the child offers an answer that is unexpected or considered wrong from an adult framework? The least degree of fine tuning to the child's sensemaking would cast the unexpected response as wrong because it is unexpected. This has been called the "negative sanctions" approach (Duchan, in press). The bottom line is that the adult regards the unexpected response as evidence that the child does not know the right answer.

The middle degree of fine tuning would say that the child's answer must come from somewhere. The adult then tries to guess by thinking what that answer would be from an adult frame of reference. The approach would result in the adult's being wrong about the child's sensemaking, but they are more accepting than if they had rejected the answer outright. Helm (1982) calls this acceptance position "strategic contextualization," and Cross and Snow call it "being semantically contingent" (Cross, 1978; Snow, 1984).

The ultimate in fine tuning would be for the adult to figure out where the child's response comes from and negotiate so that the child understands the adult position or for the adult to reframe the task to make the child's position salable to others (to strategically contextualize it) as well as in keeping with what the child intends.

Fine tuning through emphatic sensemaking leads to several sets of principles for carrying out lessons:

Principles for Adult-initiated Sequences:

Principle 1: Ask questions that you really want to know the answers to and that the child cares about.
Principle 2: Keep questions to a minimum.
Principle 3: Scale tasks and language to the language competence of the child.
Principle 4: Model, shape, and fade in keeping with the child's sense of the event.

Principles for Child-initiated Sequences:

Principle 1: Determine what events the child knows and prefers and have accouterments available for the child to initiate and carry out those events.
Principle 2: Respond contingently to the child's intent, content, and form. Give priority to the intent.
Principle 3: Minimize correction and metalinguistic rewards (e.g., "Good talking").
Principle 4: Follow the child's lead—talk to him or her about what he or she may be thinking, talk with him or her about what he or she may be meaning.
Principle 5: Accept appropriate and good answers, not just "right" answers.
Principle 6: Use intrinsic reinforcement to be in accord with the child's intent and idea of what is going on.

Principles for Routinized Sequences:

Principle 1: Use well rehearsed and mutually understandable routines to introduce new ideas (labeling routines, "Do as I do" routines).

Principle 2: Proceed from scaffolded routines to negotiated routines (from tight scripts to loose ones).

Principle 3: Use routines to mark openings and closings to the larger event, e.g., a good morning song.

Fine Tuning and Lesson Evaluation

Evaluating lesson plans is usually done by measuring performance at the beginning and at the end of a "treatment," whether it be a single lesson or series of lessons. The criterion measures for success are another indicator of the clinician's egocentricity. The criteria are chosen by the clinician according to what the clinician regards as most significant. They are also most often chosen without regard to the event structure but instead have more to do with context-stripped structures that were targeted in the lesson-plan goals. The idea behind the typical evaluation is that once the child learns the structure and can show this learning in the clinical environment, he or she will use it elsewhere and once and for all.

But language clinicians all know about the "carry-over" problem. Children do not unfailingly generalize the structures they have learned in one setting to another setting. Clinicians typically find the carry-over problem disconcerting and surprising, and they tend to lay the blame on the child's laziness, lack of motivation, or forgetfulness. They see the carry-over problem as separate from the child's learning abilities.

This sense that once the child can accomplish lessons the job is done denies the main message of the pragmatics movement: that context makes a difference. Language context makes a difference. Social context makes a difference. Intentional context makes a difference. The situational context makes a difference. If all these make a difference, how can clinicians be comfortable working toward goals that apply generally across contexts? The commitment to context dependency is made at the level of theory but is bracketed when intervention is planned to accomplish results such as remediating a "fronting" problem, teaching "requesting," or working on extending "semantic relations." This double standard of respect and disrespect for context holds even for those who conduct naturalistic therapy, in which they simulate everyday contexts. Naturalists also presume that language competence will generalize across contexts as long as the contexts are everyday ones.

In order to resolve the paradox, the question must be asked that has been asked ever since phoneme was defined: Which differences make a significant difference for the learner? Thus, we need to tune into which contexts are significant to the children and which will be influential in eliciting newly learned structures. The means for doing this is to return and rethink what has been called the "carry-over" problem or the problem of "generalization." What those terms imply is that children see certain events as the same and thereby operate in the same way in them: They generalize from one to the other. They see other events as different, thereby displaying a "carry-over" problem. When the difference between contexts that foster generalization and those that do not are analyzed, which contexts make a difference for that child are in fact determined.

In other words, generalization can be treated as part of learning and the success of clinical methods can be evaluated by examining how well they generalize the new contexts. These extensions of clinical assessment horizons lead to the following principles:

Principle 1: Analyze which contexts new learnings generalize to.
Principle 2: Assess which contexts seem to make a difference.
Principle 3: Determine the sensemaking behind stimulus generalization (i.e., what ideas lead to concepts of stimulus identity).
Principle 4: Determine the sensemaking behind response generalization (i.e., what ideas lead to response substitutability).

CONCLUSION

This chapter began with a promise to help fill the gap between language assessment and intervention and between theory and practice by delineating a conceptual framework and some principles derived from the pragmatics revolution. The notions of sensemaking and fine tuning led us to a reorganization of how language clinicians may think about what they are currently doing in both mentalistic, unstructured interventions (called "pragmatics intervention") and the more behavioral and structured approaches (dubbed "behavioral intervention"). Both approaches have the negative potential of being guided by the clinicians' egocentricity rather than being fine tuned to what the child is thinking and doing. In that way, both approaches can fall short of what they could be. Clinicians can do more than model and expand on what they take the child to mean they can be responsive to the child's intent, agenda, and overall sense of the event. They can do more than positively reinforce the child; they can also match the reinforcement to each act and to what the child wants to accomplish by it.

The principles offered for each step along the intervention process are only a beginning. The hope is that the principles will put clinicians on a new footing in their approach to research on clinical intervention—a footing that will move us away from being satisfied with demonstrations that "They got better" or "It works" and closer evaluation procedures that examine what the children learn in light of their own sensemaking and what the clinicians do in terms of how well they tune into what the children want and need in their everyday lives.

REFERENCES

Berger, P., and Kellner, H. (1981). *Sociology reinterpreted: An essay on method and vocation.* Garden City, NY: Doubleday.

Blank, M., and Franklin, E. (1980). Dialogue with preschoolers: A cognitively based system of assessment. *Applied Psycholinguistics, 1,* 127–150.

Bloom, L., and Lahey, M. (1978). *Language development and language disorders.* New York: John Wiley.

Bransford, J., and McCarrell, N. (1974). A sketch of a cognitive approach to comprehension. In W. Weimer and D. Palermo (Eds.), *Cognition and the symbolic processes.* Hillsdale, NJ: Lawrence Erlbaum.

Bromwich, R. (1981). *Working with parents and infants.* Baltimore: University Park Press.

Bruner, J. S. (1975). From communication to language: A psychological perspective. *Cognition, 3,* 255–287.

Campbell-Taylor, I. (1984). *Dimensions of clinical judgment in the diagnosis of alzheimer's disease.* Unpublished dissertation, State University of New York, Buffalo.

Chapman, R. (1983). Deciding when to intervene. In J. Miller, D. Yoder, and R. Schiefelbusch (Eds.), *Contemporary issues in language intervention* (Asha Reports No. 12, pp. 221–225). Rockville, MD: American Speech-Language and Hearing Association.

Clezy, G. (1979). *Modification of the mother-child interchange in language, speech, and hearing.* Baltimore: University Park Press.

Coggins, T., and Carpenter, R. (1981). The communicative intention inventory: A system for observing and coding children's early intentional communication. *Applied Psycholinguistics, 2,* 235–252.

Cole, P. (1982). *Language disorders in preschool children.* Englewood Cliffs, NJ: Prentice-Hall.

Cole, M., John-Steiner, V., Scribner, S., and Souberman, E. (1978). *L. S. Vgotsky: Mind in society.* Cambridge: Harvard University Press.

Craig, H. (1983). Applications of pragmatic language models for intervention. In T. Gallagher and C. Prutting (Eds.), *Pragmatic assessment and intervention issues in language.* San Diego: College-Hill Press.

Cross, T. (1978). Motherese: Its association with the rate of syntactic acquisition in young children. In N. Waterson and C. Snow (Eds.), *The development of communication.* New York: Wiley.

Dore, J. (1975). Holophrases, speech acts and language universals. *Journal of Child Language, 2,* 21–40.

Duchan, J. (1984). Language assessment: The pragmatics revolution. In R. Naremore (Ed.), *Language sciences.* San Diego: College-Hill Press.

Duchan, J. (in press). Special education for the nonhandicapped: How to interact with those who are different. P. Knoblock (Ed.), *Book on special education.* New York: Wiley.

Duchan, J., and Weitzner-Lin, B. (1984). *Nurturant and naturalistic intervention: Implications for planning lessons and tracking progress.* Unpublished manuscript.

Earle, C. (1983). Confusion resulting from misreferencing: A case study of a language-learning disabled adult. Unpublished thesis, State University of New York, Buffalo.

Englemann, S., and Osborn, J. (1976). *Distar language 1: An instructional system.* Chicago: Science Research Associates.

Frankel, R. (1982). Autism for all practical purposes: A microinteractional view. *Topics in Language Disorders, 3,* 33–43.

Gallagher, T., and Darnton, B. (1978). Conversational aspects of the speech of language disordered children: Revision behaviors. *Journal of Speech and Hearing Research, 21,* 118–136.

Garvey, C. (1979). Contingent queries and their relations in discourse. In E. Ochs and B. Schieffelin (Eds.), *Developmental pragmatics* (pp. 363–372). New York: Academic Press.

Gold, M. (1972). Stimulus factors in skill training of the retarded in a complex assembly task: Acquisition, transfer and retention. *American Journal of Mental Deficiency, 76,* 517–526.

Guess, D., Sailor, W., and Baer, D. (1978). Children with limited language. In R. Schiefelbusch (Ed.), *Language intervention strategies* (pp. 101–143). Baltimore: University Park Press.

Helm, D. (1982, August 16). *Strategic contextualization: A sensemaking practice.* Paper presented at the International Sociological Association's World Congress of Sociology, Mexico City.

Hurtig, R., Ensrud, S., and Tomblin, B. (1982). The communicative function of question production in autistic children. *Journal of Autism and Developmental Disabilities, 12,* 57–69.

Irwin, J. (Ed.). (1982). *Pragmatics: The role in language development.* Laverne, CA: Fox Point Publishing.

Johnston, J. (1982). Narratives: A new look at communication problems in older language disordered children. *Language, Speech, and Hearing Services in the Schools, 13,* 144–155.

Johnston, J. (1983). What is language intervention? The role of theory. In J. Miller, D. Yoder, and R. Schiefelbusch (Eds.), *Contemporary issues in language intervention.* (ASHA Reports No. 12, pp. 52–57). Rockville, MD: American Speech Language Hearing Association.

Jones, K., Rogerson, B., Weitzner-Lin, B., and Duchan, J. (1983, April). *The significance of conversational scaffolding in early language treatment.* Paper presented at New York Speech-Language and Hearing Association, Monticello, NY.

Kirchner, D., and Skarakis-Doyle, E. (1983). Developmental language disorders: A theoretical perspective. In T. Gallagher and C. Prutting (Eds.), *Pragmatic assessment and intervention issues in language* (pp. 215–246). San Diego: College-Hill Press.

Lubinski, R., Duchan, J. and Weitzner-Lin, B. (1980). Analysis of breakdowns in aphasic adult communication. *Proceedings of the Clinical Aphasiology Conference.* Minneapolis: BRK Publishers.

Lund, N., and Duchan, J. (1983). *Assessing children's language in naturalistic contexts.* Englewood Cliffs, NJ: Prentice-Hall.

Manolsen, A. (1983). It takes two to talk: A Hanen Early Language parent guidebook. Toronto: Hanen Early Language Resource Center.

Miller, J. (1981). *Assessing language production in children.* Baltimore: University Park Press.

Prizant, B., and Duchan, J. (1981). The functions of immediate echolalia in autistic children. *Journal of Speech and Hearing Disorders, 46,* 241–249.

Prutting, C., and Kirchner, D. (1983). Applied pragmatics. In T. Gallagher and C. Prutting (Eds.), *Pragmatic assessment and intervention issues in language* (pp. 29–64). San Diego: College-Hill Press.

Ratner, N., and Bruner, J. (1978). Games, social exchange and the acquisition of language. *Journal of Child Language, 5,* 391–402.

Rincover, A., and Koegel, R. (1975). Setting generality and stimulus control in autistic children. *Journal of Applied Behavioral Analysis, 8,* 234–246.

Sacks, H., Shegloff, E., and Jefferson, G. (1974). The simplest systematics for the organization of turn-taking for conversation. *Language, 50,* 696–735.

Shank, R., and Abelson, R. (1977). *Scripts, plans, goals and understanding.* Hillsdale, NJ: Lawrence Erlbaum.

Shriberg, L., and Kwiatkowski, J. (1982). Phonological disorders II: A conceptual framework for management. *Journal of Speech and Hearing Disorders, 47,* 242–256.

Snow, C. (1984). Parent-child interaction and the development of communicative ability. In R. Schiefelbusch and D. Bricker (Eds.), *Communicative competence: Acquisition and retardation.* Baltimore: University Park Press.

Sonnenmeier, R. (1984). *Involving parents in the language intervention process.* Unpublished thesis, State University of New York, Buffalo.

vanDijk, T. (1979). Relevance assignment in discourse comprehension. *Discourse Processes, 2,* 113–126.

Vuchinich, S. (1977). Elements of cohesion between turns in ordinary conversation. *Semiotica, 20,* 229–257.

Watson, L., and Lord, C. (1982). Developing a social communication curriculum for autistic students. *Topics in Language Disorders, 3,* 1–9.

Weisz, J. (1979). Perceived control and learned helplessness among mentally retarded and nonretarded children: A developmental analysis. *Developmental Psychology, 15,* 311–319.

Weitzner-Lin, B. (1981). *Interactive request analysis.* Dissertation, State University of New York, Buffalo.

Chapter 6

Incidental Strategies

Betty Hart and Todd Risley

Incidental teaching strategies differ from other strategies not in their nature but in their occasion: They are incidental and unplanned. The teaching occurs within an interaction that was begun for another purpose. A child may need help, information or a material, or merely social contact, or an adult may want to explain, encourage, or persuade a child to follow directions. Incidental teaching occurs when the educational aspects of the interaction are planned only to the extent that the adult has arranged an environment that stimulates interaction.

White (1978, p. 156) describes such interactions between mothers and children. The interactions were invariably initiated by the child: "the next step . . . involved the attempt by the adult to identify what it was the child was interested in at the moment." The adult prompted the child in order to identify what the child was focused on. "The adult then responded with what was needed and used some words at or above the child's apparent level of understanding, [or] incorporated a related idea . . ." The adult elaborated the child's topic.

The incidental use of teaching strategies has also been described by numerous observers of mother-infant interactions (cf. Bullowa, 1979; Schaffer, 1977; Snow, 1977). To paraphrase Schaffer (1977, pp. 12–13), the interactions generally began with spontaneous behavior from the infant, which the mother then chimed in to support, repeat, or comment on. Then the mother elaborated the child's response through modeling or repetition. The mother prompts to attract and maintain the infant's attention. She models, taking the infant's turn if necessary to keep the dialog going. As the child masters and tires of social play routines, the mother elaborates them in ways that teach organized exchanges such as peekaboo (Ratner and Bruner, 1978).

The strategies that mothers use are the same that teachers and therapists use in classrooms, clinics, and training sessions. They respond to the child's focus of attention. (Adults have usually prompted the child's focus either with materials or with their own actions or words.) Their response prompts the child to take a turn. The adult devises a prompt to accommodate the child's attention and ability level to enable the child to answer. If the child does not answer, the adult prompts again, often by modeling, taking the child's turn and then prompting the child to imitate the modeled behavior. When the child answers, the adult encourages an elaboration. The adult asks another question, provides information, or moves to the next step in a training sequence or a game and provides feedback, explicitly or through repeating the child's answering behavior.

These strategies are common to all teaching and integral to the incidental procedures used in remedial settings: delay (Halle, Baer, and Spradlin, 1981), mand-model (Rogers-Warren and Warren, 1980), and incidental teaching (Hart and Risley, 1975). These incidental procedures were each experimentally demonstrated effective in improving children's language in unstructured, extratraining situations. Their use enables teaching to occur throughout a child's day. Each procedure specifies a series of steps in teaching toward a specific goal. (See the original articles, or Hart, 1985, for specifics.)

The delay process (Halle et al., 1981) specifies that a teacher waits, expectantly maintaining eye contact for several seconds to give a child an opportunity to speak. If the child does not speak, the teacher prompts to help the child learn the cue (expectant waiting) for joining words to other social expressions of needs and wants. The teacher chooses an occasion and attracts the child's attention, perhaps by approaching the child and holding up a pitcher of juice at snack time. The prompt is comparable to the parent who approaches the infant and shakes a rattle or winds a music box, to the trainer who displays a stimulus object, or to the classroom teacher who writes a math problem on the chalkboard. In each case, the adult pauses and waits for joint focus on what is to be the topic of further interaction. The adult waits for the child to indicate a readiness to interact; for the infant to smile or reach or wave as well as to look; for a member of the class to raise a hand; for the child in language remediation to say something. If the child does not make some additional response, the adult, when teaching, again prompts the child. For an infant, the adult shakes the rattle again or moves it closer. The classroom teacher says, "Who can do this problem?" The remedial teacher asks, "What's this?" or models the behavior wanted.

The mand-model procedure (Rogers-Warren and Warren, 1980) specifies how, having achieved joint focus, a teacher prompts a child to initiate language. That is, the teacher waits for the child to focus on a material or activity (usually one the teacher has prearranged but has not specifically offered to the child). The teacher follows the child's regard, or reach, and prompts the child to speak. This is what a parent does when reading a story. If the child points, the parent stops reading momentarily to ask "What's that?" Similarly, the classroom teacher interrupts the lesson to call on a child who has raised a hand, asking "What's 2 and 2?" If the child continues to look at a stimulus object without naming it, the trainer, likewise asks, "What's this?" As the parent, trainer, and classroom teacher all do, the teacher employing the mand-model procedure models the response (takes the child's turn) if the child does not answer. The teacher or parent often waits for the child to repeat the model (Bruner, 1978; Moerk, 1972). In remedial training, the mand-model procedure, the adult always asks the child to rehearse the response and gives the child feedback.

When joint focus is achieved by a child initiating language, the incidental teaching process (Hart and Risley, 1975, 1978) specifies the steps a teacher uses to help the child elaborate through language. The adult prompts with questions that encourage the child to name, describe, or relate information. An incidental teaching interaction can be like those described by White (1978) in which a child comes to an adult and the adult prompts relative to the topic the child has chosen. A mother seeking to identify a child's topic typically uses questions, as does the incidental teacher, and models (prompts with trial repetitions of a possible child-word, for instance, for the child to confirm). Typically, when the child finally produces a topic word, the mother repeats it, as does the incidental teacher, confirming and providing feedback.

All the well-specified incidental procedures—delay, mand-modeling, incidental teaching—that have been experimentally validated as beneficial to children's language thus involve behaviors that parents and teachers naturally and spontaneously use. Parents and teachers prompt in varied ways matched to children's momentary attention and current ability level. They readily adapt if the child cannot answer. They ask an easier question, model, tell the child the answer, or rephrase a prior question. They provide feedback, confirming with repetition, praise, or materials. The strategies used incidentally are identical to those used in formal instruction, in training, and in remediation. All are individually adapted prompts for the elaboration of behavior.

But not all parents respond by teaching their children. The use of incidental strategies is apparently a characteristic of what White terms "supermothers" (White, 1971) and of Anglo-American culture (Fajardo and Freedman, 1981). Classroom and remedial teachers are given specific training in planning goals (lesson plans, training sequences) and organizing materials. Parents, too, tend to teach relative to materials (books, objects) or to routines (cf. Gleason and Weintraub, 1976) such as saying "goodbye." Thus, though procedures such as delay, mand-model, and incidental teaching replicate what parents and teachers "naturally" do, teachers must be trained to use them.

That even when thoroughly trained teachers do not naturally do incidental teaching (Cavallaro, 1982) reflects a problem in monitoring rather than in training. Formal teaching in classrooms, training situations, or clinical settings is readily monitored. Teachers submit lesson plans and work in sessions of constrained length and locale. For parents and teachers to whom teaching is not "natural" (as, for those who are not among White's "supermothers"), teaching is not likely to occur in the absence of monitoring. In addition, when the teaching itself (as in all the incidental procedures) must occur spontaneously, or unplanned occasions without specific preplanning by the adult, monitoring is likely to result in negative feedback to the adult. The adult is informed that the monitor saw an occasion on which teaching would have been appropriate or beneficial, and the monitored adult failed to recognize it.

The problem is one of directing the teacher's attention to occasions for teaching, once he or she has been trained in the teaching procedures. A teacher, for instance, who displays considerable expertise at teaching during a group time and who uses teaching strategies described in the literature, may not use these same strategies during preschool free-play periods. If teaching is not the teacher's "natural" style of interacting with children (i.e., if the teacher is not an actual or potential "supermother"), the unstructured interactions of preschool free-play do not present the cues necessary to shift the teacher into a teaching mode. She or he must be taught to recognize occasions rather than be taught how to teach.

A CORE INCIDENTAL STRATEGY

The following study concerns creating the preconditions for incidental strategies in unstructured situations. In a preschool classroom, a good teacher was encouraged to use incidental teaching because of its proven benefits to children's language (Hart and Risley, 1980). When training and feedback (largely negative, concerning missed occasions) resulted in little change in the teacher's natural style, focus was changed from teaching interactions to occasions for teaching. A core incidental strategy resulted—that of prompting a child to continue. This core strategy requires monitoring only whether a teacher responds rather than how a teacher responds.

Background: Setting and Data Collection

The training study was conducted in Turner House Preschool in Kansas City, Kansas, with twelve 4 year old black children (six of each sex) from a poverty community. The children attended a 4 day per week standard preschool program that included preacademic instruction, free play indoors and out, and lunch. During free play the children were free to move among activity areas (blocks, manipulative objects, housekeeping toys, creative activities). The three teachers were assigned to zones (LeLaurin and Risley, 1972). Their assignment to activity areas was constant throughout the study, as were the areas available to the children and their freedom to move among them.

Data collection was ongoing. Two observers recorded a 15 minute sample of each child's spontaneous speech during free play each day as part of another research project. These samples were collected and processed as described in Hart and Risley (1980). The observer wrote in longhand each utterance of the child observed. The observer noted to whom the utterance was addressed and also coded the nature of the turn (for instance, whether or not the child was responding to a listener). Those daily samples provided a description of the conversational environment in which training was undertaken and indicated changes in the behavior of both the teacher and the children.

Three aspects of the data were examined: what the children talked about, whether they elaborated their language, and in which conversational turn elaboration occurred. By examining what children talked about, we could see whether or not the conversational topic influenced the length of teacher-child exchanges and the likelihood of elaboration. Knowing in which turn children elaborated would show us the role of prompting utterances (deliberate or casual) on the part of the teacher.

In each observational sample for each child each day, each teacher-child interaction was analyzed. An interaction began whenever one party (teacher or child) was observer coded as initiating conversation to the other. Each turn in the interaction was examined until the next observer-coded initiation. The observer coded a child utterance as an initiation if more than 2 seconds elapsed with neither party speaking or if the child began to talk to someone else. Interactions were counted separately for each of the three teachers.

Each interaction was categorized in terms of what the exchange was about. Interactions were categorized as: (1) about a child's want or need, such as a material, permission, or help; (2) about the activity the child was engaged in, had just finished, or was about to begin: the "here-and-now" of preschool free play; or (3) about other topics. Other topics were those that could not be categorized as 1 or 2; often this was due to lack of information (the child said only "Yes" or "No," for instance). But many of the other topics concerned events outside the preschool, the activities of others, or natural phenomena (e.g., "It's raining").

Within each interaction each instance of elaboration was counted. The index of elaboration was a "new" vocabulary item, one that had not been recorded for the particular child previously. A list of these items for each child for each sample was output from the data for the ongoing research project. These vocabulary items were words that the children had already learned but had not used in the preschool. For instance, when woodworking was introduced, many children had occasion to use the word "nail," and it appeared as "new" in the preschool context. The child might, however, have said "nail" previously during free play but at a time when the observer was not sampling the child's speech. This effect of sampling, though, presumably affected the counts of elaboration equally across children and interactions.

Each instance of elaboration (a child's use of a "new" vocabulary item) was counted according to the turn in which it occurred in the interaction. Thus there were three categories of elaboration:

1. Initiations: a new vocabulary item that occurred in the child's opening utterance to a teacher, as in requesting a novel material such as "nail."
2. Responses: a new vocabulary item that occurred in a child's answer to a teacher's statement or question, as after a teacher asked, "What do you want?"
3. Continuations: a new vocabulary item that occurred when the child followed one utterance with another without waiting for the teacher to respond, as when a child said, "I want one. I want a nail, too."

Thirty regularly scheduled interobserver reliability recordings were made, in which the two observers recorded simultaneously but independently the utterances of the same child. Comparison of these samples yielded inter-observer agreements of 82 per cent on interactions, 88 per cent on "new" vocabulary items and 82 per cent on the turn (by the teacher) in which a new vocabulary item occurred within an interaction. For four randomly selected samples for each of the 12 children, a second coder categorized what each interaction was about. Intercoder agreement was 86 per cent.

The Pretraining Conversational Environment

The data were examined for 16 days (4 school weeks) prior to beginning to train the teacher. This was to evaluate the "conversational environment" of the preschool. The training study was planned only after the children had been attending the preschool for 6 months. They were thoroughly familiar with the activities and had established stable interaction patterns with the teachers. The researchers wanted to train teachers after they were comfortable and habituated to their roles within a group of children and wanted to evaluate the "conversational environment" after the children were well acquainted with one another, such that (in accordance with the social goals of the program) they were interacting with each other more often than with teachers.

The nature of the "conversational environment" indicated by the data accorded well with prior observational data (as Carew, 1980) and with anecdotal reports. The majority (70 per cent) of all teacher-child interactions were child initiated. This reflects the teacher-child ratio (1:4) plus the availability of teachers when assigned to zone management (LeLaurin and Risley, 1972) and the preschool rule that children ask for materials before using them. Teacher-child interactions occurred at an average of 6.5 per child per 15 minutes. This is an average of almost one interaction every third minute. Hence it is not surprising that most of these interactions (4.1 of the 6.5) contained only a single child utterance. Many of these utterances were requests for materials, answers to a teacher's questions, or some form of "Look, teacher."

The most frequent topic of interaction—when the children initiated the interaction—was the activity in which they were engaged. The children, as expected, talked most often about the here-and-now. The teachers, however, initiated talk most often to draw the children's attention to the activities of other children or to natural phenomena. The teachers' role as educators apparently led them to be, while receptive to and encouraging of children's talk of the here-and-now, mainly concerned with helping children develop appropriate social behaviors with other children and learn about things beyond their immediate activities.

This mismatch between teacher-child topics for initiation may be typical of an educational environment in which teaching language is incidental to the purpose of the interaction. Given the difference in the topics that teachers and children are most interested in talking about, it is hardly surprising that most of the interactions counted in the data consisted of a single child utterance. Though initiations (opportunities for conversation) occurred frequently in the free play situation, teacher-child conversations did not. Only slightly more than one in three (36 per cent) of all initiations was followed by subsequent teacher-child dialogue. It is apparent that the teachers were busy, given the frequency of interactions. On many occasions the children were doubtless unreceptive to conversation, wanting only a material or momentary help. Also, the teachers actively encouraged children to interact with each other rather than monopolizing a teacher.

If language development is a program goal, teachers in this situation are passing up two out of every three opportunities to help a child elaborate verbally. By far the least-used occasion for conversation was when a child asked for a material, permission, or help. At those times when a teacher clearly mediated a reinforcer for a child, it was rare for her to ask for further verbalization. Only one in ten such occasions was so used. Without a program that specified occasions and language targets, the teachers simply did not "naturally" engage in incidental teaching.

This was the case despite the finding that conversation of any sort was more than twice as likely to result in the child producing a "new" vocabulary item. On the average, per child per 15 minutes, the 4.1 interactions in which the child made a single statement led to 0.8 new vocabulary items. The child used a word new to that child's data in approximately one out of every five such interactions. Many of these interactions related to materials used or desired by the child. New materials were regularly introduced across the preschool year. In contrast, on the average per child per 15 minutes, the 2.4 interactions that continued into conversation resulted in 1.3 new vocabulary items. In almost every other teacher-child conversation, on the average, the child produced a word that had never before been recorded in the child's preschool data.

The natural, unstructured quality of the conversational environment may be reflected in the distribution of topics for conversation. As noted, neither children nor teachers conversed about the children's need and wants. The interactions the children initiated developed into conversation most often when the topic was the child's activity. The child apparently was doing something he or she wanted to talk about with the teacher. Teacher-initiated interactions that developed into conversations most often concerned other topics. The teacher wanted to talk to the child and was able to involve the child in her topic. Both teachers and children were most likely to converse about the kinds of topics they found most interesting. This may be the natural conversational environment for skilled talkers. People talk about what they are interested in at the moment.

In such an environment, training in incidental strategies is needed to focus teachers on the topics the children are most interested in and most capable of continuing into dialogue. Not all teachers are interested in children's talk about their activities. This is especially true when a teacher has not learned what prompts help the child develop the topic in interesting ways. Such teachers need the carefully structured sequences provided in procedures such as delay, mand-model, and incidental teaching. These sequences tell the teacher exactly what to say and when to say it, even though the teacher may find the process both unnatural and uninteresting.

The opportunity, as well as a need, for training was revealed when the interactions of the teachers in the preschool was compared in terms of the frequency of conversations with children. The teachers were alike in their tendency to initiate talk to children, most often about other topics, and approximately 15 per cent of these teacher-initiated interactions led to further dialog. But there was a marked contrast between Teachers A and B in terms of child-initiated interactions. The children showed a marked preference for talking with Teacher B. This was not a preference for an activity area. The data showed equal numbers of children present across activity areas each day. During preschool free play all the children usually visited each activity area each day. If any activity area remained empty, new materials were added in that area to attract children. All three teachers were equally attentive to children. The differences among the teachers in interaction styles were in accord with usual preschool practice of familiarizing children with style differences. The marked contrast between Teachers A and B may reflect the children's tendency to match a teacher's style and accentuate it over time.

The data showed that for teacher B, who had extensive experience in incidental teaching, 43 per cent of child-initiated interactions were followed by conversation; for Teacher A, 19 per cent of child-initiated interactions led to further dialog. On the whole, 61 per cent of the interactions between children and Teacher B contained a subsequent child-turn at talk. For Teacher A conversation developed in only 33 per cent of the teacher-child interactions. However, children initiated interactions with Teacher B almost three times as often as with Teacher A; hence, Teacher B had many more opportunities to talk with children about topics (the children's activities) the children were most likely to converse about. When children initiated talk with Teacher A concerning what they were doing, an average of 26 per cent of those initiations were followed by further talk from the child. For Teacher B, an average of 57 per cent of such initiations were followed by further talk from the child. However, when children initiated talk concerning other topics, a similar percentage (55 per cent) of such initiations were followed by conversation with Teacher B. Thirteen per cent of children's initiations to Teacher A about other topics were followed by further turns at talk by the children.

Teacher B, perhaps because of her experience with incidental teaching, was more successful at getting children to continue talking, regardless of topic or initiator. The children's choice of conversational partner reflected this fact. For Teacher A, the skill and responsiveness she displayed during small-group teaching sessions was not apparent during free-play periods. Apparently, the free-play setting cued a different set of responses than did the group or one-to-one instruction.

Training Use of Incidental Strategies

Teacher A became a candidate for training in incidental teaching procedures because her rate of conversing with children was so low in comparison with the other two teachers. Also, Teacher B provided an available "standard" against which to evaluate changes in Teacher A's behavior. (Teacher C, whose frequency of conversing with children was midway between the frequencies of Teachers A and B, provided yet another standard, though comparisons with her data are not discussed.) Some, though not major, benefits to children's language were expected from training Teacher A. Because new vocabulary items tended to appear in the data in approximately every other teacher-child conversation (regardless of which teacher a child was talking to), it was expected that the addressee, rather than the frequency, of new vocabulary items would change if children shifted from conversing with Teacher B to conversing with Teacher A. From observations and discussions with the three teachers it was clear that the children were conversing with teachers at will. They were just choosing one teacher more often than the others.

Teacher A was instructed in incidental teaching procedures, and specific occasions and prompts were suggested on the basis of the data and the activity area she supervised. Each day she was given feedback. In all the observer-recorded language samples the interactions were examined in terms of who initiated and whether conversation followed an initiation. Little change was seen. Though Teacher A increased her rate of prompting subsequent to children's initiations, she was not more successful in getting a child to take another turn at talk. Because no programmed incidental teaching was instituted, children were not required to elaborate before taking materials. After six months of preschool attendance, they were used to taking a material while asking to use it. This habit did not change. Children's habits of interacting with Teacher B also did not change. They did not begin to initiate more often to her. Though she increased her rate of prompting their elaboration when the children initiated, she did not discontinue initiating topics herself. The children were used to Teacher A initiating talk to them, and the more she tried to wait for them to initiate, the longer they waited for her. Without frequent initiations, Teacher A did not have enough opportunities to try out prompts and explore which were the more and less successful. She was unsuccessful in receiving conversations, such that child initiations did not increase, and her efforts to change her natural interaction style left her feeling extremely uncomfortable with the silence that prevailed in her area while she waited for children to initiate and she restrained herself from initiating to them. As she remained attentive to the children, totally silent, what she communicated was that she did not want to talk as she usually did. Thus, the children were even less likely to initiate.

The complexity of incidental teaching, it was clear, lay not in the process itself but in the conditions for its use. Incidental strategies are interactional. The child's behavior is as important as the teacher's. The children must prompt the teacher by initiating and by giving feedback (elaboration) when the teacher provides an appropriate prompt. The children must be actively engaged, doing things they want to talk about. The teacher must make clear to children her perference for listening to them rather than talking to them. This preference is shown in her differential response to child initiations. In order to learn incidental teaching, Teacher A needed more opportunities to practice.

Teacher A was told to continue, as before, prompting more talk whenever a child initiated to her. In addition, she was told to begin initiating as usual to children, but only concerning what the children were doing; that is, she could initiate only on the topic about which children were most likely to continue talking. Then if a child responded to her initiation, she was to try, as in incidental teaching, to prompt further talk. This was an adaptation of the procedures the teachers had used in the first days of the preschool year. At that time they initiated frequently to children about the children's activities in order to make clear to the children their interest and appreciation of the children's appropriate play behavior.

When Teacher A began both responding to children's initiations and initiating to them about what they were doing, her interest in talking, and especially her interest in talking about the children's activities, became apparent. Children began initiating more and more frequently. Teacher A began to feel more comfortable; by the end of the preschool year, 40 per cent, on the average, of all interactions with Teacher A contained more than one turn to talk on the part of the child. Child-initiated interactions were still the most likely to continue into conversation, suggesting that Teacher A was still learning how best to prompt. But she was regularly using children's initiations to try prompts. And the numbers of new vocabulary items in the data that were addressed to Teacher A increased, as expected. Both children and teacher benefited. The teacher was able to retain the interaction style she found comfortable; the children were able to continue to talk about what interested them.

The teacher succeeded in incorporating into her natural style the core of incidental teaching, the prompting of continued talk. She did not have to wait for child initiations, nor did she have to shift from casual conversation into a teaching mode. She did not have to evaluate the child's utterance and quickly plan a teaching goal and a sequence of prompts for elaboration. She could say whatever was natural and try again if she did not succeed in getting the child to take another turn. She and the child could shape her conversational prompts. She could develop incidental teaching on her own, with time, trial, and child feedback. The result would be identical to formal incidental teaching procedures; only the training sequence would differ.

Implications for Intervention

The core incidental strategy—that of getting a child to continue talking—is a part of all teaching. Prompting a child to take a next turn is a part of all the incidental procedures (delay, mand-model, incidental teaching) and a part of classroom, clinic, and remedial teaching. The study described here serves only to make salient the core nature of this strategy. It is essential—and apparently not simple—for a teacher to "get started" on an instructional sequence. In formal teaching in classrooms, clinics, and training sessions, teachers select materials, formulate lesson plans, and arrange an instructional setting that cues them to begin teaching. Parents use a toy, a book, or a game. They sit across or beside a child or hold an infant face to face. The cues that shift an adult into a teaching mode apparently must be deliberately arranged in free-play settings, by putting materials out of children's reach, for instance, so that the need to mediate them directly cues the teacher to teach and suggests an instructional goal.

In spite of training, teachers may not generalize procedures such as delay, mand-model, and incidental teaching or continue to use them (Cavallaro, 1982) if, as in the study described here, the shift into a teaching mode is not the teachers' natural style and the conditions in the classroom are not favorable (i.e., the children do not initiate very often but wait for the teacher to begin conversation). But even when incidental procedures cannot be successful, the core strategy can be. A teacher can always encourage a child to say something more or take another turn. The study described also showed that just taking another turn at talk was beneficial in terms of the child's language use, regardless of the topic, the initiator, or the content of the adult's responses.

Also, this core strategy is easy to instruct and easy to monitor. Rather than memorizing a sequence of instructional steps, all the teacher has to do is encourage the child to continue talking. She can be encouraged to use whatever techniques she prefers, exercising her ingenuity and imagination. Monitoring need involve only 5 minutes of observation during free play in which attempts and successes are counted. Teachers can self-record if desired. Feedback can focus on the teachers' successes. Over time, more and more of the attempts to have a child to take another turn at talk will be successful. The children will teach the teacher what the best kinds of prompts are and what the best topics are. Young children can rarely make polite conversation. If they are interested, they continue conversing; if not, they fall silent. They provide excellent feedback.

Focusing a teacher on the core strategy—getting the child to take a next turn—involves attending to the feedback children give. She or he is likely to realize that when a child is silent, expectant waiting is an effective prompt for the child to talk. She or he is likely to recognize that nonverbal behaviors such as looking at or reaching toward a material constitute a next turn, such that she can prompt again. The teacher is not trained in the succession of behaviors, prompting, modeling, and giving feedback that are essential to the incidental procedures. These are behaviors he or she already has. Rather, the use of this core strategy trains the teacher to recognize that every beginning of an interaction with a child is the beginning of a teaching moment.

REFERENCES

Bruner, J. S. (1978). Prelinguistic prerequisites of speech. In R. N. Campbell and P. T. Smith (Eds.), *Recent advances in the psychology of language: Language development and mother-child interaction.* New York: Plenum.

Bullowa, M. (Ed.) (1979). *Before speech: The beginning of interpersonal communication.* New York: Cambridge University Press.

Carew, J. V. (1980). Experience and the development of intelligence in young children, at home and in day care. *Monographs of the Society for Research in Child Development, 45,* 6–7.

Cavallaro, C. C. (1982). *Issues in the implementation of incidental teaching in preschool programs.* Paper presented at the Eighth Annual Convention of the Association for Behavior Analysis, Milwaukee.

Fajardo, B. F., and Freedman, D. G. (1981). Maternal rhythmicity in three American cultures. In T. M. Field, A. M. Soster, P. Vietze, and P. H. Liederman (Eds.), *Culture and early interactions.* Hillsdale, NJ: Lawrence Erlbaum.

Gleason, J. B., and Weintraub, S. (1976). The acquisition of routines in child language. *Language in Society, 5,* 129–136.

Halle, J. W., Baer, D. M., and Spradlin, J. E. (1981). Teacher's generalized use of delay as a stimulus control procedure to increase language use in handicapped children. *Journal of Applied Behavior Analysis, 14,* 389–409.

Hart, B. (1985). Environmental techniques that may facilitate generalization and acquisition. In A. K. Rogers-Warren and S. F. Warren (Eds.), *Teaching functional language.* Baltimore: University Park Press.

Hart, B., and Risley, T. R. (1975). Incidental teaching of language in the preschool. *Journal of Applied Behavior Analysis, 8,* 411–420.

Hart, B., and Risley, T. R. (1978). Promoting productive language through incidental teaching. *Education and Urban Society, 10,* 407–429.

Hart, B., and Risley, T. R. (1980). In vivo language intervention: Unanticipated general effects. *Journal of Applied Behavior Analysis, 13,* 407–432.

LeLaurin, K., and Risley, T. R. (1972). The organization of day care environments: "Zone" versus "man-to-man" staff assignments. *Journal of Applied Behavior Analysis, 5,* 225–232.

Moerk, E. (1972). Principles of interaction in language learning. *Merrill-Palmer Quarterly, 18,* 229–257.

Ratner, N., and Bruner, J. (1978). Games, social exchange and the acquisition of language. *Journal of Child Language, 5,* 391–401.

Rogers-Warren, A., and Warren, S. F. (1980). Mands for verbalization: Facilitating the display of newly-trained language in children. *Behavior Modification, 4,* 361–382.

Schaffer, H. R. (1977). Early interactive development. In H. R. Schaffer (Ed.), *Studies in mother-infant interaction.* New York: Academic Press.

Snow, C. E. (1977). The development of conversation between mothers and babies. *Journal of Child Language, 4,* 1–22.

White, B. (1971). An analysis of excellent early educational practices: Preliminary report. *Interchange, 2,* 71–88.

White, B. (1978). *Experience and environment (Vol. 2).* Englewood Cliffs, NJ: Prentice-Hall.

Chapter 7

A Review of Studies on Learning Disabled Children's Communicative Competence

Tanis Bryan

In a front-page newspaper article, a newly elected Chicago city alderman claimed that members of the opposition party had threatened "to set his feet on fire." The next day the opposition countercharged that they had actually said, "We will hold your feet to the fire" (Sun-Times, May 6, 1983, p. 2). Chicago columnist Mike Royko responded to the confrontation, explained how the two statements differed in meaning, and provided examples of other "political metaphors" that could be similarly misinterpreted. These included, "If we don't get your vote, we'll shoot you down," "Go along with us or we'll give you the ax," "We're going to break the back of the opposition," and "This could blow the roof off City Hall."

Did the alderman really misunderstand what was said or meant, or did he understand very well how to capture Page One headlines? Reputation aside, even Chicago politicians have not been subjected to literal translations of such threats. Rather, it seems reasonable that most people would recognize such statements as political posturing meant to impress the listener with the speaker's power and the political advisability of listener compliance.

Preparation of this manuscript was supported by a research contract from the Office of Special Education, Department of Education (US OE 300 800 62) with the Chicago Institute for the Study of Learning Disabilities, College of Education, University of Illinois at Chicago.

The confrontation generated by the presumed misunderstanding of claims to ''set'' the alderman's feet on fire to versus to ''hold'' the alderman's feet to the fire gives cause for thought when beginning a chapter on the communicative competence of the learning disabled. Whether the alderman used his opponents' hyperbole to political advantage or in fact misinterpreted the statement is not known, but surely children who have problems in language development would be at risk for failure to understand the use of the kind of language represented by such ''political metaphors.''

It would seem that such children might have particular problems in learning in-group language. Groups develop their own manner of speaking as a way to facilitate the exchange of information by group members and to mark speakers as members of that group. Language is an important key in the socialization of a group's members. If you are not a member of a group, you will not be privy to its special language, and to the extent that you do not acquire its language you are not likely to achieve group membership. Whether the language is politician's hyperbole, teenager's slang, or language specialists' jargon, comprehension and use of in-group language affects status in the group.

LEARNING DISABILITY: CHILDREN AT RISK FOR COMMUNICATION BREAKDOWN

Evidence from two distinct areas of research led to the hypothesis that learning disabled children are likely to have difficulty both in understanding in-group language and in becoming accepted as members of an in-group.

Language Deficits

One area of research has examined the language skills of the learning disabled. Although the learning disabled have been described as having attentional, perceptual, and conceptual problems, along with many other inadequacies (Bryan and Bryan, 1978), descriptions of the learning disabled and guidelines of defining learning disabled stress the presence of language problems (Federal Register, 1976). Characteristics used to define learning disabled include deficits in language comprehension and expression, oral reading and reading comprehension, and spelling and writing, each of which is a language-based skill. From early theorizing (McGrady, 1968) to recent factors analytic studies (McKinney, 1982), language problems have been among the most prevalent characteristics within learning disabled samples. Recent research is finding that subtypes within learning disabled samples may be differentiated on the basis of different types of language problems (e.g., articulation versus semantic deficits: Doehring and Hoshko, 1979; Lyon and Watson, 1981). In addition, studies comparing the learning disabled and nondisabled on specific aspects of syntax and semantics consistently show the learning disabled to be less adept than the normal achiever. (For a review, please see Donahue, Pearl, and Bryan, 1983.) Across presumably heterogeneous samples, the learning disabled consistently do more poorly than their classmates on a variety of linguistics assessments.

What is striking about these studies is that they are based on children classified as having learning disabilities, not on children identified as having language problems. Descriptions of samples in learning disabled research typically specify that these children show a discrepancy between intelligence and achievement. Children are seldom described in terms of specific problems such as language or attentional deficits. Although it may be that language problems represent a generic difficulty among children who do poorly in school, this notion is hypothetical. Classroom teachers refer children who show problems in the acquisition of academic skills and who are behavior problems; whether classroom teachers recognize that such problems may be caused or exacerbated by language difficulties is not yet known. In any case, children classified as learning disabled are more likely than normally achieving classmates to do poorly on various measures of syntactic and semantic skills.

Social Status

The second area of research that leads to the suspicion that the learning disabled are more likely than the nondisabled to experience difficulty in the acquisition of social uses of language pertains to studies of their social status. The most consistent finding in learning disability research is that these children elicit negative judgments from others. Sociometric studies show that the learning disabled are less popular and more rejected that classmates (e.g., Bruininks, 1978). Parents complain that the learning disabled are more difficult to talk to and that they feel less affection for the learning disabled than for their siblings (Owens, Adams, Forrest, Stoez, and Fisher, 1971). Teachers rate them as less desirable to have in the classroom (Keogh, Tchir, and Windeguth-Behn, 1974). Even strangers unacquainted with the child rate the learning disabled more hostile than nondisabled children after viewing a brief videotape of the children (Bryan and Sherman, 1980).

The Relationship Between Linguistic and Social Deficits

The research on learning disabled children's language deficits and social rejection led to the hypothesis that language problems are related to the social difficulties experienced by the learning disabled. Although it has been postulated that children could have deficits in but one language component, that is, syntax but not semantics (Bloom and Lahey, 1978), communicative competence requires the coordination of language and cognitive skills. Hence it seems likely that a breakdown in the acquisition of any linguistic or cognitive process could have a negative impact on the child's acquisition of communicative competence. Thus the hypothesis emerging from the language and social status research is that the rejection of the learning disabled is related to inadequate or inappropriate and deficient uses of language in social contexts. This chapter reviews research investigating the communicative competence of the learning disabled. Much of this research has been done under the sponsorship of the Chicago Institute for the Study of Learning Disabilities, established by the United States Department of Education at the University of Illinois, Chicago, 1977. However, other systematic work also has been done, particularly by researchers at the Learning Disability Research Institute, University of Kansas. This chapter includes the work of our colleagues as it relates to the communicative competence of the learning disabled.

COMMUNICATIVE COMPETENCE

The term communicative competence refers to

> [a language user's] knowledge of sentences, not only as grammatical but also as appropriate. He or she acquires competence as to when to speak, when not, and as to what to talk about with whom, when, where, in what manner. In short, a child becomes able to accomplish a repertoire of speech acts, to take part in speech events, and to evaluate their accomplishments by others. (Hymes, 1971, p. 277)

Communicative competence involves three interrelated skills:

1. The ability to produce and interpret speech-making adjustments according to the social status of listeners and situations (Ervin-Tripp, 1979a, b);
2. The ability to take into account what is and is not known to the listener and to provide adequate information (Cosgrove and Patterson, 1977); and
3. The ability to understand the rules of cooperative conversational turn-taking (i.e., know how to begin and end a conversation and how to introduce and change topics; Ochs and Schieffelin, 1979).

These three components overlap and are interrelated with social cognition. Hence, in addition to having a linguistic repertoire, the language user must produce statements that reflect an understanding of the social relations and the attitudes of participants, the purpose and setting of the interaction, and the implications of the social exchange.

Although far from complete as a corpus of data, the studies of learning disabled children's communicative competence have tapped at least to some extent into these various components of social language usage. Thus, their ability to make adjustments in response to difference listeners, their understanding of given versus new information, and their conversational turn-taking skills have been compared with those of normally achieving students in various studies. Using naturalistic and contrived situations, their persuasiveness, tactfulness, problem solving, and job-related communication skills have been assessed. Further, a few intervention studies have explored how to improve on their conversational skills and job-related language skills.

Making Adjustments in Communicative Style

To adapt speech to be appropriate to the needs, knowledge, and characteristics of a listener involves interrelated components in social cognition and language. Many studies have asked whether learning disabled children differ from normal achievers in this regard. These studies focused on children's communications to listeners who varied in the dimensions of age, intimacy (stranger versus well-known listener), and power (adult versus child listener), and one study manipulated the message content (e.g., delivering good versus bad news).

An early study examined whether learning disabled children could alter the complexity of their communications for younger versus same age peers. This study was patterned after Shatz and Gelman's (1973) finding that 4 year old children communicated differently to adults, peers, and 2 year old children. Four year old children used shorter utterances and more attention-getting statements when speaking to 2 year olds than when speaking to adults and peers. Bryan and Pflaum (1978) hypothesized that learning disabled children would fail to make age-related adjustments in the complexity and content of their communications to same age versus younger children. Fourth and fifth grade learning disabled males and females were videotaped while they taught a laboratory bowling game to a same sex classmate and to a kindergartner. A T-unit analysis was used to compare the linguistic complexity of learning disabled and nondisabled children's communications with those of their classmates and younger children. The T-unit analysis is based on each statement's independent clause with all the dependent clauses attached to it (Hunt, 1965). Children's communications were analyzed for the total number of T-units, modifiers, non–T-unit phrases and words, mean length of T-units, and the proportions of T-units that were complexities (e.g., coordinated items, additive structures, and ordering transformations). The comparisons showed that although the learning disabled did not differ from the normal achievers in the amount of talking, the learning disabled used shorter mean T-unit lengths. Smaller proportions of their T-units were complexities and they used fewer modifiers. However, learning disabled males, but not learning disabled females, accounted for group differences. Learning disabled girls and nondisabled boys used less complex syntax when instructing the younger child than they used with their classmate. However, nondisabled girls used more complex syntax in their communication to the younger children than to classmates. Only learning disabled boys showed communicative insensitivity to audience differences in age. Nondisabled girls' use of more complex syntax with younger children was interpreted as a reflection that they assume a teacher role.

A content analysis of children's statements assessed the proportion of children's statements that were instructions (how to play the game), positive social statements (personal and task-related conversation, laughter and humor), neutral feedback statements (keeping score), incompetent statements (failing to clarify or giving misinformation, inappropriate humor), or competitive and negative statements. The results showed that in general younger children received more feedback and repetitions but fewer competitive and incompetent communications than classmates. However, although learning disabled children provided about the same amount of instructions to both peers and younger children, the normal achievers provided a much higher proportion of instructions to younger children than to peers. Furthermore, learning disabled males interacting with peers and learning disabled girls interacting with younger children engaged in a higher proportion of incompetent communications than other groups.

Significant grouping by sex differences were also reported in a study of politeness and persuasiveness of requests. Donahue (1981) used a role playing paradigm to compare learning disabled and nondisabled second, fourth and sixth graders ability to vary their requests as a function of listener differences. The listener dimensions which were varied were intimacy and power because adults and children have been shown to make differential responses to these social features (Ervin-Tripp, 1979a, b; Mitchell-Kernan and Kernan, 1977; Piche, Rubin, and Michlin, 1978). Subjects were asked to pretend that they needed newspapers for a school assignment and to convince each of four imaginary listeners to give up their newspapers. The listeners varied on the dimensions of power and intimacy relative to the children: the child's father (+ power, + intimacy), the parish priest (+ power, − intimacy), a same-sex best friend

(– power, + intimacy), and a same-age and same-sex "new kid in school" (– power, – intimacy).

Children's requests were coded for politeness and persuasiveness. Politeness was analyzed using a scale developed by having adults make paired-comparison judgments of the most frequently occurring forms (e.g., "May I please have your newspaper?" versus "Could you give me your newspaper?"). The degree of persuasiveness was coded using Clark and Delia's (1976) system for ranking types of persuasive appeals along a continuum representing the degree to which the persuader adopts the listener's viewpoint. For instance, appeals that focus on speaker need (e.g., "I need it for a school project") were viewed as less listener-adapted than appeals that point out some advantages that listener compliance might generate (e.g., "Tomorrow I'll get you a paper"). Also analyzed were the total number of variety of appeal types and the number of different request forms used.

The results showed within-group sex differences similar to those reported by Bryan and Pflaum (1978). The learning disabled girls produced more polite requests and somewhat more persuasive appeals to all listeners than did the normally achieving girls. Although the learning disabled girls did not differ from their same-sex counterparts on the syntactic complexities of their statements, they differed insofar as they adopted a more deferential role.

Both learning disabled and nondisabled boys showed variations in politeness as a function of listener differences. However, nondisabled boys' requests were adjusted in response to intimacy differences, whereas learning disabled boys made adjustments responsive to power differences. Specifically, the nondisabled boys were more polite to low-intimate than to high-intimate listeners. But the learning disabled boys were more polite to low-power (peer) than to high-power (adult) listeners. The learning disabled did not differ from the nondisabled children in the number of linguistic forms they used to express politeness, yet the learning disabled boys produced fewer and a smaller variety of persuasive appeals and were less likely to produce appeals characteristic of more sophisticated levels of perspective taking.

In interpreting the group by sex differences in these studies, it is helpful to keep in mind the interdependence of the linguistic and social skills involved in listener-adapted communications: (1) discriminating between listener and situational features, (2) understanding how to vary speech in accordance with listener and situational factors, and (3) having the linguistic repertoire to do so. In both studies the normally achieving children made appropriate distinctions and responded differentially to different listeners. Although the nondisabled girls use of more complex rather than less complex utterances to younger children was unexpected,

Bryan and Pflaum (1978) suggested that the nondisabled girls assumed the role of "teacher" and "put on" their best language. Because kindergartners are much more advanced linguistically than the 2 year olds in the Shatz and Gelman (1973) study, it may be that the nondisabled girls had a good, and appropriate, sense of the communicative skill of the kindergartners. The learning disabled girls did not demonstrate deficits in their discrimination of listener features or of how to vary their speech: they had the linguistic repertoire to do so. Nonetheless, the learning disabled girls in both Bryan and Pflaum's (1978) and Donahue's (1981) studies were discrepant from their same-sex classmates. The finding that they used more "incompetent" communications and were more deferential suggests that the problems of the learning disabled females may be related to social-cognitive skills and social experiences.

Learning disabled boys show less ability to discriminate listener features and make speech adjustments accordingly. In certain respects their problems seem related to deficits in linguistic repertoire. In the Bryan and Pflaum (1978) study the learning disabled boys did not vary their syntactic complexity when communicating with younger and same-aged children. In the Donahue (1981) study the learning disabled boys had a smaller variety of persuasive appeals, and these appeared to be less mature than those used by nondisabled youngsters. However, in the Donahue study, although the learning disabled were discrepant from their peers, they did make distinctions between listeners when making requests. It cannot be determined whether their problems related to deficits in the perception of distinctive listener features or in linguistic repertoire. The results of these two studies show that the learning disabled are discrepant from same-sex classmates in the listener-adapted communications.

Pearl, Donahue, and Bryan (1983) examined listener perspective taking also, but in this case the dimension varied was the content of the message: delivering bad versus good news. A role-playing paradigm was used in which first through fourth grade learning disabled and normally achieving boys and girls were asked to tell what they would say to a classmate in response to situations that varied in whether the message conveyed was positive ("You've been chosen for the class play") or negative information ("You have not been chosen for the class play"). Children's communications were assessed for their tactfulness, that is whether they used verbal strategies to ameliorate the situation (e.g., "next time I'll choose you . . ."). Younger children and the learning disabled were found to be less tactful than older children and the nondisabled children. The learning disabled used fewer verbal strategies to soften the impact of bad news on a listener.

In sum, these data suggest that the learning disabled are discrepant in various ways from nondisabled children in their ability to make listener-related speech adjustments. Although not directly tested in these studies, these data do support the notion that social rejection may be related to lack of communicative competence. It may be that lack of communicative competence prohibits participation in intimate friendships or in-group experiences. Conversely, group rejection may limit the social experiences involved in the acquisition of communicative competence. It should also be remembered that although learning disabled children differ from nondisabled children, particularly from their same-sex counterparts in these studies, their language or speech problems are not very obvious. Their use of syntactic and semantic structures are correct, and they participate verbally as much as nondisabled youngsters.

Conveying Appropriate and Adequate Information

Choosing what to say requires understanding what the listener already knows and what information needs to be added to make a communication meaningful. The ability to choose what information to convey is another component of communicative competence and requires both linguistic and cognitive skills. Much of the research on children's ability to convey and comprehend information has used a referential communication paradigm. In this procedure, one partner describes an object or pattern so that a listener can identify or construct it. The listener is prohibited from observing that which is described so that the listener's response is based on the message alone. Referential communication tasks have been used to study the speaker and listener skills of the learning disabled.

Speaker Skills. In the speaker role the child constructs a message and then monitors the listener's response to determine whether the message is adequate. The speaker has to be able to formulate a reasonable informative message and then adjust the message if the listener appears to be confused. Noel (1980) compared learning disabled and nondisabled 9 year old boys' ability to describe ambiguous figures. Analyses of the messages showed that learning disabled boys did not differ from the nondisabled on the number of words or categories used but that the learning disabled boys were more likely to refer to the shape of the figure (e.g., "It's round") while the nondisabled were more likely to generate labels (e.g., "It looks like a tree"). In a second part of the study, another group of learning disabled and nondisabled boys had to select one of several pictures in response to these clues. The type of messages produced by nondisabled boys resulted in more correct picture selections from both learning disabled and nondisabled boys.

Spekman (1981) had dyads of learning disabled and nondisabled 9 to 11 year old boys take turns doing a referential communication task in which the listener had to construct a pattern of geometric shapes based on listener clues. Spekman reported that there were no differences in the amount of time or the amount of turns taken by dyads. However, learning disabled speakers produced less informative descriptions: dyads in which a learning disabled child was a member were less accurate in their constructions than those in which both participants were nondisabled. Both studies therefore found messages were less informative when constructed by learning disabled boys than by nondisabled boys. The learning disabled boys' descriptions of the overall pattern of designs suggest that they have difficulty selecting essential information and presenting it effectively or they cannot retrieve such information with the exactness of nondisabled boys. Although their messages are not as adequate, they do not seem to be unaware of their listener's difficulties.

Pearl, Donahue, and Bryan (1981) used a referential task to compare learning disabled and nondisabled youngsters responses with implicit and subtle messages from a listener who indicated that the clues were inadequate. In this case, learning disabled and nondisabled children were asked to describe a series of abstract figures to an adult experimenter. On certain trials the experimenter would respond with direct feedback (1) by selecting the correct figure, (2) by explicitly requesting another clue, (3) by implicitly requesting another clue (e.g., "I don't understand"), or (4) by responding with a puzzled facial expression. Children in first through eighth grades were found to respond to explicit and implicit feedback, but it was not until seventh and eighth grade that children generated another clue in response to the puzzled facial expression. Thus, the learning disabled are as likely to be sensitive to listener responses as the nondisabled.

Listener Skills. On referential communication tasks, the listener role requires the listener (1) to judge whether the message is adequate by monitoring its informational value and to ask for more information when the message is inadequate, (2) to understand the communication rules that dictate that listeners take an active stance—that is, that the listener has to let the speaker know when the message is off-base; and (3) to comprehend the message in order to make the correct choice based on the information. Learning disabled children's ability to monitor the information value of a message and request clarification was examined by Kotsonis and Patterson (1980). Seven and 10 year old learning disabled and nondisabled boys were taught the rules of a game, one rule at a time. The child was asked after each rule was presented, "Do you know how to play yet or do you need another clue?" It was found that both younger and older learning disabled boys asked for fewer game rules than did the nondisabled.

Donahue, Pearl, and Bryan (1980) evaluated the performance of first through eighth grade learning disabled and nondisabled children on a referential communication task that required skills in each of the components cited previously. In this case, the child had to select one of four pictures on the basis of experimenter clues. The adequacy of the clues, however, differed across trials. On some trials the clues were (1) fully informative: the child could eliminate three of the four choices; (2) partially informative: the child could eliminate two of the four choices; or (3) uninformative: the child could not eliminate any of the choices. In addition, an appraisal task was administered to determine whether differences were a function of perceptual problems. On the appraisal task children were shown the same pictures and asked to indicate whether a clue would be an adequate one for an imaginary listener. The results showed that there were no group differences when the children were given the fully informative clues. When the messages were partially informative or uninformative the learning disabled children asked fewer questions and then made more errors in their picture choices. Analysis of whether they had responded impulsively suggested that the learning disabled and nondisabled children were equivalent in the time they took to either make a picture choice or ask for clarification: Both groups took longer as the informational value of the messages decreased. Further, with the exception of the younger learning disabled girls, group differences did not appear related to perceptual difficulties. Only the first and second grade learning disabled girls had difficulty on the appraisal task; their failure to ask questions in response to inadequate messages seemed related to a deficit in judging the adequacy of the messages.

Noel (1980) and Spekman (1981) also included measures of learning disabled boys' listener skills. Noel judged listener skills on the basis of accuracy in selecting correct choices, whereas Spekman analyzed the ability to follow directions, the number of questions asked, and the number of needed versus redundant requests. Neither study showed differences between the learning disabled and nondisabled boys' listener skills. However, the adequacy of messages was not controlled in these studies, hence the need for listeners to request clarification could not be judged.

In sum, group differences in referential communication tasks do not consistently find the learning disabled less skilled than the nondisabled. When messages are fully informative and the situation is highly structured, the learning disabled respond as well as the nondisabled. Performance differences emerge under two conditions. The learning disabled do more poorly when given ambiguous information and when they must take active steps to obtain information. As speakers, the learning disabled produce messages that are less informative. As listeners, the learning disabled respond inappropriately to ambiguous statements because they fail to request message clarification.

None of the studies systematically varied the dimension of partner age or status in measuring referential skills. This is unfortunate, as it is possible that performance differences resulted from learning disabled children's perception of the situation. Perhaps they assume that adults would give them the information they needed to perform. With adult partners, the learning disabled child may interpret a breakdown in communication as their fault. Moreover, the learning disabled may be more willing to ask questions of peers than adults if they judge peers to be as imperfect others. This bodes ill for the learning disabled student's willingness to solicit information in the classroom. Classroom research shows that teachers increasingly dominate classroom talk and are remiss in their efforts to make sure that students comprehend instructions and assignments (Moran, 1980). Hence, as the learning disabled age, if they demean their peers as sources of information they may fail to seek clarification and help from classmates. They may be at increasingly greater disadvantages in the classroom if they are unwilling to ask questions and seek clarification from adults or peers.

Conversational Turn-Taking and Interpersonal Strategies

The third component of communicative competence relates to understanding the rules that govern the give and take of listener-speaker exchanges. When people embark in an exchange of talk, they must share a set of social rules for the initiation, maintenance, and close of the conversation. Verbal and nonverbal behaviors are used to govern how participants maintain the flow of meaning and sequence conversational turns. Children appear to acquire the rules for sustaining a conversation as they acquire the linguistic knowledge involved in establishing and sustaining a topic of conversation (Dore, Gearhart, and Newman, 1978; Keenan and Schieffelin, 1976). Data on learning disabled children's conversational turn-taking skills can be gleaned indirectly from studies done in classroom and recreational settings and directly from contrived laboratory situations.

Classroom Conversations. A number of studies that examined learning disabled children's conversational skills compared the frequency with which the learning disabled and nondisabled classmates spoke to teachers and peers. Bryan and Wheeler (1972) and Bryan (1974) compared kindergarten through sixth graders, whereas Schumaker, Sheldon-Wildgen, and Sherman (1982) evaluated junior high students. These comparisons failed to show that the learning disabled differ from the nondisabled in the frequency of classroom communications.

Differences in conversation between the learning disabled and nondisabled emerge when the content rather than the quantity of children's conversations are compared.

In search of verbal correlates of peer rejection, Bryan, Wheeler, Felcan, and Henek (1976) made verbatim recordings of learning disabled and nondisabled children's communications during summer school sessions. The learning disabled were found to make more competitive utterances and to produce fewer statements that were positive and friendly (e.g., giving a compliment). A second study collected verbatim recordings of children's statements during art and physical education classes. Bryan and Bryan (1978) found the learning disabled to make more competitive and rejecting statements to peers and to be the targets of more insults from peers than classmates. Although these results showed more hostile statements were made by the learning disabled, such statements did not occur frequently. Further, although the studies reported type of classroom activity, no more specific contextual cues are provided to explain what generated the hostile exchanges. Whether the hostile communications were initiations or responses, deserved or undeserved, involved many or few remains unknown. Until more is known about the chain of events, it is not possible to understand whether these communications are related to language proficiency.

Conversation During Recreation. The results of the classroom studies were recently confirmed in studies of learning disabled and nondisabled adolescents' communications during outdoor recreation activities. Smiley and Bryan (1983a, 1983b) videotaped groups of learning disabled and nondisabled junior high boys engaged in raft building and obstacle course activities. Videotapes of the interactions were used to analyze the boys' conversations while they were engaged in these various activities. Analyses of the boys' conversations during the raft building showed that a greater percentage of the learning disabled adolescents' statements were negative, whereas a greater percentage of nondisabled boys' statements were chitchat. Groups did not differ in the percentage of statements that were related to actual raft building. It is striking that the learning disabled made negative statements while engaged in helping behaviors. The results of the analyses of boys' conversations made during the obstacle course activities were similar. In the obstacle course study, the boys had to jump from one to another stump without falling or they had to stand on a stump and fall back into the arms of the group without "jackknifing" (i.e., bending their knees). During these activities the learning disabled in comparison to the nondisabled were less likely to make positive encouraging statements (e.g., "Good catch," "Don't be afraid") and self-disclosing statements, which are statements associated with trust and intimacy (e.g., "Are you scared?" "I don't want to do this"). They were more likely than the nondisabled boys to make negative, discouraging statements (e.g., "Look, he can't even get up there," "Better not kick me in the face").

The results of studies comparing the statements of the learning disabled and nondisabled children in sports or recreation activities differ from results based on classroom activities. It is not clear as to why the learning disabled should evidence such verbal hostility when engaged in prosocial helping, cooperative, presumably fun activities. Outside the classroom, in these nonevaluative situations, negative interactions cannot be attributed to anxiety increased by classroom stress. However, it may be that for the learning disabled, public performance in physical activities that their peers observe and ostensibly judge may well be charged with personal anxiety. Among adolescent males, peer assessment of physical prowess may well carry considerable importance. Hence, their verbal statements may be defensive and intended to protect their self-esteem. It is also possible that the learning disabled do not realize they are being verbally hostile. Given the lack of listener sensitivity shown in the earlier described studies, it may be that they believe they are being socially appropriate. This may well be their attempt at in-group peer talk. Without an assessment of respondents' feelings toward them, this is clearly speculative. Nonetheless, learning disabled youngsters' consistently poor showings on sociometrics suggest that although they may be trying to be appropriate, others may be judging their attempts negatively.

Are the learning disabled less skilled than nondisabled youngsters in conversational turn-taking? In certain respects, they are as skilled as their nondisabled classmates. They talk as much as others, and they show no problems in the give-and-take flow of conversational exchanges. Indeed, the Smiley and Bryan (1983a, 1983b) data suggest they are as skilled as any in the verbal shooting match. At the same time, however, the learning disabled are found discrepant from peers when the focus of evaluation is on the content of their communications. Although the basic structure of their communications is correct, albeit less complex (Pearl et al., 1981), it is the social-cognitive-affective components of communications that differentiate the learning disabled from the nondisabled. The learning disabled seem to be poor actors, inappropriate and discrepant from same sex peers in their responses to their peers. Let us now consider studies that focused on the conversational skills of children in more structured situations. In these studies, small-group problem solving and role-play tasks were used to isolate specific components of communicative competence. Persuasion, conversational turn-taking, problem solving, and job-related language skills were evaluated.

Conversations During Problem Solving Tasks. Bryan, Donahue, and Pearl (1981) had third through eighth graders do a problem solving task with two same-sex classmates. The triads were asked first to independently rank order 15 possible gift items for their class (e.g., movie tickets, candy). Then triads were assembled to do the task together. This study examined whether the learning disabled would be as persuasive as the nondisabled and whether their independently made first choices would be selected as first choices by the group. Also assessed was whether the learning disabled could be experimentally induced to take a persuasive stance with peers. Hence half of the learning disabled and nondisabled children were given a "pep talk" prior to the group activity. These children were told they had made really good choices on their own and that they should try to convince their peers to make the same choices. The remaining children were given neutral feedback prior to the group activity. Analyses of persuasiveness found that across grade, sex, and conditions, the learning disabled children's first choices were less likely to be among the group's first choices than those of the nondisabled children. The pep talk did not have an impact on learning disabled or nondisabled children's persuasiveness.

Analyses of children's communicative intentions during the group activity provided clarification of learning disabled children's relative lack of persuasiveness. During the course of the decision making the learning disabled were more likely to agree and less likely to disagree or try to negate classmates arguments than nondisabled peers. Nondisabled youngsters were more likely to engage in housekeeping, to emit statements which keep the group on task and hold the conversational flow (e.g., "Now, let me think," "OK, guys let's get this down"). There were no differences between learning disabled and nondisabled in the percentage of conversational turns. They engaged verbally in the interaction as much as their peers. There also were no differences in the number of initiations of suggestions made for gift choices. Furthermore, the learning disabled were more likely than the nondisabled to respond to requests for clarification. Thus whenever the learning disabled have the opportunity to say something they do so, but they seem to studiously avoid verbal disagreements which might require a chain of declaration-counterdeclaration-defense.

The results of this study led to several questions. First, what role does language proficiency play in learning disabled children's peer interactions? Clearly, to engage in an argument would require more complex communication strategies than simply agreeing. To generate an argument, counter with another suggested choice and rationale, and be prepared to defend both in the course of sometimes heated three-way interactions may be linguistically difficult for a child who lacks verbal flexibility and fluency. Studies of referential communication skills and those finding the learning disabled less skilled than the nondisabled on a wide variety of syntactic and semantic skills make this explanation quite plausible.

Nonetheless, because the learning disabled may hold only marginal social status in the group, his or her suggestions may be ignored. Perhaps knowing this, the learning disabled opt to try to ingratiate peers by behaving in an agreeable, conforming manner. On the surface this would seem a more adaptive strategy than the hostile, negative communications reported in the classroom and outdoor recreation studies. In addition, unlike the activities in the recreation and classroom observation studies, in this case children were involved in a problem solving task. If the learning disabled lack feelings of self-efficacy they may judge their opinions less worthy than those of their peers. Although an explanation based on language deficits is seductive, then alternative explanations based on social status or self-efficacy judgments are also believable. In an attempt to sort out language from social status factors, a number of studies were conducted. As a first step, mothers and learning disabled children were engaged in a problem solving task similar to the one just described (Bryan, Donahue, Pearl, and Herzog, 1984). It was hypothesized that the social constraints that may influence the learning disabled interactions with peers would be absent in mother-child interactions. For instance, it seemed likely that a child would disagree with his or her mother. Furthermore, this study asked whether mothers or learning disabled youngsters might engage in "conversational buffering." Bell and Harper (1977) employed the term "buffering" to describe how parents make adjustments that help the handicapped child to participate in social interactions. Hence, this study examined mothers' use of verbal compensatory strategies that would aid the learning disabled to participate in a verbal problem solving task.

Mother-child pairs in which the children were in grades one through six participated in a "Lost in Space" task. On this task the dyad pretends to be astronauts whose space ship crashes on the moon. The pair has to rank in order of importance a list of fifteen items that they should take in a 200-mile walk across the moon from the wounded space ship to the mother ship. The analysis of the communication strategies showed that mothers of nondisabled and learning disabled children were sensitive to the communicative skills of their children and that both groups engaged in verbal buffering. Although not reaching conventional levels of statistical significance, mothers of the learning disabled tended to initiate topics more often than mothers of nondisabled children. Second, the mothers of the nondisabled girls made a smaller proportion of conversational housekeeping statements that served to monitor the conversation. More significant differences were found between groups of children. Comparisons of learning disabled and nondisabled children's communications showed that the learning disabled made a smaller proportion of disagreements than the nondisabled. Thus, once again, the learning disabled were found to agree more and disagree less with a partner on a problem solving task. Even with their mothers, the learning disabled tend not to engage in verbal disputes.

Thus, two studies showed the learning disabled more likely than the nondisabled to agree and less likely to disagree with peers and mothers.

This suggests that learning disabled are less likely than nondisabled children to be assertive conversational partners. The question then arose as to whether the roots of this relatively passive conversational style could be identified. Although it seems likely that a passive conversational style may originate early in the preschool period, the youngest age level available for our learning disabilities research was first and second grade. It is only with reluctance that most school districts will use the term learning disability before children reach the third grade, thus learning disabled youngsters are more likely to be identified or labeled in the intermediate grades. In cooperating school districts a small sample of 12 learning disabled children was identified. Donahue and Prescott (1981) analyzed the first and second graders' communication strategies while involved in a triadic decision making task modeled after the Bryan, Donahue, and Pearl (1981) small-group study. Children were asked to cooperatively sort possible gifts for this class into three boxes representing how much they like each item. The analysis focused on the children's disagreements defined by nomination of a gift item followed by a disagreement, an optional discussion of the item's merits, and a resolution in which the item was placed in a box. The children whose opinion was complied with by the group were considered to have made the winning move in the dispute.

Analyses showed that within dispute episodes the learning disabled were as likely to take conversational turns, initiate topics, and agree and disagree with their classmates' opinions. Nonetheless, it is striking that the learning disabled were less likely to win the final move in the disputes. These results extended the finding of the Bryan and co-workers (1981) study by showing that the opinions of the younger learning disabled are less likely to be accepted by peers than are the opinions of nondisabled youngsters. In contrast to the Bryan, Donahue, and Pearl (1981) study, the young learning disabled in this case were as assertive conversational partners as their peers. These results suggest that for whatever reason the opinions of the young learning disabled are being rejected by their classmates. A lack of positive responses to their opinions may serve subsequently to extinguish their attempts to influence their peers. By middle childhood the learning disabled might give up attempting to influence others, finding it socially easier to conform with peer judgments. Whatever the reason for peer failure to abide by young learning disabled children's judgments, these data suggest that intervention efforts to increase learning disabled children's active participation in negotiations with peers may not be effective.

Because findings of conversational differences between learning disabled and nondisabled children could have been due to their having marginal social status, this next study placed the learning disabled in a social position of high status. Bryan, Donahue, Pearl, and Sturm (1981) examined learning disabled children's ability to initiate and sustain a conversation with a peer in a situation in which it was made explicit that the learning disabled were in a dominant speaker role. The children, in dyads, were asked to role-play a television talk show. Second and fourth grade learning disabled and nondisabled children were cast in the role of television talk show hosts, whereas nondisabled classmates were cast in the role of television talk show guests. The children were briefed on how to be a talk show host or guest and then videotaped during a 3 minute talk show interview. The children's statements were analyzed for their turn-taking initiations and for proportion and types of questions. Types of questions were (1) choice questions, which solicit either-or judgments; (2) product questions, which solicit information in response to ''wh'' interrogative pronouns; and (3) process questions, which elicit extended descriptions. Children's responses to questions, confirmations, and conversational devices were also analyzed. Once again the learning disabled took as many conversational turns as the nondisabled children: They participated as much. Their communication strategies differed from the nondisabled, as the learning disabled children's communications consisted of a smaller proportion of questions. Further, their questions were less likely to be process questions than those of the nondisabled children. The learning disabled were thus less likely to ask open-ended questions, which, although no more demanding in syntactic and semantic skills, are perceived as a more adaptive strategy in this context. In addition, the guests of the learning disabled differed from guests of the nondisabled. They were less likely to provide elaborative responses to questions. There was more role switching evident as the guests of the learning disabled were more likely to ask questions (choice questions) than guests of the nondisabled. Finally, guests of the learning disabled displayed more nonfunctional body touching suggestive of discomfort in the situation. Although the learning disabled were certainly cooperative conversational partners, placing them in a dominant speaker role did not lead them to be assertive conversational partners. Although the learning disabled were able to generate questions, their questions were fewer in number and of a kind less adaptive to this situation.

As in the referential communication studies, these results indicate that even when placed in a socially dominant position the learning disabled are less able than the nondisabled to control a conversation through questioning. Their partners responded to their relative lack of conversational skill by generating simpler responses to their questions than they did to those of the nondisabled and even by taking over the host's questioning role. There was social ''noise'' in the interactions between the learning disabled and nondisabled dyads that was evidenced by the greater frequency of nonfunctional body touching among this group than among the guests of the nondisabled hosts. As in the referential communication studies in which the learning disabled were placed in the speaker roles, the learning disabled appeared to lack the verbal fluency needed to formulate questions whose propositional content is easy to expand upon and to generate adequate responses to their guests' communications (Donahue, Pearl, and Bryan, 1983).

It should be noted that these findings were not confirmed in a study of junior high school learning disabled students. Assessments based on student interviews showed that learning disabled and nondisabled junior high youngsters were equivalent in their use of open-minded questions, confirming statements, requests, and relevant responses in interviews (Banikowski and Alley, note 1).

However, studies evaluating specific communication skills find the language differences between the learning disabled and nondisabled persist into adolescence. Matthews, Whang, and Fawcett (1980) compared learning disabled and nondisabled high school students performance on ten occupation-related skills, most of which involved language proficiency. Four of the ten categories found the learning disabled less skilled than the nondisabled adolescents: in participating in a job interview, in accepting criticism from an employer, in giving criticism to a co-worker, and in explaining a problem to an employer. Hazel, Schumaker, Sherman, and Sheldon-Wildgen (1982) developed a social skill assessment instrument that assessed social skills, again largely verbal skills, needed by adolescents. Students role-played eight specific social skills: giving positive feedback, giving negative feedback, resisting peer pressure, negotiating conflict situations, following instructions, conversing, and problem solving (personal). Schumaker, Hazel, Sherman, and Sheldon (1982) compared learning disabled adolescents performance on these skills to nondisabled high school students and a group of court-adjudicated juvenile delinquent adolescents who were referred for social skills training by probation officers. The comparison showed that the nondisabled youths performed better than both the learning disabled and juvenile delinquent groups on seven of the eight skills. The learning disabled did better than the juvenile delinquent on resisting peer pressure.

Summary

There appears to be an important discrepancy in the verbal behavior of the learning disabled as described in the observation versus the small-group studies. In the classroom and outdoor recreation studies, the learning disabled act verbally aggressive and hostile. In contrast, in problem solving studies the learning disabled participate equally but assume a rather deferential posture relative to peers and mother. These differences may be due to the different conceptual-linguistic demands placed on the child in these various situations. It may be that the learning disabled can be socially appropriate more easily in highly structured situations. In these tasks they allow nondisabled peers to take command while they comply. In the outdoor situations perhaps the rules governing appropriate behaviors are less obvious. It may be also that in any problem solving situation the learning disabled judge themselves less skilled and hence take the compliant, safe route.

ASSESSMENT OF COMMUNICATIVE COMPETENCE

Assuming that developmental data are forthcoming, the integration of norms into assessment devices creates particularly thorny problems in this domain. That is, in addition to the usual criteria that must be met in manufacturing tests, pragmatics has properties that make it particularly difficult to assess. One property is its enormity. There are myriads of rules governing social intercourse. The selection of which rules to assess will obviously be a critical factor in determining the usefulness of any instrument. In addition, paper-and-pencil tests may not be valid. These may identify children who have language problems, but it is likely that existing instruments may do as well. In fact, the relationship of pragmatic competence to skills in syntax and semantics or even general intelligence is not yet known. In the area of communicative competence, researchers should strive to develop formative and summative assessment techniques that could be used to identify the components that need to be taught and to assess how well the components have been taught. Paper-and-pencil measures are unattractive because they are so far removed from social interactions.

Naturalistic Observation

Assessment techniques that capture the dynamics of social interactions will clearly lend themselves more to formative and summative evaluation. However, considerable ingenuity will be required to develop assessment devices that meet the criteria of reliability, validity, and cost effectiveness. Preferred would be language assessment based on observations made in the child's natural environment. There is certainly a long, respectable history in the study of children's language development based on observations in naturalistic settings. In light of this history, speech and language therapists are likely to feel quite comfortable with using observational data to evaluate children's language. Furthermore, Public Law 94–142 mandates that diagnostic evaluations include a classroom observation made by someone other than the classroom teacher. Presumably then observational data are already being used to judge children referred for manifesting educational problems, many of which are language related. Finally, many research projects have developed observation codes to use in naturalistic settings such as the classroom. Much of the recent work on effective classroom instruction has been generated by methods involving observational data. Since these codes include measures of child and teacher language, they could be adapted for use with individual children.

There are different types of observation systems that could be adapted for the purposes of evaluating a suspected language disorder. One type, the event recording method, involves specification of particular language behaviors in advance of the observation. For instance, a child may be referred for evaluation because the teacher notes the child responds to questions with great hesitation or with bizarre, inappropriate responses. The observer may just record the child's responses to questions. A second method is based on time sampling in which any or all behaviors of the target child and others are recorded every set period, say, every 10 seconds. In time sampling, one can capture the flow of a conversation and identify the antecedents and consequences of various events more accurately than in event recording. For example, this method may be appropriate if the child is referred for using aggressive language toward others or for failing to respond to others. Thus, if a child appears to be having some kind of language-related problem, there are observational codes that can be adapted for evaluating the presence or absence of such behaviors.

The observer needs to be aware of certain problems associated with observational methods. First, it is important to evaluate both positive and negative instances of communicative competence. To record only hostile, aggressive statements and to ignore prosocial, positive statements provides an unnecessarily biased report. Because the observer is likely to hold a negative set and have the expectation of observing inappropriate rather than appropriate language, he or she must take special care to make balanced recordings. Second, it is sometimes the case that the child's language problem is exacerbated rather than facilitated by a particular classroom setting. The teacher who is very directive, demanding speedy responses from the child who is a bit shy and or inexperienced in talking to adults, may elicit less language than the child is actually capable of producing. The teacher who is disorganized and fails to make classroom assignments clear may have many children in the classroom misbehaving, not just the child who is referred. The context of the classroom, the match between the personality of the child and the teacher, and the linguistic demands placed on the child influence the child's performance. Such factors need to be taken into account when evaluating the child's language. Finally, in doing observations of specific behaviors, the researcher quickly learns that the behaviors of interest may occur very infrequently. An enormous amount of time can be spent waiting. Although naturalistic observations are very attractive to language therapists, collection and analysis of such information does have important limitations.

It is advisable that an evaluation of the effectiveness of language intervention include some observation. To have a child demonstrate newly acquired language skills in the context of one-on-one or small-group instruction is a first step in intervention. But, it is also necessary to demonstrate that these newly acquired skills are being used in the child's everyday world. This does require observing the child's communication strategies in the classroom or other appropriate settings. Again, naturalistic observations for this purpose are costly and time consuming. It is uncertain whether or not the child will demonstrate skillfulness or deficits during the course of observations.

Role Plays

A second method preferable to paper and pencil tests, but not as expensive as naturalistic observations, is role-plays. With role plays the child is asked to imagine some situation and is invited to demonstrate how or she would respond. Role plays are very attractive as a method of assessment and intervention in language disorders. The teacher or clinician can specify the specific language components and create imaginary situations in which the behavior can be demonstrated and practiced. As reviewed in this chapter, role plays have been used extensively to compare the communicative competence of elementary and high school learning disabled students. Hence we have seen their communicative competence in being polite (e.g., making requests; giving bad news to a friend) and in job-related skills (e.g., accepting and giving negative feedback). It seems reasonable that if a child cannot perform such communication acts appropriately in role plays, they will not be able to do so in the real world. Thus role plays provide a means of assessment that seem much more socially valid than paper-and-pencil tests yet not as time consuming or unreliable as observations.

As with observational methods, however, there are certain limitations in using role plays. Young children showing language deficiencies may have difficulty understanding "let's pretend," a concept necessary for role plays. With older students as well as younger, there is some question as to how valid such measures may be. Skills acquired during role play do not necessarily generalize to other situations (Schumaker and Ellis, 1982). Role plays may be of particular use in assessment with older students, unless the evaluator can be creative in communicating the idea of pretend to younger students. While Hazel and colleagues (1982) showed that role plays can be used to teach communication skills, it is not yet clear as to how to get such skills to generalize to other situations and settings.

Structured Activities

Another alternative to assessment is the use of structured activities. In this case children are engaged in small-group activities. The tasks are programmed to generate those specific components of pragmatics that the clinician wishes to assess. As such, this method should not suffer the limitations of either naturalistic observations or role plays. The assessment would be based on naturally occurring communications when the child is engaged with others in various activities. Thus the child's ability to interact with others would be assessed under more realistic circumstances than role plays, yet the tasks could be structured to assess whatever is considered problematic. Although small-group activities require some effort to execute, it is not unreasonable to conduct observations while children are engaged in specific tasks with others.

Social Validation

Any method that is developed will have to show the properties of validity, reliability, and cost-effectiveness. Although this may be difficult in pragmatics, it has been shown that it is possible to delineate the components of complex verbal behaviors for assessment and intervention purposes. For instance, adolescent girls' public speaking skills and conversational skills were assessed and taught. Furthermore, the effectiveness of the assessment as an intervention were submitted to measures of social validation (Fawcett and Miller, 1975; Minkin, et al., 1976). Research showing that certain components of communicative competence consistently discriminate the learning disabled from the normally achieving provide a reasonable starting point for the development of assessment and intervention.

In-Group Language

One final issue must be mentioned. This concerns who shall do the intervening. Likely candidates would be speech and language therapists. At the outset, however, it should be recognized that professionals, indeed any adult, may be limited in the pragmatic skills they can effectively teach. The beginning of this chapter indicated that much of the research on learning disabled children's communicative competence was stimulated by the consistent finding that they have difficulty in establishing satisfactory peer relationships. Although there have been no direct tests to establish that their social status is affected by pragmatic deficits, the results of existing research suggest that failure to acquire social language fluency may well limit the learning disabled in their social relationships. Failure to detect, understand, respond to, or generate in-group language may be contributing to their isolated or rejected status. The probable reason no one has tested learning disabled children's in-group language skills is because researchers are not privy to this language. Adults are not experts in children's in-group communication styles. Thus it is unlikely that adults can teach peer-pleasing language, beyond rather gross approximations. Adults are likely to have considerably greater success in teaching adult-pleasing language. The point is that it would be presumptive to try to teach in-group language if one is not a member of that in-group. At the outset, professionals should recognize those areas of pragmatics that can and should be effectively taught.

Although it is unlikely that adults can teach in-group language, peers can teach language. The therapist's role may be to structure instruction so that the learning disabled child is exposed to in-group language through peer interactions. No research has examined whether there is an increase in understanding and using peer in-group language as a function of mainstreaming. However, given the decreasing opportunities for children to talk in class as they age (Moran, 1980), it is likely that special programming will be required to involve the child in activities that facilitate this kind of learning. Classrooms in which teachers do most of the talking or children are engaged primarily in seat work would not promote such interactions. Thus, it is likely that for the learning disabled child to observe, learn, and imitate in-group language, special attention to the social organization of the classroom will be necessary. Although teachers cannot guarantee that learning disabled children will engage in imitative learning, the classroom can be organized to promote peer modeling. A number of studies have examined the effectiveness of various kinds of intervention for improving learning disabled children's communicative competence. A consideration of these studies, follows.

APPROACHES TO LANGUAGE INTERVENTION

In light of accumulating evidence that some children have difficulty in acquiring communicative competence, interest has been growing in developing intervention methods. These methods have been generated from a number of conceptual frameworks. As in the early history of language intervention, a number of programs have been generated by reinforcement theory. Thus, studies have shown that children's communication skills can be improved through the use of systematic rewards. In the area of communicative competence, this is a somewhat broad statement, as most of this work has been done with preschool- or kindergarten-aged children who were isolated from peers for one reason or another (e.g., children with delayed language development related to mental retardation or children who were very shy).

Interventions for the learning disabled have focused on elementary and high school aged students, and the conceptual frameworks have included modeling theory and cognitive behavior modification. In the case of modeling theory the work of Donahue and colleagues (Bryan, Donahue, Pearl, and Sturm, 1981) with elementary-aged learning disabled students will be reviewed. With the older students, Hazel and co-workers (1982) used a program in which groups of students were provided training that used cognitive behavior modification strategies (e.g., models, rehearsal, feedback). A third method is direct instruction: This is simply providing the child practice in the specific language component deemed faulty. In this next section, the results of studies using direct instruction, models, and cognitive behavior modification will be discussed.

Direct Instruction

When Donahue, Pearl, and Bryan (1980) found that the learning disabled failed to ask questions in response to inadequate clues in a referential communication task, Donahue, Pearl, and Bryan (1980) hypothesized that they lacked question-asking skills. Thus, an intervention study was designed to evaluate the effectiveness of question-asking practice on learning disabled children's requests for clarification. The referential communication task used in the Donahue, Pearl, and Bryan (1980) study was again administered to identify youngsters who failed to ask questions in response to inadequate clues. These youngsters were then assigned to one of two conditions. In the intervention condition the children played the twenty-questions game. In a control condition, the children played tick tack toe. Following this session, the referential communication task was readministered. The results showed that playing the twenty-questions game did not lead the learning disabled to increase their question asking. Children in both the experimental and the control conditions still failed to ask for more information in response to inadequate clues from the adult experimenter. Donahue interpreted these results to indicate that other factors in the situation, not the children's question-asking skills, were determining their failure to request clarification. Although the linguistic demands on syntax and semantics were constant in both situations, the twenty-question games defined question asking as appropriate and necessary, whereas the referential communication task presented ambiguous social demands. The implication is that practicing a particular verbal behavior is not sufficient if the verbal behavior is to be used in situations that differ in their social demands on the child. Not only particular verbal skills must be taught but also the parameters of the situations in which the child is expected to display these skills. In the following studies, a modeling paradigm was used to teach specific communication skills. In these studies, the behavior to be learned was demonstrated in the situation in which it was to be practiced.

Structured Situations

Modeling has been found effective for increasing the use of syntactic structures by normal and language handicapped children (Leonard, 1975; Prelock and Panagos, 1980; Rosenthal and Zimmerman, 1978). In the usual procedure, the child in instructed to listen carefully while an adult "models" the target syntactic structures in some context (i.e., while describing pictures). The child then does the same task (describes the pictures), and the frequency with which the child uses the targeted syntactic structures is measured. There have been a few studies in which a modeling paradigm was used to teach specific communication skills to the learning disabled. In light of concern for the relative effectiveness of peer versus adult models, these studies used peer models. Studies comparing the relative effects of adults versus peers have not yet been attempted.

Donahue and Bryan (1983) examined whether a modeling paradigm would be an effective method for improving the conversational competence of second through eighth grade learning disabled children. The conversational behaviors selected as targets were generated by the Bryan, Donahue, Pearl, and Strum (1981) television talk show study. In the study, second and fourth grade learning disabled and nondisabled children role played the part of a television talk show host while classmates role played a television talk show guest. A comparison of the conversational skills of the learning disabled and nondisabled children showed the learning disabled less able to maintain the conversation as a result of their asking fewer open-ended questions. Using the television talk show paradigm, Donahue and Bryan (1983) targeted open-ended questions, contingent questions and comments, and conversational devices as the conversational skills to be taught. Before role playing the television talk show, learning disabled and nondisabled subjects were exposed to one of two experimental conditions: a model or a control. In the modeling condition, the child heard a taped dialog of two children discussing television shows. One of the children modeled three conversational behaviors: process questions (e.g., "What do you think about commercials?"), conversational devices (e.g., "Uh huh," "Oh, yeah"), and questions and comments that were contingent on the other child's previous remark (e.g., "Why did you like that movie so much?" "Especially those boring ones that they show over and over"). In the control condition, the child heard a taped monolog in which one speaker presented the same content. After hearing either the model dialog or the control monolog tape, subjects did the television talk show with a classmate who did not hear the tape. Children's communications were then analyzed to determine the influence of the model. Children's statements were coded for the frequency and type of questions (choice questions, which solicit "either-or" judgments in response; product questions, which solicit information in response to "wh" interrogative pronouns; process questions, which solicit extended descriptions or explanations); responses to questions (canonical responses, which provide minimal information, and elaborated responses, which go beyond the literal meaning of the question to expand on the topic); confirmations (questions or comments that paraphrased or interpreted the previous speaker's statement or that offer an opinion); and conversational devices.

The results found the modeling condition highly effective in increasing the conversational skills of the learning disabled. The model eliminated differences between the learning disabled and nondisabled that were found in the monolog condition. Compared with the nondisabled children the learning disabled children in the monolog condition contributed less talk to the conversation, but there were no group differences in the model condition. With respect to question asking, learning disabled children in the monolog condition produced a smaller percentage of process questions than did nondisabled children. Again there were no differences between groups in the dialog condition. Learning disabled children also produced more comments in the dialog condition than did learning disabled children in the monolog condition.

Analyses were also made of guests' responses to the learning disabled and nondisabled children. The guests of nondisabled children increased their elaborated responses in the dialog condition compared with the monolog condition. In contrast, the dialog condition led to decreased use of elaborated responses by guests of the learning disabled children. The learning disabled children also elicited more requests for clarification from their guests than did the nondisabled children, and this was more likely to occur in the dialog than the monolog condition.

The results of this study demonstrated the efficacy of a modeling paradigm for enhancing the communicative competence of the learning disabled. As found in the earlier Bryan, Donahue, Pearl, and Strum (1981) study, the learning disabled in the control condition were less likely than nondisabled children to use open-ended questions. Exposure to the model dialog, however, was sufficient to increase learning disabled students' use of this type of question. However, there were no significant group differences between the learning disabled and nondisabled on the other two targeted behaviors, conversational devices and contingent responses. It appears that no training was necessary in these two skills. However, a by-product of the modeling condition was that it increased the learning disabled children's contribution of talk in the dyadic interaction.

The effectiveness of the modeling paradigm is striking for a number of reasons. First, learning disabled children were able to abstract conversational rules through listening to a model who presented very few examples of each behavior. The taped dialog was about 2 minutes in length. In addition, the children applied the modeled behaviors in the absence of direct explanations, behavioral rehearsal, or incentives. It may be that the learning disabled children already had these conversational skills in their behavioral repertoire and the modeling condition simply cued this as the appropriate time to use these skills. The model may be teaching parameters of social situations rather than language skills. On the other hand, there is no metric for how many trials children need in order to learn these communication skills. Guest responses to the learning disabled suggest that the learning disabled were in fact practicing a new skill, that they were abstracting the modeled rules and trying to apply them. The finding that guests of the learning disabled were less likely to respond with elaborated responses to the learning disabled in the dialog condition and more likely to request clarification of the learning disabled suggests that the open-ended questions generated by the learning disabled may have been vague or otherwise difficult to answer in an extended way. Mild problems in semantic and syntactic structure may have interfered with the learning disabled children's ability to formulate coherent questions. Thus, even though the modeling condition was highly effective in increasing specific conversational skills in the learning disabled, their performance still suggests they suffer subtle and significant deficits in language production. The results are nonetheless promising in indicating that modeling conversational skills may be an effective method for intervention.

Group Training Programs

Although using peer models may be an effective way to teach certain language skills to the learning disabled, using peers to teach language skills seems risky because children do not always adopt adult-pleasing means of communicating, as in the case of slang. Nonetheless, unless the child shares the communication modes of his or her contemporaries, the child may be limited in access to the peer group. Because communication skills become increasingly important in peer group membership as children age, the communicative competence that learning disabled youngsters bring to peer interactions must be addressed. Ideally, then, language intervention programs would include increasing the child's opportunities to model peer communication strategies. This requires structuring academic or nonacademic activities in which the learning disabled interact with normally achieving youngsters while engaged in activities facilitated by talking. The teacher does not control the content or quality of talk nor can the teacher control whether the learning disabled will imitate the nondisabled. A few studies have explored the impact of structured activities involving learning disabled and nondisabled students.

An extensive intervention program for assessing and teaching social skills to adolescents was developed by Hazel, and colleagues (1982).

When these investigators found learning disabled adolescents perform social skills less well than normally achieving students, they developed a training program to teach these skills. This research is included here because six of the eight social skills involved communicative skills: giving positive feedback, giving negative feedback, resisting peer pressure, negotiating conflict situations, and following instructions and conversation. The eighth skill was personal problem solving, a noninteractive task in which students had to generate and evaluate solutions to various social problems. Participants in the training program were learning disabled high school students, normally achieving classmates, and court-adjudicated juvenile delinquents referred for social skills training by probation officers. The skills selected for training were six on which the learning disabled had done poorly (Hazel and co-workers, 1981). The training consisted of skill explanations, rationales, modeling, and rehearsal with feedback. Students' acquisition of these skills was assessed using a multiple-baseline design. Training consisted of 2 hour sessions once a week for 10 weeks during school.

Analyses of group performance showed that all three groups acquired the six social skills after training. However, the learning disabled still performed the problem solving skill at lower levels than did the other two groups after training (59 per cent level compared to 77 per cent). Learning disabled benefited from training as much as other groups, although they continued to have more difficulty in this particular area.

Concerned about the generalizability of the skills acquired in the training program, Schumaker and Ellis (1982) developed contrived but unobtrusive classroom situations to test whether three of the students would use their newly acquired skills. Resource room teachers and classmates were engaged as confederates to assess whether these students would use such skills as negotiating, question asking, giving negative feedback, and resisting peer pressure. The results were mixed. Each of the students showed some improvement on some of the skills, but the gains were reportedly not large and only approximated an adequate performance level. It appears possible to improve social skills in role plays, but it is not clear that these skills will generalize to other situations. Nonetheless, there were improvements even though they were idiosyncratic.

SUMMARY

Approaches to language intervention have varied to include direct instruction, structured situations, and group training programs. Each holds some promise and each has its limitations. Implementation of programs to facilitate the learning disabled youngsters' acquisition of communicative competence should therefore be carefully considered in light of the following issues. First, it must be established that the child has a language problem. It may be that the child's difficulty rests in the area of social-cognition rather than language. It may also be that in certain situations (e.g., marginal social status in the peer group) the child is prohibited by others from using his or her language skills. Other factors, such as a lack of self-confidence, may have a significant influence on the language strategy the child opts to use. In selecting what is to be taught, the adult should recognize that what appears important to an adult may not be important to children. Although there is considerable merit in teaching adult-pleasing communication strategies to the learning disabled, the expectation that this will have a positive influence on the child's peer relationships is not warranted. At the same time, teaching such skills as those involved in obtaining and keeping a job may be the kind of language skills adults can effectively, and importantly, teach the learning disabled. In providing a training program, it is necessary to plan for generalization of the skill to the situation in which it is to be used. The learning disabled have to be able to discern how and when to use newly acquired skills. Finally, careful consideration should be given to planning interventions whereby the learning disabled will acquire the language skills necessary for peer acceptance. This may involve teaching slang or ritual insults and how to tell and understand whatever the current brand of humor. This kind of learning will probably require peers as therapists, either directly or indirectly. To help the learning disabled acquire the communication skills of their peer group may require that the peer group be involved. Situations in which the learning disabled are exposed to nondisabled peer models and both groups find positive interactions reinforcing seems most likely to facilitate the mastery of peer-related communication skills by the learning disabled. This approach to language intervention runs counter to traditional one-to-one teacher-child training, but it would free the teacher to provide intensive direct instruction that the learning disabled need in other areas.

REFERENCES

Banikowski, A., and Alley, G. (In preparation). *The verbal cognitive-socialization strategies used by learning disabled and non–learning-disabled junior high school adolescents in a peer-to-peer interview activity.* University of Kansas, Lawrence: University of Kansas Institute for Research in Learning Disabilities.

Bell, R. Q., and Harper, L. V. (1977). *Child effects on adults.* Hillsdale, NJ: Lawrence Erlbaum.

Bloom, L. and Lahey, M. (1978). *Language development and language disorders.* New York: Wiley.

Bruininks, V. L. (1978). Actual and perceived peer status of learning disabled students in mainstream programs. *Journal of Special Education, 12:* 51–58.

Bryan, J. H., and Sherman, A. (1980). Immediate impressions of nonverbal ingratiation attempts by learning disabled boys. *Learning Disability Quarterly, 3:* 19–28.

Bryan, T. (1974). An observational analysis of classroom behaviors of children with learning disabilities. *Journal of Learning Disabilities, 1:* 23–34.

Bryan, T., and Bryan, J. (1978). *Understanding learning disabilities* (2nd ed.). Sherman Oaks, CA: Alfred Publishing.

Bryan, T., Donahue, M., and Pearl, R. (1981). Learning disabled children's peer interactions during a small group problem solving task. *Learning Disability Quarterly, 4:* 13–22.

Bryan, T., Donahue, M., Pearl, R., and Herzog, A. (1984). Conversational interactions between mothers and learning disabled or nondisabled children during a problem solving task. *Journal of Speech and Hearing Disorders, 49:* 64–71.

Bryan, T., Donahue, M., Pearl, R., and Strum, C. (1981). Learning disabled children's conversational skills: The TV Talk Show. *Learning Disability Quarterly, 4:* 250–259.

Bryan, T., and Pflaum, S. (1978). Linguistic, cognitive and social analyses of learning disabled children's social interactions. *Learning Disability Quarterly, 1:* 70–79.

Bryan, T., and Wheeler, R. (1972). Perception of children with learning disabilities: The eye of the observer. *Journal of Learning Disabilities, 5:* 484–488.

Bryan, T., Wheeler, R., Felcan, J., and Henek, T. (1976). "Come on dummy": An observational study of children's communications. *Journal of Learning Disabilities, 9:* 661–669.

Clark, R., and Delia, J. (1976). The development of functional persuasive skills in childhood and early adolescence. *Child Development, 47:* 1008–1014.

Cosgrove, J., and Patterson, C. (1977). Plans and the development of listener skills. *Developmental Psychology, 13:* 557–564.

Doehring, D. G., Hoshko, I. M., and Bryan, T. (1979). Statistical classification of children with reading problems. *Journal of Clinical Neuropsychology, 1:* 5–16.

Donahue, M. (1981). Conversational competence in learning disabled children: An attempt to activate the inactive listener. *Proceedings from the Second Annual University of Wisconsin Symposium on Research in Child Language Disorders.*

Donahue, M., and Bryan, T. (1983). Conversational skills and modeling in learning disabled boys. *Applied Psycholinguistics, 4:* 251–278.

Donahue, M., Pearl, R., and Bryan, T. (1980). Conversational competence in learning disabled children: Responses to inadequate messages. *Applied Psycholinguistics, 1:* 387–403.

Donahue, M., Pearl, R., and Bryan, T. (1983). Communicative competence in learning disabled children. In I. Bialer and K. D. Gadow (Eds.), *Advances in learning and behavioral disabilities (Vol. 2)* (pp. 49–84). Greenwich, CT: JAI.

Donahue, M., and Prescott, B. (1981). *LD children's conversational participation in dispute episodes with peers.* University of Illinois at Chicago: Chicago Institute for the Study of Learning Disabilities.

Dore, J., Gearhart, M., and Newman, D. (1978). The structure of nursery school conversations. In K. Nelson (Ed.), *Children's language (Vol. 1)* (pp. 337–395). New York: Gardner.

Ervin-Tripp, S. (1979a). Children's verbal turn-taking. In E. Ochs and B. Schieffelin (Eds.), *Developmental Pragmatics.* New York: Academic Press.

Ervin-Tripp, S. (1979b). Is Sybil there? The structure of some American English directives. *Language in Society, 5:* 25–66.

Fawcett, S. B., and Miller, L. K. (1975). Training public-speaking behavior: An experimental analysis and social validation. *Journal of Applied Behavior Analysis, 8:* 125–136.

Federal Register, 41, No. 2305, November 29, 1976.

Hazel, J. S., Schumaker, J. B., Sherman, J. A., and Sheldon-Wildgen, J. (1982). Application of a group training program in social skills and problem solving skills to learning disabled and non-learning disabled youth. *Learning Disability Quarterly, 5:* 398–408.

Hunt, K. (1965). *Grammatical structures written at three grade levels.* National Council of Teachers of English (Research Report No. 3). Champaign, IL: National Council of Teachers of English.

Hymes, D. (1971). On communicative competence. In J. Pride and J. Holmes (Eds.), *Socialinguistics.* Baltimore: Penguin.

Keenan, E., and Schieffelin, B. (1976). Topic as a discourse notion. A study of topic in the conversations of children and adults. In C. Li (Ed.), *Subject and topic.* New York: Academic Press.

Keogh, B. K., Tchir, C., and Windeguth-Behn, A. (1974). Teacher's perceptions of educationally high risk children. *Journal of Learning Disabilities, 7:* 367–374.

Kotsonis, M. E., and Patterson, C. J. (1980). Comprehension-monitoring skills in learning-disabled children. *Developmental Psychology, 16:* 541–542.

Leonard, L. B. (1975). Developmental considerations in the management of language disabled children. *Journal of Learning Disabilities, 8:* 232–237.

Lyon, R., and Watson, B. (1981). Empirically derived subgroups of learning disabled readers: Diagnostic characteristics. *Journal of Learning Disabilities, 14:* 256–261.

Matthews, R., Whang, P., and Fawcett, S. (1980). *Behavioral assessment of occupational skills of learning disabled adolescents* (Research Report No. 5). University of Kansas, Lawrence: University of Kansas Institute for Research in Learning Disabilities.

McGrady, H. J. (1968). Language pathology and learning disabilities. In H. R. Myklebust (Ed.), *Progress in learning disabilities.* New York: Grune & Stratton.

McKinney, J. D. (1982). *The search for subtypes of specific learning disability.* Paper presented at the 15th Annual Gatlinburg Conference on Research in Mental Retardation and Developmental Disabilities, Gatlinburg, TN.

Minkin, N., Braukmann, C. J., Minkin, B. L., Timbers, G. D., Timbers, B. J., Fixsen, D. L., Phillips, E. L., and Wolf, M. M. (1976). The social validation and training of conversational skills. *Journal of Applied Behavior Analysis, 9:* 127–139.

Mitchell-Kernan, C., and Kernan, K. (1977). Pragmatics of directives choice among children. In S. Ervin-Tripp and Mitchell-Kernan (Eds.), *Child discourse.* New York: Academic Press.

Moran, M. A. (1980). *An investigation of the demands on oral language skills of learning disabled students in secondary classrooms* (Research Report No. 1). University of Kansas, Lawrence: University of Kansas Institute for Research in Learning Disabilities.

Noel, M. N. (1980). Referential communication abilities of learning disabled children. *Learning Disability Quarterly, 3:* 70–75.

Ochs, E., and Schieffelin, B. (Eds.). (1979). *Developmental pragmatics.* New York: Academic Press.

Owen, R. W., Adams, P. A., Forrest, T., Stoez, L. M., & Fisher, S. (1971). Learning disorders in children: Sibling studies. *Monographs of the Society for Research in Child Development. 36* (144).

Pearl, R., Donahue, M., and Bryan, T. (1983). *The development of tact: Children's strategies for delivering bad news.* University of Illinois at Chicago: Chicago Institute for the Study of Learning Disabilities.

Pearl, R., Donahue, M., and Bryan, T. (1981). Learning disabled and normal children's responses to non-explicit requests for clarification. *Perceptual and Motor Skills, 53:* 919–925.

Piche, G., Rubin, D., and Michlin, M. (1978). Age and social class in children's use of persuasive communicative appeals. *Child Development, 49:* 773–780.

Prelock, P., and Panagos, J. (1980). Mimicry vs. imitative modeling: Facilitating sentence production in the speech of the retarded. *Journal of Psycholinguistic Research, 9:* 565–578.

Rosenthal, T., and Zimmerman, B. (1978). *Social learning and cognition.* New York: Academic Press.

Schumaker, J. B., and Ellis, E. S. (1982). Social skills training of LD adolescents: A generalization study. *Learning Disability Quarterly, 5:* 409-414.

Schumaker, J., Hazel, J., Sherman, J., and Sheldon, M. (1982). Social skill performances of learning disabled, non-learning disabled and delinquent adolescents. *Learning Disability Quarterly, 5:* 388–397.

Schumaker, J., Sheldon-Wildgen, J., and Sherman, J. (1982). Social interaction of learning disabled junior high students in their regular classrooms: An observational analysis. *Journal of Learning Disabilities, 15:* 355–358.

Shatz, M., and Gelman, R. (1973). The development of communication skills: Modifications in the speech of young children as a function of listener. *Monographs of the Society for Research in Child Development, 38:* 1–36.

Smiley, A., and Bryan, T. (1983a). *Learning disabled boys' problem solving and social interactions during raft building.* University of Illinois at Chicago: Chicago Institute for the Study of Learning Disabilities.

Smiley, A., and Bryan, T. (1983b). *Learning disabled junior high school boys' motor performance and trust during obstacle course activities.* University of Illinois at Chicago: Chicago Institute for the Study of Learning Disabilities.

Spekman, N. (1981). Dyadic verbal communication abilities of learning disabled and normally achieving fourth and fifth grade boys. *Learning Disability Quarterly, 4:* 139–151.

Chapter 8

Mismatched Premises of the Communicative Competence Model and Language Intervention

Mabel L. Rice

IMPLICATIONS OF THE PREMISES OF THE COMMUNICATIVE COMPETENCE MODEL FOR LANGUAGE INTERVENTION

The current dominant model of children's language characterizes their knowledge as communicative competence. This concept, introduced by Hymes (1972) emphasizes the wide scope of underlying knowledge. It encompasses grammar, cognitive knowledge, social context, and cultural identity. The concept has generated a rich array of descriptive data documenting children's surprisingly sophisticated sociolinguistic and conversational competencies (cf. Ochs and Schieffelin, 1979; Rice, 1984; Schiefelbusch and Pickar, 1984). Additionally, it has led to cross-cultural studies of language acquisition, thereby contributing to an understanding of linguistic universals and deepening an appreciation of cultural relatively (Heath, 1983; Ochs and Schieffelin, 1982; Schieffelin and Eisenberg, 1984).

The findings are welcomed by developmentalists interested in accounting for the general mechanisms of children's language acquisition. The broad purview of the communicative competence model has been especially attractive to scholars concerned with children who have difficulty acquiring language (cf. Schiefelbusch and Pickar, 1984). It provides a comprehensive description of children's communicative repertoires that serves well as a guide for description and analysis of children's language skills and as a source of goals and activities for remediation (e.g., Prutting, 1982; Roth and Spekman, 1984a, 1984b; see also other chapters in this volume).

The notion of communicative competence emphasizes that language is a socially situated cultural form. It involves three domains of competence: linguistic, interpersonal, and cultural competence. Most of the contemporary child-language literature addresses one or both of the first two areas. The earlier concern with formal language structures per se has been superseded by an interest in the interpersonal aspects of communication. The cultural aspects of children's language acquisition are relatively unexplored.

Almost all the applied adaptations of the communicative competence model have involved the interpersonal area of competence. Recent formulations of language assessment procedures (e.g., Lund and Duchan, 1983), therapy goals (e.g., Roth and Spekman, 1984a, 1984b), and intervention planning and activities (e.g., the earlier chapters in this volume by Dore, Hart and Risley, and Duchan), stress the interactional context of language use. It is now recognized that the language-disordered child must adjust communication to the demands of the social situation.

What is less recognized is that interpersonal communication is embedded in a broader social context, that each participant in a communicative interaction is a member of a cultural community that brings to the situation attitudes and values about the interaction. Ethnographic studies of children acquiring language in naturalistic circumstances, set in the broad cultural context, are beginning to appear in the normative literature (e.g., Heath, 1983; Ochs and Schieffelin, 1982) but have yet to work their way into studies of language-disordered children.

Even though Hymes's description of communicative competence is widely advocated by interventionists, the model is only partially adopted. Without consideration of the full cultural context of the development of communication, the model is incomplete. The consequences of selective borrowing are apparent when the underlying assumptions of intervention practices are compared with the premises of the model. Nontrivial discrepancies are evident and have powerful implications for how to provide intervention for language-disordered children.

This chapter argues that consideration of a child's discourse competencies, while a very important advance for language interventionists, inevitably brings clinicians face to face with the import of the cultural context of intervention and the assumptions, attitudes, beliefs, and values associated with it. Although the perspective has recently been expanded, the frame is still narrowly defined. Examination of underlying assumptions can be a helpful means of identifying the parameters of frameworks and possible sources of tension between competing assumptions. These concerns supplement rather than contradict efforts to delineate the interpersonal and discourse dimensions that are discussed elsewhere in this volume.

In the following discussion, the issues are brought up in the following order: delineation of the reasons for considering the implications underlying intervention and the model of communicative competence, discussion of the cultural context of language intervention, identification of some key premises of language intervention and parallel premises of the communicative competence model, implications of the model for language intervention, and conclusions about the efficacy of the implications.

The Rationale for Exploring Underlying Premises

The educational and social policy implications of the adoption of a particular model for language intervention are considerable, given the large numbers of children involved. In short, what interventionists believe to be the most appropriate way to help youngsters makes a major difference in the lives of the many individuals and families who receive services. Although precise prevalence figures are unavailable, a frequent estimate is that 10 per cent of elementary school aged children have communication disorders of various types and severity (Owens, 1984). In the United States, during the 1982 to 83 school year, 1,134,165 children (ages 3 to 21) received special education services for "speech impairment." In addition, 1,745,791 received services for "learning disabilities," which often include communication disorders. The prevalence of language disorders in preschool children is reported to be between 2 and 3 per cent. (Leske, 1981). In the 3 to 5 year age range, 71 per cent of children who receive special services from the schools are "speech-impaired" (Karr and Punch, 1984). The concern with language problems is also evident in the typical caseload of speech-language pathologists: the mean proportion of clients with language disorders is 54 per cent and an additional 26 per cent have articulation disorders.

Although there is widespread acceptance of the communicative competence theoretical model among language clinicians, there is great diversity in intervention activities. As Johnston (1983) observed, there are many different ways of providing instruction for facilitating language acquisition. Activities, settings, and instructors vary. Sometimes language intervention is carried out in a small room with one child and one clinician and sometimes in the home or classroom with the teacher or the parent directing the activities. Some procedures emphasize the passive nature of children's learning, whereas others assume an active, rule-inducting, hypothesis-testing change mechanism.

The diversity of intervention programs can be attributed to the influence of differing theoretical points of view (Johnston, 1983). The existence of several competing theoretical models is a consequence of the rapid shifts in the normative literature during the last decade. By the time new models are incorporated into language intervention activities, they are superseded in the normative studies by a revised version or a competing account. As interventionists have assimilated the numerous changes in perspective, some have adopted one version of a model and others have adopted other versions or a competing model. The present situation resembles the jumble of rocks at the foot of a hill after a series of landslides. There is a jumble of alternative models of language acquisition, each with an influence on therapy activities. Among the boulders are operant-behavioral training, formal syntactic training, cognitive knowledge-processing strategies, communicative competence-social functionalism, and discernible traces of traditional classroom pedagogy.

Although there is obvious diversity, the widespread acceptance of the notion of communicative competence is a unifying theme. Interventionists of widely divergent theoretical persuasions have adopted the communicative competence model of children's knowledge. For example, behaviorists find the model to be consistent with their concern with generalization of trained behaviors to new settings and unfamiliar persons (Hart and Rogers-Warrent, 1978). Cognitivists apply the model to a concern with meaningful therapy contexts (MacDonald, 1976). Advocates of social functionalism argue for new approaches to assessment and therapy (Duchan, 1984).

There are several inconsistencies in the current state of affairs. These differences are illustrated in Figure 8–1. On the surface, there are differences in therapy activities that are ostensibly related to underlying differences in theoretical models. For example, therapy procedure *A* may have its roots in behaviorism, therapy procedure *B* in cognitivism, and *C* in social functionalism. Yet all three share a commitment to the goal of developing children's communicative competence. At the same time shared adherence to fundamental premises is also present; that is a distinctive set of operating principles that characterizes the work of speech and language therapists exists. The professional commonality of perspective is indicated by the background texture in Figure 8–1. Furthermore, these basic premises of intervention are often unlike the premises that undergird the ethnographic perspective of the notion of communicative competence, as indicated by a different background texture in the figure. On the one hand, there is a variety of therapy approaches, each embracing the comprehensive communicative competence model. On the other hand, these different approaches all reflect adherence to a common set of underlying premises that differ from the basic premises of the communicative competence model.

There are reasons to examine the substrata of initial premises just as there is value in the consideration of the immediate theoretical constructs that guide intervention (Johnston, 1983). The premises involve

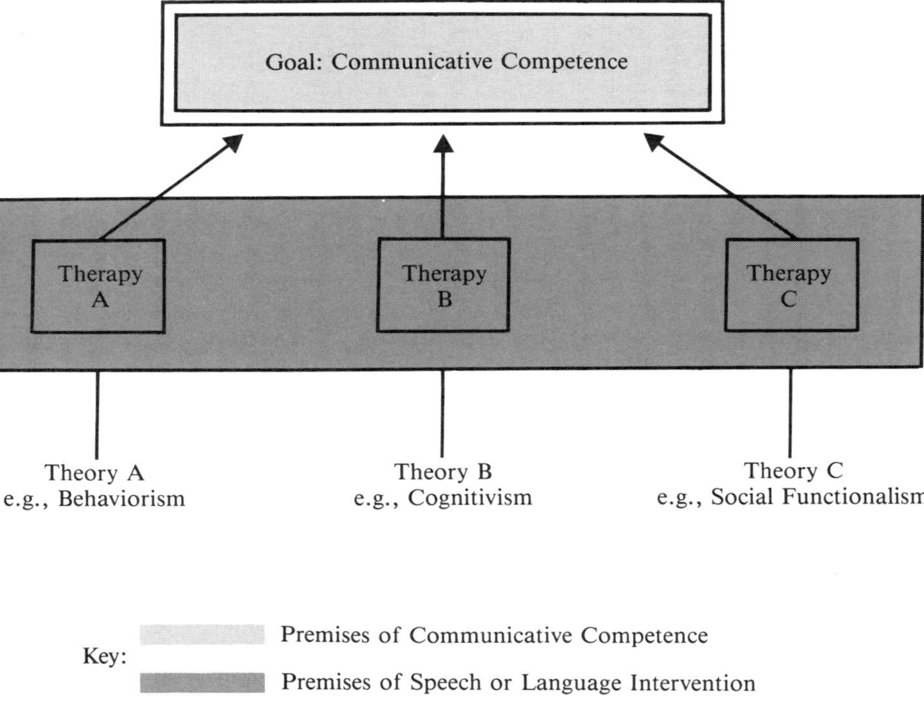

Figure 8–1. Inconsistencies among theory, practice, and operating assumptions for language intervention.

notions about the nature of the problem, appropriate sources of information about the problem, the nature of language, what to teach children (the goals of intervention), the nature of language learning, and appropriate means of facilitating change in children's language or communicative competence. These premises determine how a clinician or teacher views the overall purpose of intervention, the clinician or teacher views the overall purpose of intervention, the clinician's role in the process, the role and responsibilities of the individual enrolled in therapy, and expected outcomes.

It is possible for the surface goals and activities of therapy to be drawn from the communicative competence model and implemented with a different set of operating assumptions. In that situation, the effectiveness of therapy is compromised to the extent that the activities and general context of therapy are inconsistent with fundamental premises. For example, counting the number of topic initiations in a conversation is inconsistent with the premise that topic initiations are contextually embedded and are therefore not equivalent from one instance to another.

The Cultural Context of Language Intervention

The recent functional, interactive approaches to intervention highlight the child's linguistic knowledge and interaction skills but do not stress the significance of the general cultural context. The focus is on developing the child's ability to select among available linguistic alternatives for responses that are appropriate to the situation and the interlocutor and in furthering the child's ability to participate in discourse. What can be overlooked in this perspective is the compelling influence of cultural context. On the one hand, each individual who receives therapy is a native of a cultural milieu and brings to therapy his or her own attitudes, values, and premises about the intervention goals and activities. On the other hand, the interventionist also brings two cultural perspectives: (1) his or her personal cultural identification and (2) the general cultural assumptions and attitudes of the professional group.

An awareness of cultural discrepancies between the recipient and the provider of services was heightened in the late 1960s and early 1970s in the discussion of black dialect (Baratz, 1969; Taylor, Stroud, Hurst, Moore, and Williams, 1969). Current concerns focus on the problems of cultural difference in the case of bilingual individuals (Cummins, 1984; Miller, 1984; Omark and Erickson, 1983) and minority groups (Cole, 1985). Cultural differences are most apparent when representatives from markedly different groups interact. yet when cultural assumptions are carefully considered, it is apparent that any interactions between individuals can involve cultural differences. As Betty Hart once remarked,

"The minimal number of families needed for a cross-cultural study is two." Each child's family constitutes a cultural entity.

Professional premises can also be considered as a kind of cultural knowledge. The interventionist's accumulated knowledge and affinity for certain theoretical perspectives provides a cognitive map or schema for how to approach the intervention process, and a shared network of information, formal literature, and professional policies and ethnics provide a social structure that defines the profession's role and activities. Values and attitudes reflect professional training and a dominant mainstream culture. Finally, language clinicians participate in an enculturation process of transmission of knowledge and skills via formal educational experiences.

Because of the intrinsic nature of clinicians' perspectives, identification of the basic premises of professional behavior can be a difficult task. Ethnographers have recognized the difficulty of participant-observation in one's own culture. Ethnographers emphasize the need for diverse and converging sources of information, direct participation in the culture's activities, and acknowledgement of sources. In this effort, descriptions of ethnographic methods (Hymes, 1962, 1964; Lemish and Lemish, 1982; Levine, Gallimore, Weisner, and Turner, 1979; Saville-Troike, 1982; Slobin, 1967) and recent reports of ethnographic studies (Heath, 1983; Ochs and Schieffelin, 1982) have been drawn upon and contrasted with the contemporary literature on language acquisition, disorders, and remediation and the author's own extensive clinical work with young children in public school and hospital settings and ongoing discussions with colleagues who provide therapy in and out of university settings.

Premises of Language Intervention

The following premises are extracted from the author's observations of and participation in the usual practices for language intervention. In order to achieve a clear contrast, a prototypic exemplar, or a stereotype, has been developed. As with most stereotypes, the full set of identifying features (premises) are unlikely to be evident in a particular individual, although across all individuals the set of features is believed to occur frequently enough to define the common premises.

1. *The child lacks certain language skills.* A deficit of some sort requires remediation or tutorial assistance (cf. with Duchan's "fit the deficit" approach mentioned in Chapter 5). The initial step is the identification of the problem, that is, the manner in which a child does not conform to the normative expectations for his or her peer group. The emphasis is on the evaluation of an individual child. Identification of a problem is followed by categorization of the child as "language disordered." This designation makes the child eligible for services designed

for "language-disordered children," ranging from scheduled regular clinic appointments to individual tutorial sessions in the public schools to special classrooms to consultation with the child's parents for advice about appropriate home activities.

2. *Certain behaviors are targeted as the goals of language change.* In this time of individualized education programs for each child enrolled in public school language intervention, it is essential that specifiable behaviors or events are targeted as the goals of language change. Usually these are the behaviors designated as atypical, below age norms, or somehow inadequate for the child. For example, if it is determined that Johnny does not mark plural nouns with a final /s/ and most children his age do, then the /s/ plural morpheme becomes a therapy goal. In the area of discourse skills, examples of discrete goals are turn-taking, responding to questions, and maintaining a topic (e.g., Friel-Patti and Lougeay-Mottinger, 1985).

3. *Goal behaviors are determined by the clinician.* The determination of which behaviors to try to change is a matter of the clinician or teacher observing an a priori set of language performances of the child and evaluating which are adequate and which are not. Sometimes the behaviors are selected according to a checklist of targeted behaviors (often drawn from descriptions of normal children's language skills), and sometimes standardized tests are used. It is usually necessary to control for context in order to ensure that children are evaluated across comparable contexts.

4. *Language is viewed as a set of discrete, hierarchically arranged skills.* An isolated language skill, such as a plural morpheme, is regarded as part of an overall hierarchically organized set of skills, such that some are easier than others and such that there are organized fields of skills (response classes). Part of the selection of therapy goals entails the identification of the point at which language troubles begin, selection of a skill precursor to the targeted skill, and selection of a skill or behavior likely to generate maximal generalization to related skills.

5. *Learning is assumed to draw upon discrete processes.* Three processes central to the design of many intervention procedures are imitation, comprehension, and production. Other important processes include attention, memory, auditory processing, and mental representation (cf. Leonard, 1981).

6. *Learning is maximized in dyadic interactions,* in which the adult provides an occasion or request for a behavior from the child, the child responds, and the adult in turn reacts to the child's response with an altered or adjusted response. Almost all the langauge intervention programs presume an adult-directed interactional context, sometimes on a literal response-by-response basis and sometimes in less structured but nevertheless contrived circumstances.

7. *Preferred measures of growth or change are magnitude or consistency of response* (i.e., the number of times the child uses a correct form). The usual basic units of change are total number of correct or percentage of correct responses. Data are collected for each session and regularly reported on progress charts (e.g., Strong, 1983). Language interventionists rarely conclude that their job is done when a child produces a targeted behavior once. Embedded in tallies of responses is the assumption that one instance of a response is equivalent to another. There is no place for the moment of insight, the "light-bulb phenomenon," or the "a-ha" experience.

8. *"Teacher-proof" materials are desirable.* It is possible to devise a powerful set of procedures independent of the adult-child relationship, procedures that can be used by any teacher with any child that are a basic outline of sequenced materials and strategies for responding to the child. In the multitude of commercial products available for language therapy, there are no caveats about individual teachers' styles of teaching or personality or preferences or about individual children's styles of learning or personality or preferences. Instead the procedures, vocabulary lists, and sequence of grammatical skills are standardized across children and teachers.

Summary

The premises can be summarized conceptually as follows:

1. The nature of the problem resides in the individual child.
2. The focus of language change is a discrete, specifiable language skill.
3. The primary source of relevant information is the clinician or teacher's immediate observations of the child.
4. Language is regarded as a set of hierarchically organized skills, with some horizontal linkages.

Language change is implemented in dyadic interactions between an adult and a child. The child draws on discrete processes, such as imitation, comprehension, and production, when learning new forms. Change is measured in terms of consistency or amount of response. Procedures for change can be developed independently of the dynamics of particular contexts.

Premises of the Communicative Competence Model

The same caveats apply to this list of premises as to the preceding one: they were extracted from various sources; they form a prototypic set of features; and other scholars would probably arrive at slightly different but greatly similar lists.

1. *A language "deficit" or difference does not reside in an individual child.* Instead, the communication pattern may reflect the conventions of a social community unlike the standard white, middle-class comparison group or the attitudes and values of a particular home setting. Included in the differences in social context are definitions of what constitutes a "deficit." If the standards for communication in the child's immediate social milieu differ from the mainstream standards and the child has mastered the conventions of his or her own setting, it is a matter of cultural difference rather than an individual problem. One of the differences in perspectives that may influence the determination of the problem is that of parental expectations for children's communication. In some cultures, such as Japan's, the parents accept baby talk as a child register. In such cases, the child may appear to be delayed relative to mainstream American norms but within expected competencies relative to home or local cultural norms.

2. *Communication is an integrated composite of social and individual factors.* The social factors include interrelated patterns of attitudes, behaviors, and interactions. The individual factors include social role and status, formal linguistic knowledge, cognitive abilities, and accumulated experiences. The two domains are intrinsically and inextricably interwoven. A child's selection of what to say and how to say it depends on how the child is perceived by others in his or her group as well as how the child understands the situation and his or her own role.

3. *The teacher or clinician is an information gatherer.* The sources of information include observations of the child's performance in specified situations relative to certain pedagogical goals, such as the use of the plural /s/ morpheme when counting objects, or in different communicative contexts, including dyadic interactions with an unfamiliar adult, classroom settings with teachers and peers, home situations, and informal play circumstances. The emphasis is on communication-in-context. Therefore, context-controlled standardized tests or checklists are not the primary source of information. In addition to the child, key informants include the classroom teachers, the parents, and, if the teacher is not a member of the child's social group, other members of the child's community (cf. Heath, 1978). A vital piece of information is the community definition of adequate communication. Saville-Troike states: "Any study of language pathologies outside of one's own speech community must include culture-specific information on what is considered 'normal' and 'aberrant' performance within the other group" (1982, p. 9).

4. *The child's behavior consists of variable sets of rules,* as patterns of "ways of speaking" (Saville-Troike, 1982, p. 13). The concern is not only with pronunciation and grammatical form but also with

context-governed variations. The contextual influences may be interlinguistic or interpersonal or intersituational. Linguistic knowledge is not regarded as a discrete entity independent of context. Instead, the rules are adjusted to the linguistic context (e.g., the use of pronouns depends on preceding text or discourse), the interpersonal context (e.g., register-selection depends on the relative status of the persons involved in the interaction), and the situational context (e.g., some situations call for a minimal amount of verbiage, whereas others allow for a great deal of spontaneous output).

5. *The teacher or clinician is a representative of the dominant cultural group.* In this role, the teacher or clinician acts as a socializer of the mainstream cultural context. The language interventionist is not an inherently objective observer, even when counting observable responses. Instead, the reliance on counting discrete events is a reflection of the teacher's cultural perspective.

6. *Common-sense knowledge of a well-informed teacher is valuable.* The teacher is the best judge of which activities and goals are most appropriate for a particular child at a given time. There are no a priori procedures or sequences more powerful than the teacher's immediate judgment about what to do next, when a child has mastered a targeted goal, and when an activity has lost its effectiveness. In order to do this, the teacher calls upon an understanding of many subtle aspects of communication and performance, such as nonverbal communication, gaze patterns, moments of silence, omitted information or topics of conversation, latency of response, affective reactions, and inflectional patterns.

7. *Children can learn language in a variety of ways.* "Children are essentially participant-observers of communication, like small ethnographers, learning and inductively developing the rules of their speech community through processes of observation and interaction" (Saville-Troike, 1982, p. 205). Language is a part of the communicative interactions that are integral to children's enculturation. They are not dependent on child-centered dyadic interactions with an adult in order to infer the rules of formal grammar (cf. Heath, 1983; Ochs and Schieffelin, 1982). The cognitive mechanisms of language change include observational processes (Rice, 1984).

8. *Naturalistic settings are appropriate contexts for language intervention.* Parents and other family members are potential teachers. The home setting allows for language-related activities embedded in the flow of daily events, and involvement of the parent increases the parent's awareness of the child's language development and the possible contribution of the parent (cf. Heath, 1984; Heath and Branscombe, 1984).

9. *Responses of the same form are not necessarily equivalent.* Underlying communicative functions can alter the meaning of surface forms. The well-known examples of indirect requests are instances of the

same form but unequivalent meanings: In some circumstances, "Do you think it's too hot in here?" calls for a "yes" or "no" answer and in others calls for movement to open the window. Another example of unequivalence across forms is children's linguistic errors. Children learn early on the meanings of words such as "put" and "give." These meanings subsequently become interrelated and overlap as children realize the close semantic associations between the words. The overlap is evident in utterances like "Whenever Eva doesn't need her towel she gives it on my table and when I'm done with it I give it back to her" (Bowerman, in press). The first give has the meaning of put, whereas the second give has the meaning of give.

Summary

The premises of the communicative competence model can be conceptually summarized as follows:

1. The language problem may reside in cultural conventions or expectations unlike the mainstream standards. If so, the problem is not located in the child but in sociocultural variablility. The focus of language change is communicative competence, an interrelated composite of social conventions and individual linguistic repertoires.
2. The sources of relevant information are varied, including the child's performance in various settings and under differing circumstances, the child's attitudes toward communication and remediation, adults in the child's social milieu at school and at home, and participants in the child's community.
3. A child's communicative competence rests on an underlying network of variable, context-sensitive rules. The knowledge is wholistic in nature, instead of discrete and hierarchically organized.
4. Language change can be implemented in a variety of ways: dyadic interactions, group contexts with individual participation, and group contexts with observational opportunities. An array of settings and "teachers" are appropriate: isolated one-to-one interactions, classroom activities, and interactions embedded in the routines of the home and the community. Qualitative judgments by the teacher of the child's progress are suitable measures of the child's change and of determinants of appropriate activities.

Implications of the Model for Language Intervention

When the two sets of premises are juxtaposed, fundamental differences are apparent regarding the nature of language problems and differences, the nature of language, the nature of language acquisition, appropriate sources of relevant information, what to teach, and how to facilitate language change. These differences are summarized in Table 8-1. A major implication is that the goal of teaching communicative competence may be jeopardized by inconsistent assumptions of how to go about facilitating language change and by overly constrained and formalized teaching procedures.

The Role of Enculturation

The major differences center on the role of enculturation in the development of communicative competence, in naturalistic circumstances, and in remediation and teaching contexts. If intervention programs were to incorporate the assumptions of the communicative competence model, the following additions would appear.

1. *Assessment includes information about parental attitudes and values regarding communication, language, and speech.* This information is central in determining if a child has a language problem. It is usually assumed that the parents are more likely to conclude that the child's communication skills are adequate than to agree with the judgment of a problem by a representative of a mainstream institution. This is not always the case, however. For example, the author once worked with a 5 year old daughter of a minister who was concerned about her oral recitation of prayers at the dinner table. Her articulation was somewhat slurred during prayers, possibly because of a reduced intensity of presentation and a general self-consciousness. On all formal tests her performance was at or above age norms. Yet as far as her father was concerned, she had a serious communication problem, and the author believed that if her father thought she had a problem, then she did have one. Her time in therapy was brief and productive. Therapy included practice in prayer recitation and the pronunciation of key words, and her skills improved to match her father's standards.

2. *Assessment includes information about the child's attitudes toward communication and remediation or intervention.* This is especially critical with children in the middle elementary school age group or older. Intervention is a difficult business if the child regards it as a waste of time, or worse, as a major embarrassment (cf. Prather, 1984). At the very least, there must be a joint agreement between the child and the clinician or teacher about the nature of the problem and the desirability of change. Under the best of circumstances, the child can become a full partner in the determination of therapy goals and activities that are consistent with the younger's immediate communicative needs.

3. *Planning of intervention goals, procedures, and activities involves the parent or other interested adults in the child's home setting.* The parental involvement envisioned within the communicative compe-

Table 8–1. Summary of Premises of Language Intervention Versus Premises of the Communicative Competence Model

	Language Intervention	Communicative Competence
Nature of Language Problems or Differences	Resides in the individual child. A problem of inadequate or incomplete learning.	May reside in cultural conventions or expectations unlike mainstream standards. Often is a combination of sociocultural variability and individual limitations.
Nature of Language	A set of hierarchically organized linguistic and sociolinguistic skills, with some horizontal linkages.	A wholistic network of variable, context-sensitive linguistic rules for reference and communication.
Nature of Language Acquisition	Child draws on discrete psychological processes such as limitation, comprehension, and production when learning new forms.	Child functions as member of the social milieu, drawing on wholistically interrelated psychological and social processes. Language is an integral part of child's social roles, self-esteem, attitudes, values, and motivations.
Appropriate Sources of Relevant Information	Professional's (clinician's or teacher's) immediate observations of the child's verbal behaviors.	A variety of observations and sources are required for a valid description, including child's performance in various settings, child's attitudes, associated adults' attitudes, and adults' performance in child's milieu.
What to Teach	Discrete, specifiable language skills.	Communicative competence, an interrelated composite of social conventions and individual linguistic repertoires, which are dependent upon the social realities of an individual.
How to Facilitate Language Change	In dyadic interactions between an adult and a child. Change is measured in terms of consistency or amount of response. Procedures for change can be developed independent of the dynamics of particular contexts.	Dyadic interactions, group contexts with individual participation, or observational opportunities. An array of possible settings and "teachers": isolated one-to-one interactions, classroom activities, interactions embedded in the routines of the home and community. Qualitative judgments by the teacher are suitable measures of a child's change and determinants of appropriate activities.

tence model goes beyond the current requirements of the Education for All Handicapped Children Act (PL 94–142, enacted in 1975), which stipulates that parents must be notified of all educational plans for their child. Within the communicative competence model, the parents are regarded as important sources of information about their child's language functioning. Parents can agree to allow the clinician to collect observations in the child's home and natural settings, to serve as participant-observers and collect their own notes about the child's communicative competence, and to collaborate on the selection of therapy goals that are consistent with home realities and mainstream standards. Within this scenario, the burden of responsibility is fully shared between the teacher or clinician and the parents. Times of visits, conferences, and observations are determined by what is convenient for all parties involved, which may not necessarily be during the regular institutional business hours or at the institutional location.

4. *The interventionist inspects his or her own behaviors, attitudes, and values for cultural biases.* Such culturally linked attitudes as tolerance for dirt, unstructured activities, and counterfactual statements can influence the communicative interactions between adult and child. It can be difficult for an adult who expects children to be clean, play in a structured rule-defined manner, and tell the truth to work with a child whose expectations are otherwise.

5. *Selection of intervention goals and activities requires evaluation of the cultural biases of the existing normative literature and therapy materials.* For example, much of the normative literature describing mother-child interactions is drawn from observations of white, middle-class families, usually with a mother who is a full-time caregiver of a single child. Observations of children in other circumstances (e.g., Heath, 1983) reveal a wide range of differences in mother-child interactions. The school materials and routines constitute a cultural situation that may be significantly unlike that of a child's home (Heath, 1983). What may appear to be a problem with an individual child's performance or abilities may be an unfamiliarity with the assumptions inherent in the use of pictured materials, toy objects, or interaction routines. For example, if children are accustomed to playing with toys until they are tired of them, a set time allocated for toy play may prove to be frustrating to the child who has not tired of his play when play time is over (as Heath observed in certain cultural groups, 1983).

6. *Therapy goals include development of the ability to switch from home codes to mainstream codes.* Inherent in this goal is recognition of the existence of communicative alternatives, each suited to the immediate social context. Of course, in order to facilitate this ability the clinician must be familiar with both communicative codes.

Other Differences

In addition to the differences between the two sets of premises regarding the role of cultural context, there are important disparities in the *nature of language* and the *role of the teacher* in intervention. Incorporation of the communicative competence perspective would entail the following:

1. *Language training involves more than discretely defined formal linguistic structures and conversational rules.* Activities and circumstances would be provided to allow for simultaneous practice of interrelated components of communicative competence. For example, pronouns would be introduced in the context of conversational text, along with rules for turn-taking during a conversation, or new word meanings would be introduced in the social register in which they are found, such as formal terms for animals in the context of scientific descriptions or slang terms in the context of street talk. It is not necessary within the communicative competence model to relegate the formal language system to peripheral status, as Duchan advocates in her ''hot version of the pragmatics movement'' (Duchan, 1984). Instead, formal language can remain central, although wholistically conceived and intimately interrelated with sociocultural context.

2. *The clinician or teacher is regarded as a sensitive, innovative, and powerful agent of communicative change.* It is perhaps more accurate to characterize the teacher as a coordinator of experiences that allow the child to change. As such, the teacher draws both on formal, explicit knowledge of how to teach and on intuitive, common-sense understandings of the individual child and the immediate circumstances. A wide variety of activities and contexts are possible. Some can draw on the child's observational learning, some may be designed to facilitate children's cognitive heuristics, and others may involve rote, repetitive, imitative activities. Flexibility and variety are valued over structure and uniformity.

Conclusions

Although language interventionists have adopted the model of communicative competence as a description of children's linguistic repertoires, they have not incorporated the premises of the model into therapy designs. The premises do imply some adjustments in assumptions, activities, roles for the clinician or teacher, and therapy procedures.

There are some impediments, however, to a straightforward transfer of the implications of the communicative competence model to current modes of operation. A major one is that the model does not specify the particulars of how children acquire language. It provides an appealing model of the components of communicative knowledge and makes a strong case for the interrelatedness of the components. What is not available, however, are answers to some critical questions, such as the following: Does a general language acquisition mechanism underlie the whole bundle of competencies or are certain processes linked with some aspects and not others? For example, is observational learning sufficiently powerful to account for all aspects of communicative competence or only some? How does the model predict which children are at risk for language acquisition? Do the assumptions of the acquisition process apply to children having difficulty acquiring language or children who do not master one or more of the aspects of communicative competence in naturalistic circumstances? To what extent are the parts interrelated? If a youngster has not mastered one, such as formal grammar, does that limit mastery of another aspect, such as sociolinguistic alternations? If language is embedded in the enculturation process, what is the role of the individual child? How do personal attributes, such as cognitive abilities and personal social style, interact with the cultural milieu to produce individual differences in communicative competence? Do all components of communicative competence develop in synchrony, or are there times in the developmental sequence when there are disproportionate gains in one but not the others? Are some aspects of communicative competence more fundamental than others or "easier" than others? Which aspects are culture specific and which are universal?

These questions, among others, challenge contemporary scholars and are the subject of current study. One way of testing the predictions of the communicative competence model, and of specifying the particulars of children's acquisition, is to incorporate the premises into language therapy. The requirements of teaching provide on-line tests of the power of models and the underlying assumptions. Descriptions of the knowledge profiles of language-disordered children and their response to therapy activities and sequences can contribute to an understanding of language acquisition in three ways: by "grounding" explanations (i.e., moving explanation beyond simple description), by testing connections among the various components of communicative competence, and by highlighting particular aspects of communicative structures (e.g., determining that formal linguistic structures are more difficult for language-disordered children than are discourse rules) (cf. Menn and Obler's (1982) list of three reasons why exceptional language data are useful as linguistic evidence).

The communicative competence model does not provide a specific blueprint for therapy, but there is value in testing its premises in the therapy context. There are, however, additional constraints on the adoption of the implications. A major one is the institutionalization of some of the premises of previous models. For example, current laws require the formulation of Individualized Educational Plans (IEPs) for each child receiving language therapy in the public schools. A central notion in the requirement of IEPs is accountability, in the form of specified goals and well-defined activities. Although the intent of this requirement is laudable, the implementation restricts the flexibility of programming and discourages a reliance on the immediate judgment of the clinician or teacher. It would not look good on an IEP to state that the teacher plans to improvise activities to encourage a child to converse. Other institutional conventions that constrain implementation of the sort of therapy activities implied by the communicative competence model include a set time and place for therapy, predetermined procedures for assessment, institutional policies for contacting parents and visiting in children's homes, and set hours for work.

It is most reasonable to predict that it is possible for an individual clinician or teacher to incorporate parts of the communicative model into language intervention programming if he or she is creative. Some innovative programs have been able to do so by working with the classroom teachers (e.g., Fujiki and Brinton, 1984) and parents (e.g., MacDonald, 1976; Rice, 1973).

Implementation of the implied model of therapy brings with it major ethical responsibilities. Among them are the need to maintain confidentiality and an awareness of the rights and welfare of the children and families (see Heath, 1978).

The overall conclusion is that while a full implementation of the premises of communicative competence into language intervention is unlikely, given present institutional constraints and incomplete specification within the model, there is good reason to evaluate carefully the premises of current practices. Where those premises are inconsistent with the goals of therapy, the parallel premises from the communicative competence model offer a promising alternative.

REFERENCES

Baratz, J. C. (1969). Language and cognitive assessments of Negro children: Assumptions and research. *ASHA, 11,* 87–91.

Bowerman, M. (in press). Beyond communicative adequacy: From piecemeal knowledge to an integrated system in the child's acquisition of language. In K. Nelson (Ed.), *Children's language* (Vol. 5). Hillsdale, NJ: Lawrence Erlbaum.

Cole, L. (1985). Interview. *ASHA, 27,* 23–25.

Cummins, J. (1984). *Bilingualism and special education: Issues in assessment and pedagogy.* Clevedon, Avon, England: Multilingual Matters.

Duchan, J. F. (1984). Language assessment: The pragmatics revolution. In R. C. Naremore (Ed.), *Language science.* San Diego: College-Hill Press.

Friel-Patti, S., and Lougeay-Mottinger, J. (1985). Preschool language intervention: Some key concerns. *Topics in Language Disorders, 5*(2), 46–57.

Fujiki, M., and Brinton, B. (1984). Supplementing language therapy: Working with the classroom teacher. *Language, Speech, and Hearing Services in the Schools, 15,* 98–109.

Hart, B., and Rogers-Warren, A. (1978). A milieu approach to teaching language. In R. L. Schiefelbusch (Ed.), *Language intervention strategies.* Baltimore: University Park Press.

Heath, S. B. (1978). *Outline for the ethnographic study of literacy and oral language from schools to communities.* Philadelphia: University of Pennsylvania Press.

Heath, S. B. (1983). *Ways with words: Language, life, and work in communities and classrooms.* Cambridge: Cambridge University Press.

Heath, S. B. (1984). The achievement of preschool literacy for mother and child. In H. Goelman, A. Oberg, and F. Smith (Eds.), *Awakening to literacy.* Exeter, England: Heinemann Educational Books.

Heath, S. B., and Branscombe, A. (1984). The book as narrative prop in language acquisition. In B. Schieffelin and P. Gilmore (Eds.), *The acquisition of literacy: Ethnographic perspective.* Unpublished manuscript.

Hymes, D. (1962). The ethnography of speaking. In T. Gladwin and W. C. Sturtevant (Eds.), *Anthropology and human behavior* (pp. 13–53). Washington, DC: American Anthropological Association.

Hymes, D. (1964). Formal discussion. In U. Bellugi and R. Brown (Eds.), The acquisition of language. *Monographs of the Society for Research in Child Development, 29*(Serial No. 92), pp. 107–112.

Hymes D. (1972). On communicative competence. In J. B. Pride and J. Holmes (Eds.), *Sociolinguistics.* Harmondsworth, England: Penguin.

Johnston, J. R. (1983). What is language intervention: The role of theory. In J. Miller, D. Yoder, and R. L. Schiefelbusch (Eds.), *Contemporary issues in language intervention.* ASHA Reports 12. Rockville, MD: American Speech-Language-Hearing Association.

Karr, S., and Punch, J. (1984). PL 94–142: State child counts. *ASHA, 26,* 33.

Lemish, P. S., and Lemish, D. (1982). A guide to the literature of qualitative research. *Journal of Broadcasting, 26,* 839–846.

Leonard, L. B. (1981). Facilitating linguistic skills in children with specific language impairment. *Applied Psycholinguistics, 2*(2), 89–118.

Leske, M. C. (1981). Speech prevalence estimates of communicative disorders in the U.S. *ASHA, 23,* 229–237.

Levine, H. G., Gallimore, R., Weisner, T. S., and Turner, J. L. (1979). Teaching participant-observation research methods: A skills-building approach. *Anthropology and Education Quarterly, 11,* 38–54.

Lund, N. J., and Duchan, J. F. (1983). *Assessing children's language in naturalistic contexts.* Englewood Cliffs, NJ: Prentice-Hall.

MacDonald, J. D. (1976). Environmental language intervention programs for establishing initial communication in handicapped children. In F. B. Withrow and C. J. Nygren (Eds.), *Language curriculum and materials for the handicapped learner.* Columbus: Merrill.

Menn, L., and Obler, L. K. (1982). Exceptional language data as linguistic evidence: An introduction. In L. Obler and L. Menn (Eds.), *Exceptional language and linguistics.* New York: Academic Press.

Miller, N. (1984). *Bilingualism and language disability: Assessment and remediation.* San Diego: College-Hill Press.

Ochs, E., and Schieffelin, B. B. (Eds.). (1979). *Developmental pragmatics.* NY: Academic Press.

Ochs, E., and Schieffelin, B. B. (1982). *Language acquisition and socialization: Three developmental stories and their implications.* (Sociolinguistic Working Paper No. 105). Austin, TX: Southwest Educational Development Laboratory.

Omark, D. R., and Erickson, J. G. (1983). *The bilingual exceptional child.* San Diego: College-Hill Press.

Owens, R. E. (1984). *Language development: An introduction.* Columbus, OH: Merrill.

Prather, E. M. (1984). Developmental language disorders: Adolescents. In A. Holland (Ed.), *Language disorders in children.* San Diego: College-Hill Press.

Prutting, C. A. (1982). Pragmatics as social competence. *Journal of Speech and Hearing Disorders, 47,* 123–134.

Rice, M. (1973). A rural preschool language development program based upon parent programming. *Journal of Minnesota Speech and Hearing Association, 12*(1), 37–44.

Rice, M. L. (1984). Cognitive aspects of communicative development. In R. L. Schiefelbusch and J. Pickar (Eds.), *Communicative competence: Acquisition and intervention.* Baltimore: University Park Press.

Roth, F. P., and Spekman, N. J. (1984a). Assessing the pragmatic abilities of children: Part 1. Organizational framework and assessment parameters. *Journal of Speech and Hearing Disorders, 49,* 2–11.

Roth, F. P., and Spekman, N. J. (1984b). Assessing the pragmatic abilities of children: Part 2. Guidelines, considerations, and specific evaluation procedures. *Journal of Speech and Hearing Disorders, 49,* 12–17.

Saville-Troike, M. (1982). *The enthnography of communication.* Oxford: Basil Blackwell.

Schiefelbusch, R. L. and Pickar, J. (Eds.). (1984). *Communicative competence: Acquisition and intervention.* Baltimore: University Park Press.

Schieffelin, B. B., and Eisenberg, A. R. (1984). Cultural variation in dialogue. In R. L. Schiefelbusch and J. Pickar (Eds.), *Communicative competence: Acquisition and intervention.* Baltimore: University Park Press.

Slobin, D. I. (Ed.). (1967). *A field manual for cross cultural study of the acquisition of communicative competence.* Berkeley: A. S. U. C. Bookstore.

Strong, J. (1983). *Language facilitation.* Baltimore: University Park Press.

Taylor, O. L., Stroud, R. V., Hurst, C. G., Moore, E. J., and Williams, R. (1969). Philosophies and goals of the ASHA black caucus. *ASHA, 11,* 221–225.

Author Index

C

D

E

F

G

H

I

J

K

L

M

N

O

P

R

S

Subject Index

D

E

F

G

H

R

S

T

V

W